Essential Manual on Perfect 24-hour Blood Pressure Management from Morning to Nocturnal Hypertension: Up-to-date for Anticipation Medicine

For Tomoko

Essential Manual on Perfect 24-hour Blood Pressure Management

from Morning to Nocturnal Hypertension:
Up-to-date for Anticipation Medicine

Kazuomi Kario MD, PhD, FACC, FACP, FAHA, FESC
Professor and Chairman, Division of Cardiovascular Medicine, Department of Medicine,
Jichi Medical University School of Medicine, Tochigi, Japan

3311-1, Yakushiji, Shimotsuke, Tochigi 329-0498, JAPAN
Tel: +81-285-58-7538; Fax: +81-285-44-4311; E-mail: kkario@jichi.ac.jp

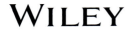

This edition first published by Wiley Publishing Japan K.K. 2018
© 2018 by Wiley Publishing Japan K.K.

Registered office: Wiley Publishing Japan K.K. – Koishikawa Sakura Bldg. 4F, 1-28-1
Koishikawa Bunkyo-ku, Tokyo 112-0002, Japan.
Tel: +81 3 3830 1221

For details of our editorial offices, for customer services and for information about how to apply for permission to reuse the copyright material in this book please see our website at www.wiley.co.jp.

All rights reserved. No part of this publication may be reproduced, stored in a retrieval system, or transmitted, in any form or by any means, electronic, mechanical, photocopying, recording or otherwise, without the prior permission of the publisher.

Designations used by companies to distinguish their products are often claimed as trademarks. All brand names and product names used in this book are trade names, service marks, trademarks or registered trademarks of their respective owners. The publisher is not associated with any product or vendor mentioned in this book. It is sold on the understanding that the publisher is not engaged in rendering professional services. If professional advice or other expert assistance is required, the services of a competent professional should be sought.

The contents of this work are intended to further general scientific research, understanding, and discussion only and are not intended and should not be relied upon as recommending or promoting a specific method, diagnosis, or treatment by health science practitioners for any particular patient. The publisher and the author make no representations or warranties with respect to the accuracy or completeness of the contents of this work and specifically disclaim all warranties, including without limitation any implied warranties of fitness for a particular purpose. In view of ongoing research, equipment modifications, changes in governmental regulations, and the constant flow of information relating to the use of medicines, equipment, and devices, the reader is urged to review and evaluate the information provided in the package insert or instructions for each medicine, equipment, or device for, among other things, any changes in the instructions or indication of usage and for added warnings and precautions. Readers should consult with a specialist where appropriate. The fact that an organization or Website is referred to in this work as a citation and/or a potential source of further information does not mean that the author or the publisher endorses the information the organization or Website may provide or recommendations it may make. Further, readers should be aware that Internet Websites listed in this work may have changed or disappeared between when this work was written and when it is read. No warranty may be created or extended by any promotional statements for this work. Neither the publisher nor the author shall be liable for any damages arising herefrom.

Printed in Japan

ISBN 978-4-939028-48-9 C3047 Y6500E

Publication date: 2 April 2018

Contents

Author biography, x
Preface, xii
Acknowledgments, xvii

CHAPTER 1 **Out-of-clinic BP,** **1**
SPRINT and automated office BP, 1
Different clinical BP measurements, 1
Diagnosis of hypertension and subtypes, 4

CHAPTER 2 **Morning and nocturnal hypertension as therapeutic targets,** **7**
Definition of morning hypertension, 7
Definition of nocturnal hypertension, 7
Shift of the prevalence of morning hypertension by
    2017 AHA/ACC guidelines, 10
When to use home and ambulatory BP monitoring, 11
Staged management of morning and nocturnal hypertension, 14

CHAPTER 3 **Home BP monitoring and morning hypertension,** **17**
How to measure home BP, 17
Evidence for morning hypertension control, 21
Subtypes of morning hypertension, 27

CHAPTER 4 **Ambulatory BP monitoring,** **29**
ABPM parameters, 29
Normal and typical patterns of ambulatory hypertension subtypes, 32
Development of ICT-based multisensor-ABPM (IMS-ABPM), 32
New ABPM indices, 33
Anticipation of ambulatory BP, 44
Multi-sensors and the real-time hybrid Wi-SUN/Wi-Fi
    transmission system, 46
HI-JAMP registry, 49

CHAPTER 5 **Morning surge in BP,** **51**
Definition of MBPS, 51
Cardiovascular events with MBPS, 52
Organ damage with MBPS, 54
    Hypertensive heart disease, 55
    Vascular disease and inflammation, 56
    Silent cerebrovascular disease, 58
    Chronic kidney disease, 59

v

Determinants of MBPS,   61
   "Thermosensitive hypertension" and MBPS,   61
   Mechanism of morning risk,   63
   Haemostatic abnormality and MBPS,   68
   Vascular mechanism of exaggerated MBPS,   71

CHAPTER 6   Nocturnal hypertension,   75
   Circadian rhythm of BP,   75
   Non-dipper/risers of nighttime BP,   75
      Cardiovascular risk,   76
      Organ damage and frailty,   80
   Definition and risk of nocturnal hypertension,   83
   Mechanism of nocturnal hypertension,   87
   Associated conditions of nocturnal hypertension,   89
      Diabetes,   89
      Chronic kidney disease,   90
      Sleep apnoea syndrome,   90
   Extreme dipper,   93

CHAPTER 7   Development of nighttime home BP monitoring,   95
   Cutting-edge of home BP monitoring,   95
   Recommendation for nighttime home BP measurement,   95
      Basic nighttime home BP monitoring (Medinote),   97
      Trigger nighttime BP monitoring (TNP),   102
      IT-based trigger nighttime BP monitoring system,   107
   CPAP adherence and nighttime BP surge,   110
   Antihypertensive medication on nighttime BP surge,   115

CHAPTER 8   Development of wearable beat-by-beat (surge) BP monitoring,   119

CHAPTER 9   BP surge,   125
   BP variability with different time phase,   125
   The resonance hypothesis of BP surge,   125
      Evidence and mechanism of BP variability,   127
      Visit-to-visit variability in clinic BP,   128
      Ambulatory BP variability,   132
      Home BP variability,   132
      Maximum home SBP,   134
      Standard deviation of morning home BP,   136
      Morning-evening difference (ME-dif),   137
      Morning orthostatic hypertension,   138

CHAPTER 10   What is systemic haemodynamic atherothrombotic syndrome?,   145

A typical case of SHATS, 145
Clinical relevance of SHATS, 148
Pathological target of SHATS, 150
Mechanism of vicious cycle of SHATS, 152

CHAPTER 11 Biomarker of SHATS, 157
Vascular biomarkers, 157
   1) CAVI/PWV, 157
   2) Central pressure, 162
   3) Flow-mediated dilatation (FMD), 163
Cardiac biomarkers, 163
   1) NT-proBNP, 163
   2) High-sensitivity troponin T (hs-TNT) and growth differentiation factor 15 (GDF-15), 167
   3) Electrocardiography (ECG), 167
Microalbuminuria, 168
Brain, 168
Baroreflex sensitivity, 173

CHAPTER 12 Antihypertensive strategy, 175
Chronotherapy, 175
Salt restriction, 177
Drug treatment, 177

CHAPTER 13 24-hour BP-lowering characteristics of drugs, 181
Diuretics, 181
Calcium channel blockers, 181
   Amlodipine, 181
   Nifedipine, 185
   Cilnidipine, 187
   Azelnidipine, 188
Angiotensin-converting enzyme inhibitors, 188
Angiotensin-receptor blockers (ARBs), 190
   Valsaratan, 190
   Telmisartan, 190
   Candesartan, 190
   Olmesartan, 192
   Azilsartan, 197
Alpha-adrenergic blockers and beta-adrenergic blockers, 199
Sacubitril/valsartan, 201
SGLT2 inhibitor, 205

CHAPTER 14 Combination therapy: Home and ambulatory BP-profile-based combination strategy, 211

First-line therapy, 211
Second-line therapy, 211
   Arterial stiffness type, 211
   Volume retention type, 212
Third-line therapy, 214
Evidence of RAS inhibitor-based combination, 214

CHAPTER 15 Resistant hypertension and renal denervation, 227
The strategies for the management of resistant hypertension, 227
Fourth-line therapy, 227
Era of renal denervation, 230
Hypothesis of perfect 24-hour BP control by renal denervation, 231
Evidence for renal denervation, 231
   Morning BP, 234
   Nighttime BP, 234
   Sleep apnoea, 235
   Isolated systolic hypertension, 235
   Potential beyond-BP effect, 235
   The Symplicity Spyral™ and evidence, 236
Current potential candidates, 239
Responders and future indication of renal denervation, 242

CHAPTER 16 HOPE Asia Network, 245
HOPE Asia Network formation, 245
Characteristics of cardiovascular disease in Asia, 249
Obesity and salt intake in Asia, 249
24-hour ambulatory BP profile in Asia, 255
Facilitation of a home BP-guided approach in Asia, 256
Asia BP@Home study, 258

CHAPTER 17 Disaster hypertension and ICT-based home BP monitoring, 259
Disaster hypertension, 259
Disaster cardiovascular prevention (DCAP) network, 259
ICT-based BP control: successful model of telemedicine, 266

CHAPTER 18 Anticipation telemedicine, 269
Anticipation medicine, 269
Concept of event management, 269
Innovation technology, 271
Telemedicine and telecare, 272

References, 275
Index, 303

Author biography

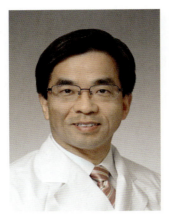

Kazuomi Kario MD PhD FACC FACP FAHA FESC

Professor
Division of Cardiovascular Medicine, Department of Medicine,
Center of Excellence, Cardiovascular Research and Development
(JCARD),
Jichi Medical University School of Medicine
Hypertension Cardiovascular Outcome Prevention and Evidence
(HOPE) Asia Network/World Hypertension League

3311-1, Yakushiji, Shimotsuke, Tochigi 329-0498, JAPAN
Tel: +81-285-58-7538; Fax: +81-285-44-4311;
E-mail: kkario@jichi.ac.jp

Dr Kazuomi Kario graduated from Jichi Medical School in 1986. He is currently Professor and Chairman of Cardiovascular Medicine, Jichi Medical University School of Medicine, Japan; Staff Visiting Professor, Institute of Cardiovascular Science, University College London, London, UK; Visiting Professor, Shanghai Jiao Tong University School of Medicine, Shanghai, China; Adjunct Professor, Yonsei University School of Medicine, Seoul, Korea and Distinguished Professor, *Fu Wai Hospital*, National Center for Cardiovascular Diseases, Chinese Academy of Medical Sciences, Beijing, China.

In 2003, Dr Kario and his team were the first to demonstrate **'morning surge' in blood pressure** (BP) as an independent risk factor for cardiovascular disease (Kario et al. Circulation 2003) [1,2]. He first used 'morning hypertension' with the definition of morning BP ≥135/85 mmHg, regardless of clinic BP, and stressed its clinical relevance in his book *Clinician's Manual on Early Morning Risk Management in Hypertension* in 2004 (Science Press, London, UK, 2004) [3]. He is proposing the **'resonance hypothesis' of BP surge** [4], and the concept of **systemic haemodynamic atherothrombotic syndrome** (SHATS) as a vicious cycle of BP variability and vascular disease [5]. He is the author of the recently published *Essential Manual on Perfect 24-hour Blood Pressure Management from Morning to Nocturnal Hypertension* (Wiley Blackwell, UK, 2015).

Professor Kario's research includes the research and development of new technology-based BP monitoring such as **IT-based home nocturnal BP mon-**

itoring (Hypertension 2013) and **hypoxia-triggered home sleep BP monitoring (TSP)** (Hypertension Research 2013); **wearable surge BP monitoring (WSP)** and **IT-based multisensor ambulatory BP monitoring (IMS-ABPM)** to clarify the clinical relevance of 24-hour BP control (Progress in Cardiovascular Disease 2016, 2017). He is the principal investigator of several clinical studies, such as the *Japan Morning Surge-Home Blood Pressure (J-HOP); Japan Ambulatory BP Monitoring (JAMP); Home-activity ICT-based Japan Ambulatory Blood Pressure Monitoring Prospective (HI-JAMP); Sleep BP and disordered breathing in REsistant hypertension And cardiovascular Disease (SPREAD)* and *The Home BP measurement with Olmesartan Naive patients to Establish Standard Target blood pressure (HONEST)*, the largest prospective observational study involving >20,000 patients.

He has served as Editor-in-Chief of *Curr Hypertens Rev* and is past Executive Editor of *Hypertens Res*. He is an editorial board member of more than 15 international journals including *Hypertension, J Hypertens, Circ J, J Clin Hypertens, J Am Soc Hypertens, Am J Hypertens, Blood Press Monit, Curr Hypertens Rep,* and *Curr Cardiol Rev*. Professor Kario has published more than 700 academic papers during his distinguished career. He founded the *Hypertension Cardiovascular Outcome Prevention and Evidence in Asia (**HOPE Asia Network**)"* in 2016.

References

1. Kario K, Pickering TG, Umeda Y, Hoshide S, Hoshide Y, Morinari M, Murata M, Kuroda T, Schwartz JE, Shimada K. Morning surge in blood pressure as a predictor of silent and clinical cerebrovascular disease in elderly hypertensives: a prospective study. *Circulation*. 2003; 107: 1401-1406. http://circ.ahajournals.org/
2. Kario K, Ishikawa J, Pickering TG, Hoshide S, Eguchi K, Morinari M, Hoshide Y, Kuroda T, Shimada K. Morning hypertension: the strongest independent risk factor for stroke in elderly hypertensive patients. *Hypertens Res.* 2006; 29: 581-587.
3. Kario K. *Clinician's Manual on Early Morning Risk Management in Hypertension*. Science Press, London, UK, pp.1-68, 2004.
4. Kario K. New insight of morning blood pressure surge into the triggers of cardiovascular disease - synergistic resonance of blood pressure variability. *Am J Hypertens.* 2016; 29: 14-16.
5. Kario K. Orthostatic hypertension - a new haemodynamic cardiovascular risk factor. *Nat Rev Nephrol.* 2013; 9: 726-738.

Preface
- Direction to perfect 24-hour blood pressure control

Cardiovascular events do not establish in a day, but the onset is non-linear. Over a lifetime, blood pressure (BP) plays two key roles as a central risk factor for cardiovascular disease (**Figure 0.1**) [1,2]. The first is as chronic risk factor advancing vascular disease and the second is as acute risk factor triggering cardiovascular events.

The essential benefit of the management of hypertension is derived from BP lowering per se, highlighting the importance of BP control throughout a 24-hour period. Recent guidelines stressed the importance of an out-of-clinic BP-guided approach for the diagnosis and management of hypertension [3,4]. Recently published 2017 American Heart Association/American College of Cardiology (AHA/ACC) guidelines for the management of hypertension proposed "universal BP goal" of 130/80 mmHg for BP measured in all settings (clinic, home and daytime ambulatory) for the new definition of hypertension and as the BP target for all patients, regardless of comorbidities (**Figures 0.2, 0.3**) [4]. The direction of BP management is the earlier and the lower throughout a 24-hour period, the better. This is the essential pathway for the management of hypertension [5].

"Perfect 24-hour BP control" is the ideal BP status, lowering the average 24-hour BP, maintaining adequate circadian rhythm, and stabilising BP variability (**Figure 0.4**) [6]. In the near future, the new haemodynamic biomarker-initiated "anticipation medicine" approach using the real-time information and communications technology (ICT)-based cardiovascular risk prediction and alert system over 24-hours would ideally prevent adverse cardiovascular events,

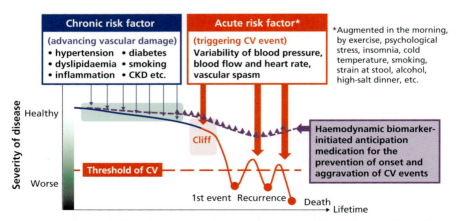

Figure 0.1 Differential effect of acute verus chronic risk factors and haemodynamic biomarker-initiated cardiovascular anticipation medicine. CV, cardiovascular. *Source:* Kario. 2016 [1]

BP Category	SBP		DBP
Normal	<120 mmHg	and	<80 mm Hg
Elevated	120–129 mmHg	and	<80 mmHg
Hypertension			
Stage 1	130–139 mmHg	or	80–89 mmHg
Stage 2	≥140 mmHg	or	≥90 mmHg

*Individuals with SBP and DBP in 2 categories should be designated to the higher BP category. BP indicates blood pressure (based on an average of ≥2 careful readings obtained on ≥2 occasions); DBP, diastolic blood pressure; and SBP, systolic blood pressure.

Figure 0.2 Categories of BP in adults*. Reprinted from *J Am Coll Cardiol*, Whelton PK et al., 2017 ACC/AHA/AAPA/ABC/ACPM/AGS/APhA/ASH/ASPC/NMA/PCNA guideline for the prevention, detection, evaluation, and management of high blood pressure in adults: a report of the American College of Cardiology/American Heart Association task force on clinical practice guidelines., in press. Copyright (2017), with permission from Elsevier [4]

Clinic	HBPM	Daytime ABPM	Nighttime ABPM	24-hour ABPM
120/80	120/80	120/80	100/65	115/75
130/80	130/80	130/80	110/65	125/75
140/90	135/85	135/85	120/70	130/80
160/100	145/90	145/90	140/85	145/90

ABPM indicates ambulatory blood pressure monitoring; BP, blood pressure; DBP, diastolic blood pressure; HBPM, home blood pressure monitoring; and SBP, systolic blood pressure.

Figure 0.3 Corresponding values of SBP/DBP for clinic, HBPM, daytime, nighttime, and 24-hour ABPM measurements. Reprinted from *J Am Coll Cardiol*, Whelton PK et al., 2017 ACC/AHA/AAPA/ABC/ACPM/AGS/APhA/ASH/ASPC/NMA/PCNA Guideline for the Prevention, Detection, Evaluation, and Management of High Blood Pressure in Adults: A Report of the American College of Cardiology/American Heart Association Task Force on Clinical Practice Guidelines., in press. Copyright (2017), with permission from Elsevier [4]

resulting in a healthy life [1,2].

Practically, the first target is morning hypertension [7,8]. BP has been shown to increase over the period from night to early morning, and cardiovascular events occur more frequently in the morning. The second target is uncontrolled nocturnal hypertension, control of which is a limitation of current hypertensive medication. (**Figure 0.5**) [9]. Stabilizing BP variability at the physiological oscillation level is the final goal for achieving zero cardiovascular events.

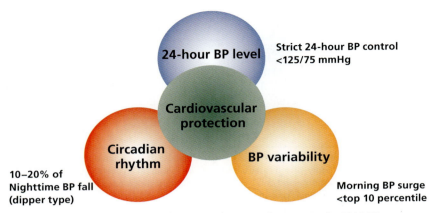

Figure 0.4 Triad of perfect 24-hour BP control. *Source:* Kario. 2004 [6]

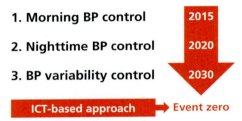

Figure 0.5 ICT-based staged strategy for "CV Event Zero." *Source:* Kario. 2015 [1]

In this book, I would like to show the recent evidence on morning hypertension and nocturnal hypertension, and the technology that will support the at-home BP-guided individual approach. I believe the "perfect 24-hour BP control" strategy using the health information technology (HIT)-based non-pharmacological approach, medication (changing the dose, the class, and timing of administration of drugs) and/or neuromodulation device treatment [10] will achieve the most effective cardiovascular and renal protection.

I hope this book will provide good practical advice for the up-dated treatment of hypertension on a day-to-day basis.

Kazuomi Kario, MD, PhD, FACC, FACP, FAHA, FESC
Division of Cardiovascular Medicine
Department of Medicine
Jichi Medical University School of Medicine
Tochigi,
Japan

References

1. Kario K. Evidence and perspectives on the 24-hour management of hypertension: hemodynamic biomarker-initiated 'anticipation medicine' for zero cardiovascular Event. *Prog Cardiovasc Dis*. 2016; 59: 262-281.
2. Kario K, Tomitani N, Kanegae H, Yasui N, Nishizawa M, Fujiwara T, Shigezumi T, Nagai R, Harada H. Development of a new ICT-based multisensor blood pressure monitoring system for use in hemodynamic biomarker-initiated anticipation medicine for cardiovascular disease: the national IMPACT program project. *Prog Cardiovasc Dis*. 2017; 60: 435-449.
3. Shimamoto K, Ando K, Fujita T, Hasebe N, Higaki J, Horiuchi M, Imai Y, Imaizumi T, Ishimitsu T, Ito M, Ito S, Itoh H, Iwao H, Kai H, Kario K, Kashihara N, Kawano Y, Kim-Mitsuyama S, Kimura G, Kohara K, Komuro I, Kumagai H, Matsuura H, Miura K, Morishita R, Naruse M, Node K, Ohya Y, Rakugi H, Saito I, Saitoh S, Shimada K, Shimosawa T, Suzuki H, Tamura K, Tanahashi N, Tsuchihashi T, Uchiyama M, Ueda S, Umemura S; Japanese Society of Hypertension Committee for Guidelines for the Management of Hypertension. The Japanese Society of Hypertension guidelines for the management of hypertension (JSH 2014). *Hypertens Res* 2014; 37: 253–387.
4. Whelton PK, Carey RM, Aronow WS, Casey DE Jr, Collins KJ, Dennison Himmelfarb C, DePalma SM, Gidding S, Jamerson KA, Jones DW, MacLaughlin EJ, Muntner P, Ovbiagele B, Smith SC Jr, Spencer CC, Stafford RS, Taler SJ, Thomas RJ, Williams KA Sr, Williamson JD, Wright JT Jr. 2017 ACC/AHA/AAPA/ABC/ACPM/AGS/APhA/ASH/ASPC/NMA/PCNA guideline for the prevention, detection, evaluation, and management of high blood pressure in adults: a report of the American College of Cardiology/American Heart Association task force on clinical practice guidelines. *J Am Coll Cardiol*. 2017. Nov 7. pii: S0735-1097(17)41519-1. [in press]
5. Kario K. Global impact of 2017 AHA/ACC hypertension guidelines: a perspective from Japan. *Circulation*. 2018; 137: 543-545. http://circ.ahajournals.org/
6. Kario K. *Clinician's Manual on Early Morning Risk Management in Hypertension*. Science Press, London, UK, pp.1-68, 2004.
7. Wang JG, Kario K, Park JB, Chen CH. Morning blood pressure monitoring in the management of hypertension. *J Hypertens*. 2017; 35: 1554-1563. https://journals.lww.com/jhypertension/
8. Kario K, Chen CH, Park S, Park CG, Hoshide S, Cheng HM, Huang QF, Wang JG. Consensus document on improving hypertension management in Asian patients, taking into account Asian characteristics. *Hypertension*. 2018; 71: 375-382. http://hyper.ahajournals.org
9. Kario K, Hoshide S, Haimoto H, Yamagiwa K, Uchiba K, Nagasaka S, Yano Y, Eguchi K, Matsui Y, Shimizu M, Ishikawa J, Ishikawa S; J-HOP study group. Sleep blood pressure self-measured at home as a novel determinant of organ damage: Japan Morning Surge Home Blood Pressure (J-HOP) study. *J Clin Hypertens (Greenwich)*. 2015; 17: 340-348.
10. Townsend RR, Mahfoud F, Kandzari DE, Kario K, Pocock S, Weber MA, Ewen S, Tsioufis K, Tousoulis D, Sharp ASP, Watkinson AF, Schmieder RE, Schmid A, Choi JW, East C, Walton A, Hopper I, Cohen DL, Wilensky R, Lee DP, Ma A, Devireddy CM, Lea JP, Lurz PC, Fengler K, Davies J, Chapman N, Cohen SA, DeBruin V, Fahy M, Jones DE, Rothman M, Böhm M; SPYRAL HTN-OFF MED trial investigators*. Catheter-based renal denervation in patients with uncontrolled hypertension in the absence of antihypertensive medications (SPYRAL HTN-OFF MED): a randomised, sham-controlled, proof-of-concept trial. *Lancet*. 2017; 390(10108): 2160-2170.

Acknowledgments

I would particularly like to thank the three academic fathers of my research, Kazuyuki Shimada, Takefumi Matsuo and the late Thomas G Pickering, who continuously supported me. I would also like to thank other senior researchers in this field and my colleagues who provided many helpful academic comments and criticism on the contents of this book. They include Ryozo Nagai, Michael Weber, Bryan Williams, Gianfranco Parati, George Stergiou, Jiguang Wang, Satoshi Hoshide, Tomoyuki Kabutoya, Hiroyuki Mizuno, Takeshi Fujiwara, Naoko Tomitani, Hiroshi Kanegae, Masafumi Nishizawa, Tetsuro Yoshida, Yuichiro Yano, Masahisa Shimpo, Yasushi Imai, Takahide Kohro, Hiroshi Funayama, Kenji Harada, Ken Kono, Yukiyo Ogata, Toshinobu Saito, Takahiro Komori, Katsuaki Yokota, Motoki Fukutomi, Tomonori Watanabe, Masao Takahashi, Yoshioki Nishimura, Hayato Shimizu, Ayako Yokota, Shinichi Toriumi, Kennichi Katsurada, Hiroaki Watanabe, Mizuri Taki, Yusuke Oba, Tsunashi Kozaki, Yukako Ogoyama, Hajime Shinohara, Kana Kubota, Kazuyo Ishibashi, Hirotaka Waki, Takahiro Watanabe, Yusuke Ishiyama, Seigo Arima, Takafumi Okuyama, Hisaya Kobayashi, Daisuke Kaneko, Yusuke Suzuki, Yuki Imaizumi, Yasuhiro Yokoyama, Tadayuki Mitama, Yutaka Aoyama, Masafumi Sato, Shunsuke Saito, Satoshi Niijima, Keita Negishi, Sirisawat Wanthong, Praew Kotruchin, Kazuo Eguchi, Joji Ishikawa, Yoshio Matsui, Michiaki Nagai, Shizukiyo Ishikawa, Seiichi Shibasaki, Motohiro Shimizu, Mitsunori Sugiyama, Mikio Iwashita, Toshikazu Shiga, Noboru Shinomiya, Mitsuo Kuwabara, Nobuhiko Yasui, Shinobu Ozaki, Kyohei Fukatani, Takashi Kuwayama. Last but not least, I would like to thank Kimiyo Saito, Noriko Sugawara, Hiromi Ueno, Haruna Hamasaki, Yuri Matsumoto, Yukie Okawara, Ryoko Nozue, Risa Furusawa, Hiromi Suwa, Rika Toyoda, Yukiko Suzuki, Keiko Sato, Chie Iwashita, Emiko Takahashi, Fumiaki Nakamura, Hideki Tamura, Tomoko Morimoto, Tomoko Shiga, Noriko Harada for their research coordination, and Asuka Kobayashi, Kaori Morita, Yosuke Sato, Ayumi Kasahara and Ayako Okura for their editorial support, without whom this book would not have been possible.

Studies described in this manuscript was partly supported by the ImPACT Program of Council for Science, Technology and Innovation (Cabinet Office, Government of Japan); Japan Agency for Medical Research and Development (AMED) under Grant Number JP17he1102002h0003; JSPS KAKENHI, Grant-in-Aid for Scientific Research B (Grant Number JP26293192); JSPS KAKENHI, Grant-in-Aid for Scientific Research S (Grant Number 17H06151) from Japan Society for the Promotion of Science; a grant from the Foundation for Development of the Community (Tochigi); MSD Life Science Foundation, Public Interest Incorporated Foundation.

CHAPTER 1
Out-of-clinic BP

SPRINT and automated office BP

The most striking evidence directly influencing the 2017 AHA/ACC guidelines [1] is the results of the SPRINT study [2]. This trial clearly demonstrated the benefit of strictly lower BP control targeting systolic BP <120 mmHg in hypertensive patients. The incidence of cardiovascular events and all-cause mortality were lower in the strict BP control group than in the standard BP control group (systolic BP <140 mmHg) (**Figure 1.1**). After this intervention study, the direction of BP management has been clearly set. However, the evidence from SPRINT was obtained using automated office BP (AOBP) measurement, which is different from clinic BP measured by routine clinic BP measurement. The AOBP is measured by automated BP monitoring in the sitting position 5 minutes after the doctor leaves the office. The AOBP for systolic BP is lower by 10–15 mmHg than clinic BP measured by routine measurement. This measurement may exclude the doctor-induced white-coat effect, but cannot eliminate the pressor effect of the clinic setting [3].

Different clinical BP measurements

There are four different BP measurements available in clinical practice (clinic, AOBP, home BP monitoring [HBPM], and ambulatory BP monitoring [ABPM]) (**Figure 1.2**) [3]. Each approach induces different pressor effects (**Figure 1.2**), and detects BP variability over short and longer time periods (**Figure 1.3**) [4]. However, all these BP measurements are superior to routine clinical BP measurements for predicting cardiovascular events. After the universal BP goal of 130/80 mmHg is achieved, the ideal goal of white-coat effect-excluding BP may be <125 mmHg.

All the recent guidelines, including the 2017 AHA/ACC guidelines [1], the Japanese Society of Hypertension (JSH 2014) guidelines [5], European Society of Hypertension/European Society of Cardiology (ESH/ESC 2013) guidelines [6] and NICE 2011 guidelines (UK) [7] recommend the practical use of out-of-clinic BP for the diagnosis and management of hypertension. The JSH 2014 guidelines recommend the HBPM-guided approach as the first step for the management of hypertension [5]. At the practice level, recent HBPM could measure night-

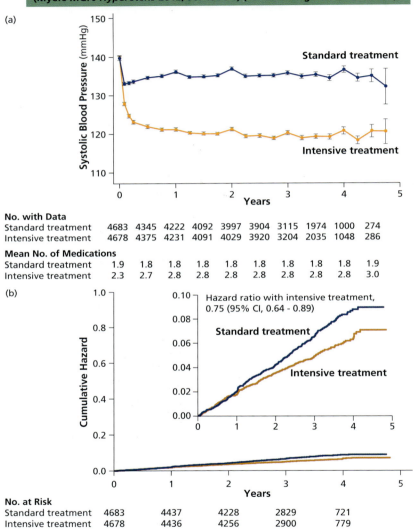

Figure 1.1 SPRINT. (a) Systolic blood pressure (BP) during follow-up (automated office BP). Throughout the 3.26 years of follow-up, the mean systolic BP was 121.5 mmHg in the intensive-treatment group and 134.6 mmHg in the standard-treatment group (mean number of antihypertensive medications was 2.8 and 1.8 respectively). (b) Primary outcome (a composite of myocardial infarction, acute coronary syndrome, stroke, heart failure, or death from cardiovascular causes). CKD, chronic kidney disease; CVD, cardiovascular disease.
Source: (a, b) SPRINT Research Group. 2015 [2]. Copyright © (2015) Massachusetts Medical Society. Reprinted with permission from Massachusetts Medical Society.

Out-of-clinic BP

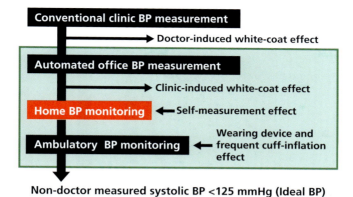

Figure 1.2 Different approaches to BP measurement and influencing factors. BP, blood pressure. *Source:* Kario. 2016 [3]. Copyright © (2017) Bentham Science Publishers Ltd. Republished with permission of Bentham Science Publishers Ltd.

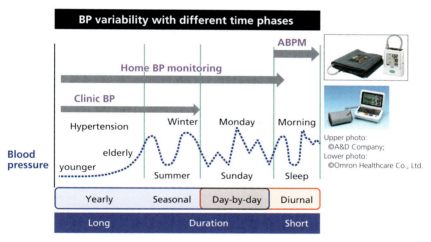

Figure 1.3 Blood pressure measurements in clinical practice. ABPM, ambulatory blood pressure monitoring. *Source:* Kario. 2016 [4]

time BP during sleep, and recent ABPM could be used as home BP monitoring (**Figures 1.3** and **1.4**) [4, 8, 9]. The research and development of continuous beat-by-beat "surge" BP monitoring has started, but it is still in the research stage (**Figure 1.4**) [8, 9].

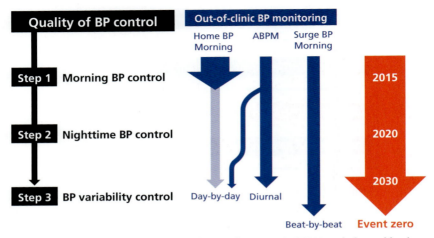

Figure 1.4 ICT-based strategy for "Zero Cardiovascular Events". ABPM, ambulatory blood pressure monitoring; BP, blood pressure. *Source:* Kario. 2017 [8]

Blood pressure (mmHg)	Systolic	Diastolic
clinic	130	80
(Automated office)	(130)	(80)
Home		
Morning	130	80
Daytime (awake)	130	80
Evening	130	80
Nighttime (sleep)	110	65
Ambulatory		
24-hour	125	75
Daytime	130	80
Nighttime	110	65
Morning	130	80

Figure 1.5 Different thresholds of BP level for diagnosis of hypertension. *Source:* modified from Kario. 2015 [10]

Diagnosis of hypertension and subtypes

Figure 1.5 [10] demonstrates the different thresholds of clinic, home, and ambulatory BP values for the definition of hypertension. Masked hypertension is defined as normotension for clinic BP and hypertension for out-of-clinic BP, while white-coat hypertension is defined as normotension for out-of-clinic BP

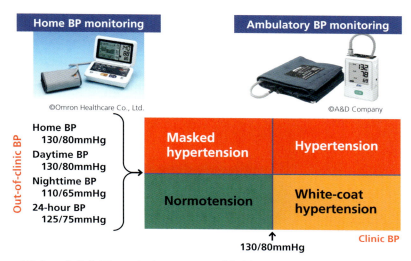

Figure 1.6 Out-of-clinic BP monitoring. *Source:* modified from Kario. 2015 [10]

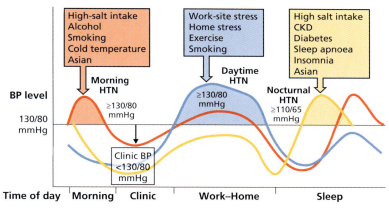

Figure 1.7 Three forms of masked hypertension and influencing factors - masked morning, daytime, and nocturnal (uncontrolled) hypertension. BP, blood pressure; HTN, hypertension; CKD, chronic kidney disease. *Source:* Kario. 2018 [11]

and hypertension for clinic BP (**Figure 1.6**) [10]. There are three subtypes of masked hypertension, namely morning hypertension, daytime (stress-induced) hypertension, and nocturnal hypertension (**Figure 1.7**) [11]. Factors influencing the pressor effect on BP values are different among these three subtypes. Of these masked hypertension subtypes, only morning hypertension could be definitively detected by the routine measurement of HBPM.

CHAPTER 2
Morning and nocturnal hypertension as therapeutic targets

Morning is the most important period for cardiovascular diseases [12, 13]. Cardiovascular events occur most frequently in the morning just after awakening, at the time of peak ambulatory blood pressure (BP) (**Figure 2.1**) [13]. Exaggerated morning BP surge (MBPS) and morning hypertension are risks for cardiovascular events (**Figure 2.2**), and are associated with advanced organ damage (**Figure 2.3**) [14-18]. Morning BP level is more closely associated with organ damage to the brain, heart and kidney, and the risk of cardiovascular and cerebrovascular events (**Figure 2.4**) and disability in the elderly than clinic BP level both in hypertensive patients and community-based normotensive populations [19, 20]. Finally, recent evidence demonstrates that uncontrolled morning hypertension is a strong predictor of cardiovascular events in medicated hypertensive patients [21].

Definition of morning hypertension

The broad definition of "morning hypertension" is having an average morning BP of ≥130 mmHg for systolic BP (SBP), and/or ≥80 mmHg for diastolic BP (DBP), regardless of clinic BP (**Figure 2.5**) [12]. In addition, strict definition of "morning hypertension" is those with a morning–evening difference (ME-dif; morning SBP – evening SBP) in home BP ≥15 mmHg [12, 16]. Morning hypertension (ambulatory morning hypertension) can also be diagnosed using ABPM [16]. Masked morning hypertension is defined as morning hypertension when clinic BP is <130/80 mmHg.

Definition of nocturnal hypertension

Nocturnal hypertension is defined as average nighttime SBP ≥110 mmHg systolic and/or DBP ≥65 mmHg (**Figure 2.6**). Nighttime BP is that measured from bedtime to rising or over the period 1 am to 6 am. by ABPM or by home BP monitoring (HBPM) (at least three readings per night for at least two days).

Clinic-masked nocturnal hypertension is defined as nocturnal hypertension with clinic BP <130/80 mmHg, while morning-masked nocturnal hypertension is defined as nocturnal hypertension with morning home BP <130/80 mmHg. Isolated nocturnal hypertension is defined as nocturnal hypertension with both clinic and morning home BP values <130/80 mmHg.

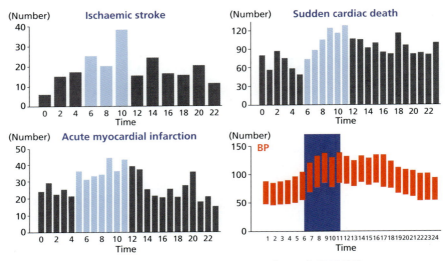

Figure 2.1 Onset time of cardiovascular events. *Source:* Muller et al. 1989 [13]

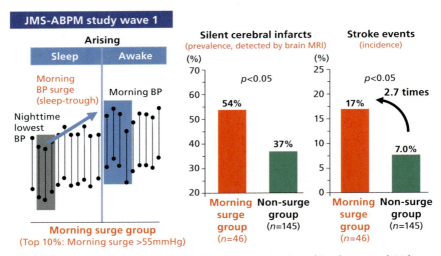

Figure 2.2 Morning BP surge and stroke risk in hypertension (matching for age and 24-hour systolic BP). ABPM, ambulaory blood pressure monitoring; BP, blood pressure. *Source:* Kario et al. 2003 [14]

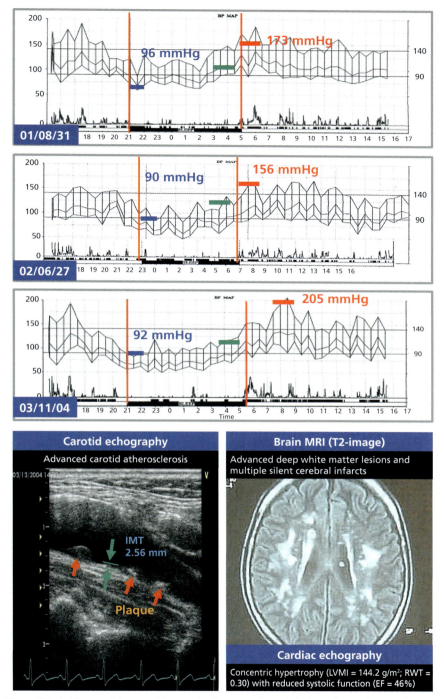

Figure 2.3 A 69-year-old man with morning hypertension exhibiting advanced organ damage. Cardiac echography demonstrated that concentric hypertrophy (left ventricular mass index [LVMI]=144.2 g/m^2; relative wall thickness [RWT]=0.30) with reduced systolic function (ejection fraction [EF]=46%). IMT, intima media thickness. *Source:* Kario. 2015 [10]

JMS-ABPM study wave 1		
Cox regression analysis for clinical stroke events		
Covariates	Relative risk (95%CI)	p-value
Clinic SBP (10 mmHg)	not selected	
24-hour SBP (10 mmHg)	not selected	
Daytime SBP (10 mmHg)	not selected	
Evening SBP (10 mmHg)	not selected	
Nighttime SBP (10 mmHg)	not selected	
Pre-awake SBP (10 mmHg)	not selected	
Morning SBP (10 mmHg)	1.44 (1.25–1.67)	<0.0001

Morning SBP is the 2-hour average of ABPM-measured SBPs after rising.
After controlling for age, gender, body mass index, smoking status, diabetes, hyperlipidaemia, silent cerebral infarct, and antihypertensive medication status at the final follow-up, all SBP variables (clinic, 24-hour, daytime, evening, nighttime, pre-awake, and morning) were added in the model, and were analysed by stepwise Cox regression analysis. ABPM, ambulatory blood pressure monitoring; CI, confidence interval; SBP, systolic blood pressure.

Figure 2.4 Morning BP is the strongest independent predictor of stroke events. *Source:* Kario et al. 2006 [16]

Morning hypertension (home BP monitoring)	
Wide definition	Average of self-measured morning home BPs ≥130 mmHg systolic and/or ≥80 mmHg diastolic
Specific definition	Above definition plus ME difference (morning BP minus evening BP) ≥15 mmHg systolic
Ambulatory morning hypertension (ABPM)	
	Average of ambulatory BPs during 2-hours after rising ≥130 mmHg systolic and/or ≥80 mmHg diastolic
Masked morning hypertension	
	Morning hypertension with clinic BP <130/80 mmHg

Figure 2.5 Definition of morning hypertension; BP, blood pressure. *Source:* Kario K. *Essential Manual on Perfect 24-hour Blood Pressure Management from Morning to Nocturnal Hypertension: Up-to-date for Anticipation Medicine.* Wiley, 2018.

Shift of the prevalence of morning hypertension by 2017 AHA/ACC guidelines

Figure 2.7 [11] shows the shift in morning hypertension prevalence patterns based on the new AHA/ACC 2017 guidelines [1] (shown in red) compared with those classified by the previous Seventh Report of the Joint National Committee on Prevention, Detection, Evaluation and Treatment of High Blood Pressure (JNC7) guidelines [22] (shown in black) from our general practice-based

Nocturnal hypertension Average of nighttime BP readings* ≥110 mmHg systolic and/or >65 mmHg diastolic
Clinic-masked nocturnal hypertension Nocturnal hypertension with clinic BP <130/80 mmHg
Morning-masked nocturnal hypertension Nocturnal hypertension with morning home BP <130/80 mmHg
Isolated nocturnal hypertension Nocturnal hypertension with both clinic and morning home BP <130/80 mmHg

*Nighttime BP is the average of BP readings measured from bedtime to rising or from 1 am to 6 am by ABPM or by HBPM (at least 3 readings per night, and over at least 2 days).

Figure 2.6 Definition of nocturnal hypertension. ABPM, ambulatory blood pressure monitoring; BP, blood pressure; HBPM, home BP monitoring. *Source:* Kario K. *Essential Manual on Perfect 24-hour Blood Pressure Management from Morning to Nocturnal Hypertension: Up-to-date for Anticipation Medicine.* Wiley, 2018.

national registry of home BP, the Japan Morning Surge-Home Blood Pressure (J-HOP) study (4,310 patients with treated hypertension: mean age 64.9 years, 47% male).

The prevalence of normotension, white-coat hypertension, masked morning hypertension and sustained morning hypertension changed from 31%, 15%, 19%, 36% by the previous definition using the previous JNC7 [22] definition (140/90 mmHg for clinic BP and 135/85 mmHg for home BP) to 14%, 17%, 10%, 58%, respectively, based on the new AHA/ACC 2017 definition (130/80 mmHg for both clinic and home BP) (**Figure 2.7**) [1, 11]. Under the new criteria, the prevalence of uncontrolled, sustained (uncontrolled) morning hypertension is increased, while that of masked (uncontrolled) morning hypertension is decreased. This lower single BP threshold of 130/80 mmHg for both clinic and home BP values could be acceptable for two reasons. First, in general, the difference between clinic and out-of-clinic BP values decreases to reach a similar level to that shown in (**Figure 2.7**) [11]. Second, clinically, the decrease in masked morning hypertension and the increase in sustained morning hypertension provides doctors with the opportunity to strictly treat hypertension without underestimation of cardiovascular risk, because doctors would not detect masked morning hypertension. The lower morning BP (SBP <125 mmHg) may be ideal for minimisation of cardiovascular risk, regardless of clinic BP level [21].

When to use home and ambulatory BP monitoring

The clinical use of HBPM and ABPM increases the quality of hypertension management. In clinical practice, HBPM and ABPM should not be considered as sep-

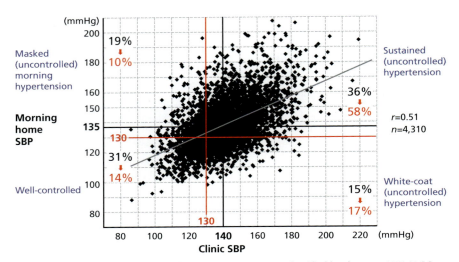

Figure. 2.7 Shift of the prevalence of hypertension patterns classified by the new AHA/ACC 2017 guidelines (shown in red) from those classified by the previous Seventh Report of the Joint National Committee on Prevention, Detection, Evaluation and Treatment of High Blood Pressure (JNC7) guidelines (shown in black) in subjects in the Japan Morning Surge-Home Blood Pressure (J-HOP) study (4,310 patients with treated hypertension: mean age 64.9 years, 47% male). SBP, systolic blood pressure. *Source:* Kario. 2018 [11]

arate but instead used in combination [5].

Morning BP can be measured using both HBPM and ABPM. HBPM is self-measured at home while the patient is seated, while ABPM measures BP regularly at 15- to 30-minute intervals throughout each 24-hour period. Clinical use of HBPM is superior to ABPM because it is convenient, without discomfort. However, the BP profiles evaluated by these two methods are different. HBPM only measures BP at a specific time (morning and/or evening) and in a specific condition (resting while sitting), while ABPM measures dynamic ambulatory BP changes during the day and nighttime BP during sleep periods. This allows detection of both dynamic nighttime BP changes and masked nocturnal hypertension. However, recent HBPM device design advances mean that they have the potential to measure nighttime BP during sleep.

HBPM is recommended to all medicated hypertensive patients, those with elevated BP (clinic SBP 120–129 mmHg and DBP <80 mmHg), or prehypertensive subjects with an estimated 2-year risk of new-onset hypertension ≥40% (calculated by the Genki-Jichi hypertension prediction simulator (Kanegae H, Oikawa T, Kario K) (**Figures 2.8** and **2.9**).

ABPM is recommended to high-risk hypertensive patients with: 1) home BP

Morning and nocturnal hypertension as therapeutic targets

Patients for whom out-of-clinic BP monitoring is recommended	
Home BP monitoring	• All medicated hypertensive patients • Subjects with clinic BP ≥120/80 mmHg • Prehypertensive subjects with estimated 2-year risk of new-onset hypertension ≥40%*
Ambulatory BP monitoring	High-risk hypertensive patients with • home BP ≥120/80 mmHg • history of cardiovascular events • organ damage (ECG-LVH, albuminuria, NT-proBNP >125 pg/mL, etc.) • nocturnal hypertension-suspected comorbidities (SAS, diabetes, CKD)

*Based on the Genki-Jichi hypertension prediction simulator (Kanegae, Oikawa, Kario).
BP, blood pressure; ECG-LVH, electrocardiogram-left ventricular hypertrophy; NT-proBNP, N-terminal pro-B-type natriuretic peptide; SAS, sleep apnoea syndrome; CKD, chronic kidney disease.

Figure 2.8 Subjects for recommendation of home and ambulatory BP monitoring. *Source:* Kario K. *Essential Manual on Perfect 24-hour Blood Pressure Management from Morning to Nocturnal Hypertension: Up-to-date for Anticipation Medicine.* Wiley, 2018.

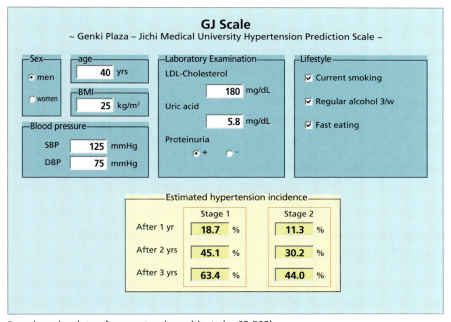

Based on the data of normotensive subjects (*n*=93,303) examined at Genki Plaza health check examination in 2005

Figure 2.9 GJ Hypertension prediction simulation. *Source:* Kario K. *Essential Manual on Perfect 24-hour Blood Pressure Management from Morning to Nocturnal Hypertension: Up-to-date for Anticipation Medicine.* Wiley, 2018.

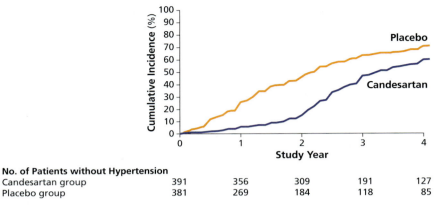

Figure 2.10 Incidence of new-onset stage 2 hypertension in patients with stage 1 hypertension (clinic BP 130–140/85–90 mmHg) for 4 years in the TROPHY study. *Source:* Julius et al. 2006 [23]. Copyright © (2006) Massachusetts Medical Society. Reprinted with permission from Massachusetts Medical Society.

≥120/80 mmHg; 2) history of cardiovascular events; 3) organ damage (e.g. ECG-LVH, albuminuria, N-terminal pro B-type natriuretic peptide [NT-proBNP] >125 pg/mL); and 4) nocturnal hypertension-suspected comorbidities (sleep apnoea syndrome, diabetes, chronic kidney disease).

In the TROPHY study [23], the incidence of new-onset Stage 2 hypertension in patients with Stage 1 hypertension (clinic BP 130–140/85–90 mmHg) was 40.4% at the 2-year follow-up, and 63.0% at the 4-year follow-up (**Figure 2.10**). However, the average home BP at baseline was 134/83 mmHg, indicating that at least half of the subjects had hypertension as diagnosed by home BP. In addition, in patients with elevated BP (clinic 120–129/<80 mmHg), the risk of Stage 2 hypertension has been shown to be >3 times higher than in those with normal (optimal) BP (**Figure 2.11**) [24].

Staged management of morning and nocturnal hypertension

Morning hypertension evaluated by HBPM should be the first target of antihypertensive treatment (Step 1) (**Figure 2.12**) [10]. After morning home BP is well-controlled (<130/80 mmHg on antihypertensive treatment), nighttime BP should be measured by ABPM or nighttime BP-capable HBPM. When nighttime BP is ≥110 mmHg systolic or ≥65 mmHg diastolic, this residual, uncontrolled nocturnal hypertension is the next target of antihypertensive treatment (Step 2).

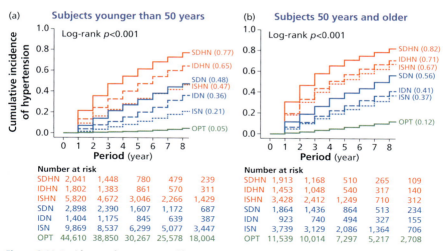

Figure 2.11 Incidence of new onset of hypertension in normotensive subjects in the Genki Plaza Medical Center for Health Care. BP was divided into seven categories: (1) Optimal BP (OPT), SBP/DBP <120/80 mmHg; (2) Isolated systolic normal BP (ISN), 120–129/<80 mmHg; (3) Isolated diastolic normal BP (IDN), <120/80–84 mmHg; (4) Systolic diastolic normal BP (SDN), 120–129/80–84 mmHg; (5) Isolated systolic high-normal BP (ISHN), 130–139/<85 mmHg; (6) Isolated diastolic high-normal BP (IDHN), <130/85–89 mmHg, and (7) Systolic diastolic high-normal BP (SDHN), 130–139/85–89 mmHg. The label of each line is the BP category and (in parentheses) the cumulative incidence of hypertension. The log-rank test was used to calculate p-values. Reproduced with permission, from Kanegae H, Oikawa T, Okawara Y, Hoshide S, Kario K. Which blood pressure measurement, systolic or diastolic, better predicts future hypertension in normotensive young adults? *J Clin Hypertens (Greenwich)*. 2017; 19: 603-610.

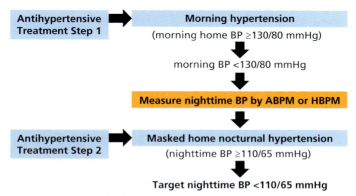

Figure 2.12 Staged home BP-guided management of morning to nocturnal hypertension. ABPM, ambulatory blood pressure monitoring; BP, blood pressure; HBPM, home BP monitoring. *Source:* modified from Kario. 2015 [10]

CHAPTER 3
Home BP monitoring and morning hypertension

Home blood-pressure-guided management of hypertension is the best approach in clinical practice. The Ohasama study first demonstrated that home blood pressure (BP) is superior to clinic BP for predicting cardiovascular prognosis [25]. The Japanese Society of Hypertension Guidelines for the Management of Hypertension (JSH 2014) recommends the home BP-guided approach [5].

How to measure home BP

Figure 3.1 shows the standard method of self-measured home BP monitoring (HBPM). **Figure 3.2** demonstrates the difference in home BP measurements among international and Japanese guidelines. The timing of morning BP measurement is the same but timing of the evening measurement is different [26]. European Society of Hypertension (ESH) guidelines [6] recommend measuring evening BP before dinner, while AHA/ASH guidelines recommend measuring evening BP before going to bed [27]. There is no significant difference in the morning BP and evening BP measured before dinner. However, bathing and

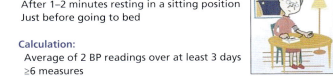

Home BP measurement is performed as follows
Morning BP
Twice
After 1–2 minutes resting in a sitting position
Within 1 hour after waking up
After urination
Before breakfast
Before taking pills

Evening BP
Twice
After 1–2 minutes resting in a sitting position
Just before going to bed

Calculation:
Average of 2 BP readings over at least 3 days
≥6 measures

Figure 3.1 Home BP measurement. BP, blood pressure.

	Timing	Frequency/occasion	Duration
AHA/ACC 2017	• Morning (before taking medications) • Evening (before supper)	≥Twice (1 min apart)	• Ideally 7 days
ESH/ESC 2013	• Morning (before taking medications) • Evening (before supper)	Twice (1–2 min apart)	• ≥3–4 days • Ideally 7 days
NICE/BHS 2011	• Twice daily • Ideally morning and evening	Twice (≥1 min apart)	• ≥4 days • Ideally 7 days
AHA/ASH/PCNA statement on HBPM (Pickering TG et al. [27])	• Morning before drug intake • Evening (at bedtime)	Twice to three times (1 min apart)	• 7 days
JSH 2014	• Morning (within 1 hr after waking up, after urination, before dosing in the morning, before breakfast) • Evening (at bedtime) Additional information: Timing of dinner, bathing, alcohol intake, evening dosing of drugs Others: At the time of symptoms, during the daytime on holidays, during sleep at night	Twice	• ≥5 days
HOPE Asia Network*	• Morning (before taking medications) • Evening (at bedtime)	Twice (≥2 min apart)	• ≥3 days

AHA, American Heart Association; ACC, American College of Cardiology; ESH, European Society of Hypertension; ESC, European Society of Cardiology; JSH, Japanese Society of Hypertension; NICE, National Institute for Clinical Excellence; BHS, British Hypertension Society; HOPE Asia Network, Hypertension Cardiovascular Outcome Prevention and Evidence in Asia. *See Chapter 16.

Figure 3.2 Comparison of Eastern and Asian guidelines: HBPM. HBPM, home blood pressure monitoring. *Source:* Kario K. *Essential Manual on Perfect 24-hour Blood Pressure Management from Morning to Nocturnal Hypertension: Up-to-date for Anticipation Medicine.* Wiley, 2018.

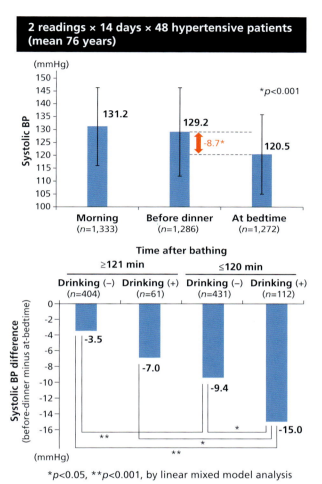

Figure 3.3 Different evening home systolic BP readings before dinner and at bedtime. BP, blood pressure. *Source:* Fujiwara et al. 2017 [26]

alcohol consumption significantly decrease evening BP measured at bedtime (**Figure 3.3**) [26]. In addition, reproducibility of home BP is better for morning BP than for evening BP. There is no significant correlation between morning home BP and clinic BP self-measured in the waiting room before examination (waiting-room BP), and clinic BP measured by the doctor (examining-room BP) (**Figure 3.4**) [28]. Thus, to simplify home BP measurement in clinical practice, we recommend morning BP measurement.

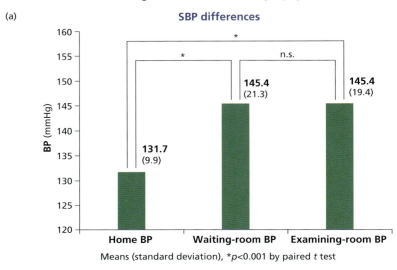
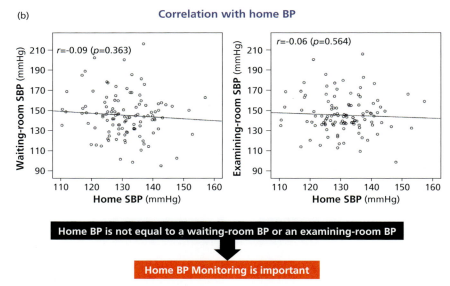

Figure 3.4 Home BP versus waiting-room and examining-room BP. BP, blood pressure; SBP, systolic BP. *Source:* Fujiwara et al. 2017 [28]

Home BP monitoring and morning hypertension

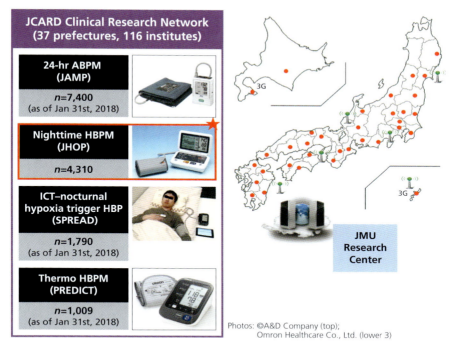

Photos: ©A&D Company (top);
Omron Healthcare Co., Ltd. (lower 3)

Figure 3.5 Jichi Medical University, Center of Excellence, Community Medicine Cardiovascular Research and Development (JCARD). ABPM, ambulatory blood pressure monitoring; ICT, information and communication technology; JMU, Jichi Medical University; HBPM, home blood pressure monitoring. *Source:* Kario K. *Essential Manual on Perfect 24-hour Blood Pressure Management from Morning to Nocturnal Hypertension: Up-to-date for Anticipation Medicine.* Wiley, 2018.

Evidence for morning hypertension control

The Ohasama study of a general population-based cohort first demonstrated that home BP is a better predictor of cardiovascular prognosis than clinic BP. In the J-HOP (Japan Morning Surge-Home Blood Pressure) study, one of the nationwide general practitioner-based cohorts of patients with cardiovascular risk (**Figure 3.5**) demonstrated morning home BP is a better predictor of stroke than evening home BP (**Figure 3.6**) [29].

On-treatment morning home BP was also a stronger predictor of cardiovascular events than clinic BP in the HOMED-BP (Hypertension Objective treatment based on Measurement by Electrical Devices of Blood Pressure) study [30] and the HONEST (Home blood pressure measurement with Olmesartan Naive

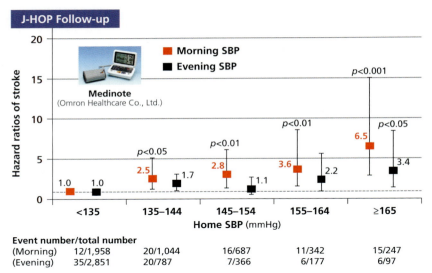

Figure 3.6 Home BP and stroke risk (*n*=4,103). BP, blood pressure; SBP, systolic BP. *Source:* Hoshide et al. 2016 [29].

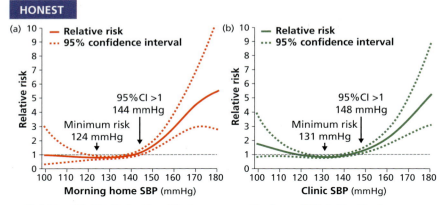

Relative risk 1 indicates the risk at mean morning home SBP during the 2-yr follow-up period (a); the risk at mean clinic SBP during the 2-yr follow-up period (b).

Adjusted for sex, age, family history of cardiovascular disease, dyslipidaemia, diabetes mellitus, chronic kidney disease, history of cardiovascular disease, and smoking status. Primary endpoint: stroke event; coronary event; sudden death.

Figure 3.7 Minimum and statistical significant increase in cardiovascular risk of morning home BP by spline regression analysis. We did a spline regression analysis using continuous BP values. The morning BP value associated with minimum risk was 124 mmHg. The morning BP value at which the lower limit of 95% confidence interval exceeded relative risk 1 was 144 mmHg. This finding was consistent with the results of the Cox proportional hazard model. Likewise, the clinic BP associated with minimum risk was 131 mmHg. The clinic BP value at which the lower limit of 95% confidence interval exceeded relative risk 1 was 148 mmHg. BP, blood pressure; SBP, systolic BP. *Source:* Kario et al. 2014 [21]

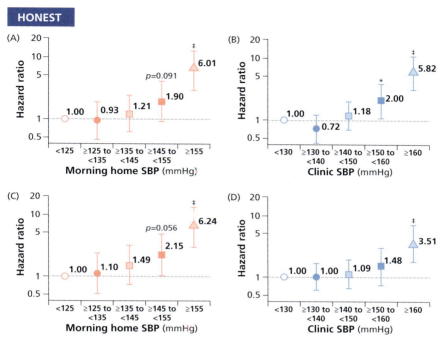

Figure 3.8 On-treatment BP and coronary/stroke events. Panel A and B: HRs for stroke events; Panel C and D: HRs for CAD events. The Cox proportional hazards model was used, adjusting for sex, age, family history of cardiovascular disease, dyslipidaemia, diabetes mellitus, chronic kidney disease, history of cardiovascular disease, and smoking status. *$p<0.05$; ‡$p<0.001$. CAD, coronary artery disease; SBP, systolic blood pressure. Reprinted from *J Am Coll Cardiol*. vol. 67, Kario K et al. Morning home blood pressure is a strong predictor of coronary artery disease: the HONEST study. p1519-1527 [31]. Copyright (2016), with permission from Elsevier. Ref. [31]

patients to Establish Standard Target blood pressure) study [21]. The HONEST trial is the largest real-world prospective study in the field, and included >21,000 patients with hypertension. The results showed that morning systolic BP (SBP) of 145 mmHg was the threshold for a statistically significant increase in cardiovascular risk in medicated hypertensive patients. In addition, the morning SBP associated with minimum risk was 124 mmHg (**Figure 3.7**) [21]. Furthermore, morning home BP could detect the risk of coronary artery disease similarly to that of a stroke, while clinic BP underestimated the risk of coronary artery disease (**Figure 3.8**) [31]. There was no significant J-curve of morning home SBP until 110 mmHg, both for stroke and coronary events (**Figure 3.9**) [31]. When on-treatment morning home SBP was well-controlled (<125 mmHg) during

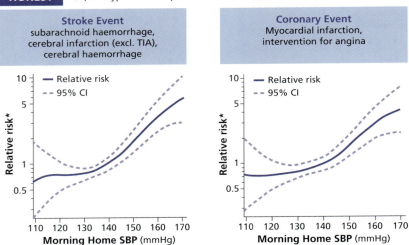

*Adjusted for age, sex, family history of CVD, complications (dyslipidaemia, diabetes, CKD), history of CVD, smoking habit.

Figure 3.9 Relationship between morning home systolic BP and stroke/coronary event (Spline regression analysis). BP, blood pressure; CKD, chronic kidney disease; CVD, cardiovascular disease; TIA, transient ischaemic attack. *Source:* Kario et al. 2016 [31]. Reprinted from *J Am Coll Cardiol*. vol. 67, Kario K et al. Morning home blood pressure is a strong predictor of coronary artery disease: the HONEST study. p1519-1527. Copyright (2016), with permission from Elsevier.

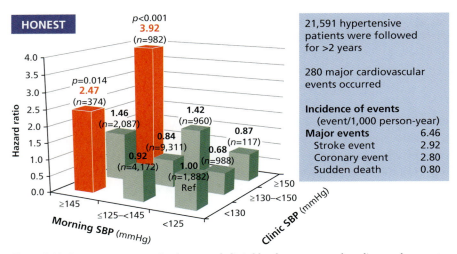

Figure 3.10 On-treatment morning home and clinic blood pressures and cardiovascular events in medicated hypertensive patients (HONEST study). Adjusted for sex, age, family history of cardiovascular disease, dyslipidaemia, diabetes mellitus, chronic kidney disease, history of cardiovascular disease, and smoking status. SBP, systolic blood pressure. *Source:* Kario et al. 2014 [21]

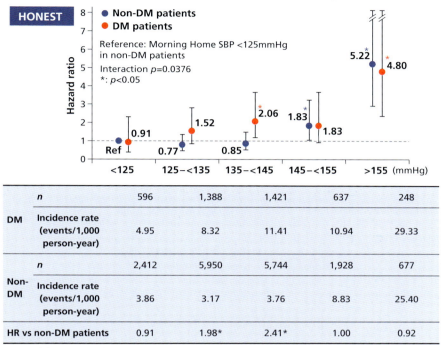

Figure 3.11 Relationship between CV events and morning home SBP in ARB-medicated patients with and without DM (HONEST study). ARB, angiotensin-receptor blocker; CKD, chronic kidney disease; CV, cardiovascular; DM, diabetes mellitus; HR, hazard ratio; SBP, systolic blood pressure. *Source:* Kushiro et al. 2017 [32]

2-year-follow-up, there was no increase in cardiovascular events even in those with clinic SBP maintained at ≥150 mmHg (**Figure 3.10**) [21].

In a subanalysis in patients with diabetes, those with morning home SBP 125–134 or 135–144 mmHg showed a tendency for, or a significant increase in, the risk of cardiovascular events compared with the well-controlled group (morning home SBP <125 mmHg) (**Figure 3.11**) [32]. In the HONEST study, patients were asked to measure morning home BP twice. There was an interesting V-shape association of the difference between the first reading and the second reading, and cardiovascular events (**Figure 3.12**) [33]. Risk was higher in those with the greatest variability between the first and second home BP measurements compared with patients whose BP readings were more stable.

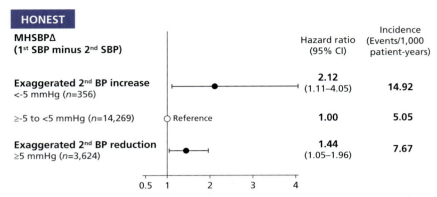

Adjusted for sex, age, family history of cardiovascular disease, dyslipidaemia, diabetes mellitus, chronic kidney disease, history of cardiovascular disease, smoking status, and averaged morning home systolic blood pressure during the follow-up period.

Figure 3.12 Home blood pressure variability within one occasion measurement and cardiovascular prognosis. Relationship between MHSBPΔ during the follow-up period and hazard ratio for cardiovascular events (reference, MHSBPΔ ≥-5 to <5 mmHg). MHSBPΔ, difference between first and second measurements of morning home systolic blood pressure; SBP, systolic blood pressure; CI, confidence interval. *Source:* Saito et al. 2016 [33]

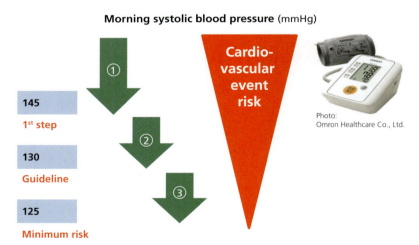

Figure 3.13 Home BP-based antihypertensive strategy for morning hypertension. BP, blood pressure. *Source:* Modified from Kario. 2015 [10]

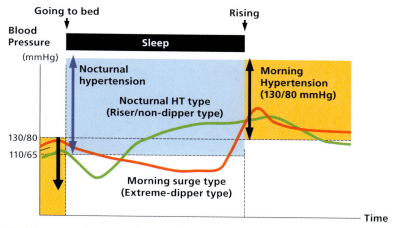

Figure 3.14 Two types of morning hypertension. *Source:* Modified from Kario. 2005 [15]

These real-world findings from the HONEST study emphasise the importance of HBPM in clinical practice. This evidence suggests that it is essential to control morning home SBP to <145 mmHg as a first step, even in patients with controlled clinic BP. The second step is to target morning home SBP <130 mmHg as per the guidelines, then a target of around 125 mmHg is the ultimate goal of home BP-guided management of hypertension (**Figure 3.13** and **3.14**) [10, 15].

Subtypes of morning hypertension

Two types of morning hypertension are detected by HBPM [1, 4]. One is the "morning surge" type exhibiting exaggerated morning BP surge, and the other is "sustained nocturnal hypertension" type with continuous hypertension from nocturnal hypertension (non-dipper/riser type) (**Figure 3.14**). Both types have different associated conditions, and both are associated with increased risk of cardiovascular and renal diseases through different pathogenic mechanisms. To differentiate these two types, morning-evening BP difference calculated using home BP values conventionally measured in the morning and in the evening is not useful. Only direct measurement of nighttime BP during sleep, traditionally by ambulatory BP monitoring, and by recently developed home nighttime BP monitoring with timer, could differentiate the two subtypes.

CHAPTER 4

Ambulatory BP monitoring

ABPM parameters

Ambulatory blood pressure monitoring (ABPM) offers the ability to more extensively assess the 24-hour ambulatory BP profile of individual patients, including BP variability. **Figures 4.1**, **4.2**, **4.3**, **4.4**, and **4.5** show the ambulatory BP and BP variability parameters calculated from ambulatory BP measurements obtained from one ABPM recording [10, 14].

24-hour BP is the average of BP readings during a 24-hour period and is the most important BP parameter in terms of cardiovascular risk [34].

Daytime BP and nighttime BP are calculated from the average of daytime BP and nighttime BP measurements, respectively. The time periods used to define daytime, nighttime, and morning ambulatory BP values are based on a diary of the individual patient's behaviour, or based on 24-hour clock time

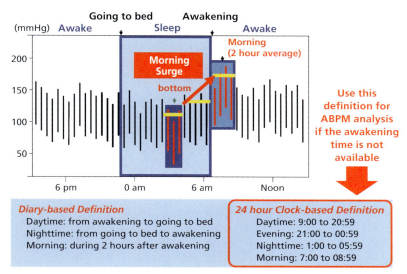

Figure 4.1 Definition of time period for calculating ABPM parameters. ABPM, ambulatory blood pressure monitoring. *Source:* Kario et al. 2003 [14]

Morning BP parameters	
Average morning SBP	= 2-hour average of morning SBPs during 2 hours after rising
Moving peak morning SBP	= Highest 1-hour moving average of consecutive SBPs during 2 hours after rising
Maximum morning SBP	= Maximum morning SBP (one SBP) during 2 hours after rising
Nighttime BP parameters	
Average nighttime SBP	= Average of nighttime SBPs from going to bed to rising
Average peak nighttime SBP	= Average of highest three different nighttime SBPs from going to bed to rising
Maximum nighttime SBP	= Maximum nighttime SBP (1 SBP) from going to bed to rising
Minimum nighttime SBP	= Minimum nighttime SBP (1 SBP) from going to bed to rising
Moving lowest nighttime SBP	= Lowest 1-hour moving average of consecutive SBPs from going to bed to rising
Pre-wakening nighttime SBP	= 2-hour average of nighttime SBPs during 2 hours before rising
Daytime BP parameters	
Average daytime SBP	= Average of daytime SBPs from rising to going to bed

Figure 4.2 Diary-based definition of morning and nighttime BP parameters. BP, blood pressure; SBP, systolic BP. *Source:* Kario. 2015 [10]

(**Figures 4.1**, **4.2**, **4.3**, **4.4**, and **4.5**) [10, 14]. The diary-based definition of daytime and nighttime BP is superior to the 24-hour clock time definition because the majority of ambulatory BP values are determined by the patient's timing of getting up in the morning and going to bed.

Morning BP parameters are defined as follows: average morning systolic BP (SBP) (2-hour average of morning SBP values during the two hours after rising or between 7 am and 9 am), moving peak morning SBP (highest 1-hour moving average of consecutive SBPs during the two hours after rising, or between 6 am and 10 am), and maximum morning SBP (maximum morning SBP [one reading] during the two hours after rising or between 6 am and 10 am).

Nighttime BP parameters are defined as follows: average nighttime SBP (average of nighttime SBP values), average peak nighttime SBP (average of three highest different nighttime SBP values), maximum nighttime SBP (one SBP reading), minimum nighttime SBP (one SBP reading), moving lowest nighttime SBP (lowest 1-hour moving average of consecutive nighttime SBP values), and pre-wakening nighttime SBP (2-hour average of nighttime SBP values during the two hours before rising).

MBPS parameters: Sleep-trough morning surge is calculated as the aver-

Morning BP surge parameters	
Sleep-trough morning surge	= Average morning SBP minus moving lowest nighttime SBP
Dynamic morning surge	= Moving peak morning SBP minus moving lowest nighttime SBP
Maximum dynamic morning surge	= Maximum morning SBP minus minimum nighttime SBP
Pre-wakening morning surge	= Average morning SBP minus pre-wakening morning SBP
Nighttime BP surge parameters	
Average nighttime surge	= Average peak nighttime SBP minus average nighttime SBP
Dynamic nighttime surge	= Average peak nighttime SBP minus moving lowest nighttime SBP
Maximum dynamic nighttime surge	= Maximum nighttime SBP minus minimum nighttime SBP
Nighttime BP dipping parameters	
Nighttime dipping (%)	= (1 minus average nighttime SBP/average daytime SBP) × 100
Subgroup classification based on nighttime SBP dipping (%)	= Extreme-dipper: >20%; Dipper: ≤20%, >10%; Non-dipper: ≤10%, >0%; Riser: ≤0%

Figure 4.3 Diary-based definition of morning and nighttime BP surge parameters. BP, blood pressure; SBP, systolic BP. *Source:* Kario. 2015 [10]

age morning SBP minus the moving lowest nighttime SBP; pre-wakening morning surge is calculated as the average morning SBP minus pre-wakening morning SBP. Dynamic morning surge is calculated as the moving peak morning SBP minus moving lowest nighttime SBP, and maximum dynamic morning surge is calculated as the maximum morning SBP minus minimum nighttime SBP. The pre-wakening morning SBP (diary) or minimal (or moving pre-wakening) morning SBP (clock base) between 5 am and 9 pm is used to calculate the pre-wakening morning SBP surge.

Nighttime BP surge parameters: Average nighttime surge is calculated as the average peak nighttime SBP minus the average nighttime SBP, dynamic nighttime surge as the average peak nighttime SBP minus moving lowest nighttime SBP, maximum dynamic nighttime surge as the maximum nighttime SBP minus minimum nighttime SBP. In addition to an increase in nighttime BP, increased BP variability during sleep (standard deviation of nighttime SBP) is an independent and synergistic risk factor for cardiovascular events.

Nighttime BP dipping parameters: Nighttime SBP dipping (%) is calculated as (1 minus average nighttime SBP/average daytime SBP) × 100. Subgroups are classified as follows: extreme dipper: >20%; dipper: ≤20%, >10%; non-dipper: ≤10%, >0%; riser: ≤0% [35, 36].

Morning BP parameters	
Average morning SBP	= 2-hour average of morning SBPs between 7 am and 9 am
Moving peak morning SBP	= Highest 1-hour moving average of consecutive SBPs between 6 am and 10 am
Maximum morning SBP	= Maximum morning SBP (one SBP) between 6 am and 10 am
Minimum morning SBP	= Minimum morning SBP (one SBP) between 6 am and 10 am before maximum morning SBP
Moving lowest pre-wakening morning SBP	= Lowest 1-hour moving average of consecutive SBPs between 6 am and 10 am before moving peak morning SBP
Nighttime BP parameters	
Average nighttime SBP	= Average of nighttime SBPs between 1 am and 6 am
Average peak nighttime SBP	= Average of highest 3 different nighttime SBPs between 1 am and 6 am
Maximum nighttime SBP	= Maximum nighttime SBP (1 SBP reading) between 1 am and 6 am
Minimum nighttime SBP	= Minimum nighttime SBP (1 SBP reading) between 1 am and 6 am
Moving lowest nighttime SBP	= Lowest 1-hour moving average of consecutive SBP reading between 1 am and 6 am

Figure 4.4 24-hour-clock-based definition of morning and nighttime BP parameters. BP, blood pressure; SBP, systolic BP. BP, blood pressure; SBP, systolic BP. *Source:* Kario. 2015 [10]

Normal and typical patterns of ambulatory hypertension subtypes

Figure 4.6 shows a normotensive dip in patients with white-coat hypertension. Both this and a normal pattern show normal diurnal BP rhythm with a nighttime BP fall of 10–19% compared with daytime BP. **Figure 4.7** shows a hypertensive extreme-dipper pattern, showing an excessive nighttime fall in BP of at least 20%, and a hypertensive dipper with adequate BP fall (10–19% reduction). **Figure 4.8** shows patients with nocturnal hypertension: a non-dipper with reduced nighttime BP fall (0–9% decrease), and a riser with higher nighttime BP than daytime BP (10% or more increase). In addition, ABPM could detect the isolated stress-induced daytime BP surge during a stressful event even when home BP and ambulatory BP during other periods were well-controlled (**Figure 4.9**).

Development of ICT-based multisensor-ABPM (IMS-ABPM)

The change in ambulatory BP is closely related to the level of physical activity. The sensitivity of BP surge (slope of the degree of BP surge against physical

Morning BP surge parameters	
Average morning surge	= Average morning SBP minus average nighttime SBP
Dynamic morning surge	= Moving peak morning SBP minus moving lowest nighttime SBP
Dynamic pre-wakening morning surge	= Moving peak morning SBP minus moving lowest pre-wakening morning SBP
Maximum dynamic morning surge	= Maximum morning SBP minus minimum nighttime SBP
Maximum pre-wakening morning surge	= Maximum morning SBP minus minimum morning SBP
Nighttime BP surge parameters	
Average nighttime surge	= Average peak nighttime SBP minus average nighttime SBP
Dynamic nighttime surge	= Average peak nighttime SBP minus moving lowest nighttime SBP
Maximum dynamic nighttime surge	= Maximum nighttime SBP minus minimum nighttime SBP
Daytime BP parameters	
Average daytime SBP	= Average of daytime SBPs between 9 am and 9 pm

Figure 4.5 24-hour-clock-based definition of morning and nighttime BP surge parameters. BP, blood pressure; SBP, systolic BP. *Source:* Kario. 2015 [10]

activity) may reflect the characteristics of individual cardiovascular properties (**Figure 4.10**) [18, 37]. Based on this concept of "trigger-specific BP sensitivity", we developed a new information and communication technology (ICT)-based multi-sensor home and ABPM device (i.e. ICT-based multi-sensor ABPM [IMS-ABPM]; A&D Company., Tokyo) equipped with (1) a high-sensitivity actigraph that can detect the wearer's fine-scale physical movements in three directions, (2) a thermometer, and (3) a barometer (**Figure 4.11**). This ABPM device has a good atrial fibrillation algorithm based on pulse wave intervals (**Figures 4.12** and **4.13**) [38].

Figure 4.14 shows the 24-hour ambulatory BP profile measured by this device (77-year-old female with hypertension) [9]. Using these data, we can examine three haemodynamic properties under resting-home and active-ambulatory conditions: (1) BP variability, (2) central haemodynamics, and (3) trigger-specific BP sensitivity (**Figure 4.11**) [9].

New ABPM indices

(1) BP variability. The IMS-ABPM device can be used for both ABPM and home BP monitoring. The device is initially used in 24-hour ABPM mode, and

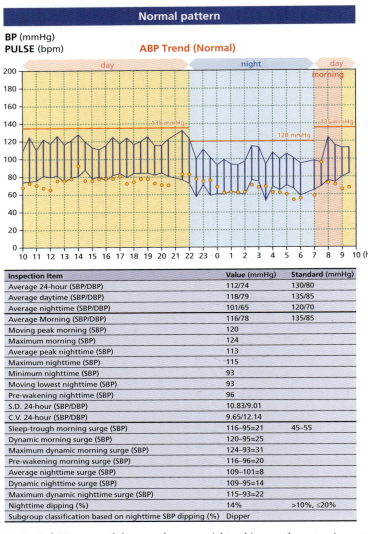

Inspection Item	Value (mmHg)	Standard (mmHg)
Average 24-hour (SBP/DBP)	112/74	130/80
Average daytime (SBP/DBP)	118/79	135/85
Average nighttime (SBP/DBP)	101/65	120/70
Average Morning (SBP/DBP)	116/78	135/85
Moving peak morning (SBP)	120	
Maximum morning (SBP)	124	
Average peak nighttime (SBP)	113	
Maximum nighttime (SBP)	115	
Minimum nighttime (SBP)	93	
Moving lowest nighttime (SBP)	93	
Pre-wakening nighttime (SBP)	96	
S.D. 24-hour (SBP/DBP)	10.83/9.01	
C.V. 24-hour (SBP/DBP)	9.65/12.14	
Sleep-trough morning surge (SBP)	116−95=21	45–55
Dynamic morning surge (SBP)	120−95=25	
Maximum dynamic morning surge (SBP)	124−93=31	
Pre-wakening morning surge (SBP)	116−96=20	
Average nighttime surge (SBP)	109−101=8	
Dynamic nighttime surge (SBP)	109−95=14	
Maximum dynamic nighttime surge (SBP)	115−93=22	
Nighttime dipping (%)	14%	>10%, ≤20%
Subgroup classification based on nighttime SBP dipping (%)	Dipper	

Figure 4.6 Typical BP pattern (left: normal pattern; right: white-coat hypertension pattern) evaluated by ABPM. ABPM, ambulatory blood pressure monitoring, BP, blood pressure; C.V., coefficient of variation; DBP, diastolic BP; SBP, systolic BP; S.D., standard deviation.
Source: Kario K. *Essential Manual on Perfect 24-hour Blood Pressure Management from Morning to Nocturnal Hypertension: Up-to-date for Anticipation Medicine.* Wiley, 2018.

Ambulatory BP monitoring

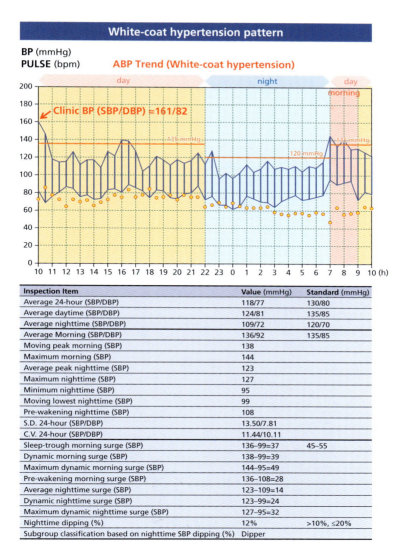

Figure 4.6 (continued)

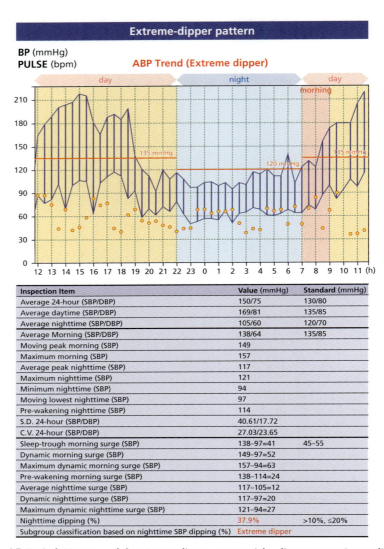

Figure 4.7 Typical BP pattern (left: extreme-dipper pattern; right: dipper pattern[normal]) evaluated by ABPM. ABPM, ambulatory blood pressure monitoring; BP, blood pressure; C.V., coefficient of variation; DBP, diastolic BP; S.D., standard deviation; SBP, systolic BP.
Source: Kario K. *Essential Manual on Perfect 24-hour Blood Pressure Management from Morning to Nocturnal Hypertension: Up-to-date for Anticipation Medicine.* Wiley, 2018.

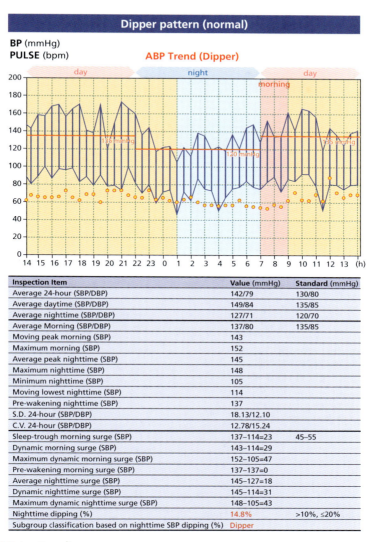

Inspection Item	Value (mmHg)	Standard (mmHg)
Average 24-hour (SBP/DBP)	142/79	130/80
Average daytime (SBP/DBP)	149/84	135/85
Average nighttime (SBP/DBP)	127/71	120/70
Average Morning (SBP/DBP)	137/80	135/85
Moving peak morning (SBP)	143	
Maximum morning (SBP)	152	
Average peak nighttime (SBP)	145	
Maximum nighttime (SBP)	148	
Minimum nighttime (SBP)	105	
Moving lowest nighttime (SBP)	114	
Pre-wakening nighttime (SBP)	137	
S.D. 24-hour (SBP/DBP)	18.13/12.10	
C.V. 24-hour (SBP/DBP)	12.78/15.24	
Sleep-trough morning surge (SBP)	137−114=23	45−55
Dynamic morning surge (SBP)	143−114=29	
Maximum dynamic morning surge (SBP)	152−105=47	
Pre-wakening morning surge (SBP)	137−137=0	
Average nighttime surge (SBP)	145−127=18	
Dynamic nighttime surge (SBP)	145−114=31	
Maximum dynamic nighttime surge (SBP)	148−105=43	
Nighttime dipping (%)	14.8%	>10%, ≤20%
Subgroup classification based on nighttime SBP dipping (%)	Dipper	

Figure 4.7 (continued)

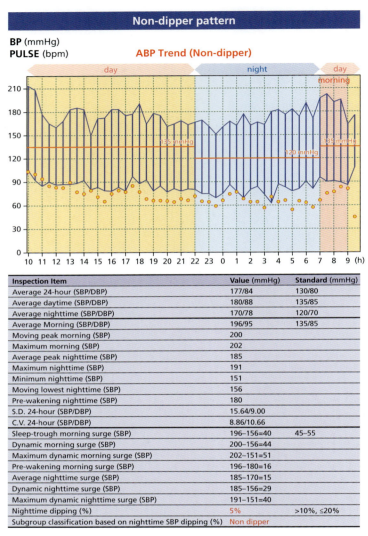

Inspection Item	Value (mmHg)	Standard (mmHg)
Average 24-hour (SBP/DBP)	177/84	130/80
Average daytime (SBP/DBP)	180/88	135/85
Average nighttime (SBP/DBP)	170/78	120/70
Average Morning (SBP/DBP)	196/95	135/85
Moving peak morning (SBP)	200	
Maximum morning (SBP)	202	
Average peak nighttime (SBP)	185	
Maximum nighttime (SBP)	191	
Minimum nighttime (SBP)	151	
Moving lowest nighttime (SBP)	156	
Pre-wakening nighttime (SBP)	180	
S.D. 24-hour (SBP/DBP)	15.64/9.00	
C.V. 24-hour (SBP/DBP)	8.86/10.66	
Sleep-trough morning surge (SBP)	196−156=40	45–55
Dynamic morning surge (SBP)	200−156=44	
Maximum dynamic morning surge (SBP)	202−151=51	
Pre-wakening morning surge (SBP)	196−180=16	
Average nighttime surge (SBP)	185−170=15	
Dynamic nighttime surge (SBP)	185−156=29	
Maximum dynamic nighttime surge (SBP)	191−151=40	
Nighttime dipping (%)	5%	>10%, ≤20%
Subgroup classification based on nighttime SBP dipping (%)	Non dipper	

Figure 4.8 Typical BP pattern (left: non-dipper pattern; right: riser pattern) evaluated by ABPM. ABPM, ambulatory blood pressure monitoring, BP, blood pressure; DBP, diastolic BP; SBP, systolic BP. *Source:* Kario K. *Essential Manual on Perfect 24-hour Blood Pressure Management from Morning to Nocturnal Hypertension: Up-to-date for Anticipation Medicine*. Wiley, 2018.

Ambulatory BP monitoring

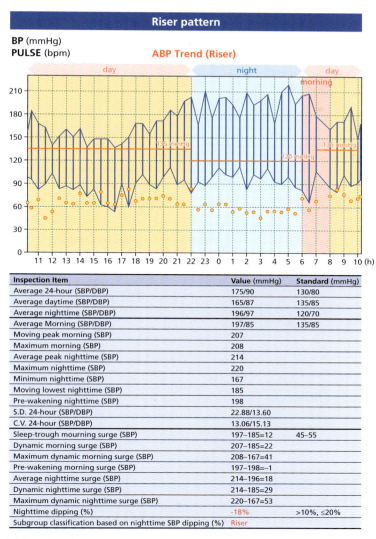

Inspection Item	Value (mmHg)	Standard (mmHg)
Average 24-hour (SBP/DBP)	175/90	130/80
Average daytime (SBP/DBP)	165/87	135/85
Average nighttime (SBP/DBP)	196/97	120/70
Average Morning (SBP/DBP)	197/85	135/85
Moving peak morning (SBP)	207	
Maximum morning (SBP)	208	
Average peak nighttime (SBP)	214	
Maximum nighttime (SBP)	220	
Minimum nighttime (SBP)	167	
Moving lowest nighttime (SBP)	185	
Pre-wakening nighttime (SBP)	198	
S.D. 24-hour (SBP/DBP)	22.88/13.60	
C.V. 24-hour (SBP/DBP)	13.06/15.13	
Sleep-trough mourning surge (SBP)	197−185=12	45−55
Dynamic morning surge (SBP)	207−185=22	
Maximum dynamic morning surge (SBP)	208−167=41	
Pre-wakening morning surge (SBP)	197−198=−1	
Average nighttime surge (SBP)	214−196=18	
Dynamic nighttime surge (SBP)	214−185=29	
Maximum dynamic nighttime surge (SBP)	220−167=53	
Nighttime dipping (%)	−18%	>10%, ≤20%
Subgroup classification based on nighttime SBP dipping (%)	Riser	

Figure 4.8 (continued)

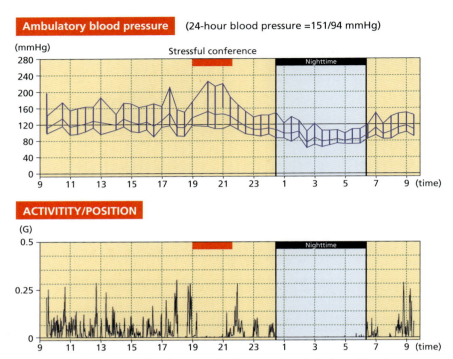

Figure 4.9 Worksite stress-induced uncontrolled hypertension. Ambulatory blood pressure (even when physical activity is almost zero) is markedly increased during a very important 2-hour stressful conference for a 47-year-old woman taking 50 mg losartan daily. Home morning BP was 132/87mmHg. *Source:* Kario K. *Essential Manual on Perfect 24-hour Blood Pressure Management from Morning to Nocturnal Hypertension: Up-to-date for Anticipation Medicine.* Wiley, 2018.

then the mode is automatically changed to home BP monitoring. Thus, the IMS-ABPM can evaluate ambulatory and home BP variability simultaneously using the same device and the same algorithm of oscillometric BP measurement. For example, the combination of exaggerated ambulatory morning BP surge and increased day-by-day home morning BP variability may be associated with a higher risk of triggering cardiovascular disease events than either of these factors alone [18].

(2) Central haemodynamics. Using intra-cuff pressure data and each of the waveforms obtained by time-series oscillometric BP measurement, we are currently analysing the shape of the envelope of intra-cuff pressure and the waveform of estimated central BP.

(3) Trigger-specific BP sensitivity. The trigger-specific BP sensitivities according to the ambulatory and home BP reactivity based on the slope of the BP

(a)
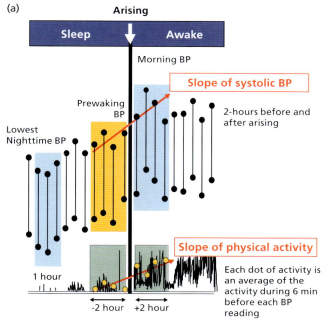

(b)
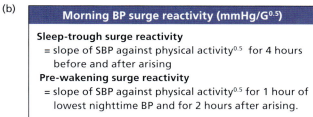

(c)
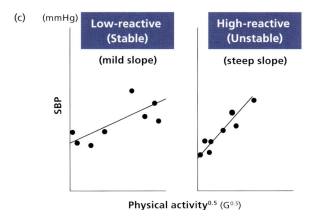

Figure 4.10 Morning BP surge reactivity by ABPM. ABPM, ambulatory BP monitoring; BP, blood pressure; SBP, systolic BP. *Source:* Kario et al. 1999 [37]; Kario. 2010 [18]

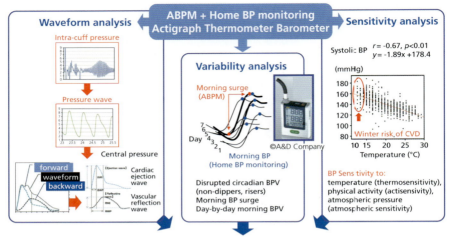

Figure 4.11 Development of ICT-based multisensor BP monitoring to access three haemodynamic properties ABPM, ambulatory BP monitoring; BP, blood pressure; BPV, BP variability; CVD, cardiovascular disease. *Source:* Kario. 2017 [39]; Reproduced by permission of Oxford University Press.

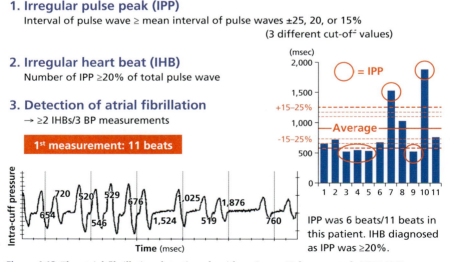

Figure 4.12 The atrial fibrillation detection algorithm. *Source:* Kabutoya et al. 2017 [38]

Patient characteristics			
	Sinus rhythm (n=20)	AF (n=16)	p
Age (years)	63±11	66±10	0.36
Men (%)	75	88	0.49
Systolic BP (mmHg)	127±17	128±12	0.82
Diastolic BP (mmHg)	77±11	82±9	0.23
Pulse rate (bpm)	65±11	78±14	0.003
Accuracy of the monitor for diagnosing AF			
Monitor detection AF +/−	Sensitivity	Specificity	Kappa
IPP 25% 14/22	0.88	1.00	0.89
IPP 20% 15/21	0.94	1.00	0.94
IPP 15% 16/20	1.00	1.00	1.00

AF, atrial fibrillation; IPP, irregular pulse peak.

Figure 4.13 Diagnostic accuracy of a new algorithm to detect atrial fibrillation. *Source:* Kabutoya et al. 2017 [38]

change against the triggers are as follows: (1) actisensitivity, defined as the slope of BP change against the physical activity before the BP measurement; (2) thermosensitivity, defined as the slope of BP change against the temperature; and (3) atmospheric sensitivity, defined as the slope against atmospheric pressure [9, 18, 39]. The negative (inverse), absent or exaggerated trigger-specific sensitivity should be pathological. Using the pathological threshold of these haemodynamic biomarkers, we identify specific high-risk patients as those with thermosensitive, actisensitive, or atmospheric hypertension or hypotension, who may have increased cardiovascular risk in the specific situation (**Figure 4.11**) [39].

Actisensitivity. As shown in **Figure 4.15**, the actisensitivity was different in each patient [9]. One regression line is calculated from six or more ambulatory BP readings with a corresponding 5-minute average of physical activity just before each BP measurement. The individual differences were large, indicating that actisensitivity would be a very useful marker for identifying high-risk patients with different BP sensitivities to physical activity. The actisensitivity is significantly steeper in winter than in summer (**Figure 4.15**) [9]. Our hypothesis is that hyperactisensitive patients are likely to have increased daytime BP variability, resulting in exertional onset of cardiovascular disease, and negative actisensitive (inverse slope) patients may have severe cardiac dysfunction or severe coronary artery disease (**Figure 4.16 left**) [9].

Thermosensitivity. Similarly, cold hyperthermosensitivity is thought to identify patients at risk of cardiovascular events in cold locations in winter, while summer hyperthermosensitivity may be associated with hypotensive episodes at

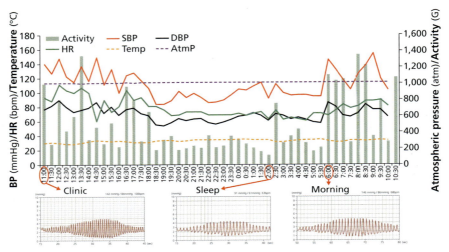

Figure 4.14 The 24-hour ambulatory blood pressure profile measured by ICT-based multisensor ambulatory BP monitoring (77-year-old woman with hypertension). Upper figure: 24-hour trend of ambulatory BP and the trigger parameters measured by devices contained within the ABPM device. Lower figures: envelopes of the intra-cuff pressures during oscillometric BP measurement at 3 time points, i.e., at the clinic, during sleep (when physical activity is at a minimum), and in the morning just after arising (when activity is high). All these envelopes and waveforms are stored in the device. Act, activity (summation of the physical activity detected by 3 direction-high sensitive actigraph); BP, blood pressure; SBP, systolic BP; DBP, diastolic BP; HR, heart rate; Temp, temperature; AtmP, atmospheric pressure. Reprinted from *Prog Cardiovasc Dis.*, Kario K. et al., Development of a new ICT-based multisensor blood pressure monitoring system for use in hemodynamic biomarker-initiated anticipation medicine for cardiovascular disease: the national IMPACT program project [9]. Copyright (2017), with permission from Elsevier.

hot locations in summer (**Figure 4.16 right**) [9]. In summer, negative thermosensitivity (i.e. a significant increase in BP in hot temperatures) may be at least partially responsible for poor sleep quality. In addition, negative thermosensitivity may be associated with autonomic nervous dysfunction. The clinical implications and the pathological threshold of these trigger-specific BP sensitivity indices should be investigated in a prospective clinical study.

Anticipation of ambulatory BP

The mixed-model analysis of the association of daytime ambulatory SBP with physical activity, temperature, atmospheric pressure, and season (4,699 data points obtained from 79 patients in summer and 72 patients in winter) demon-

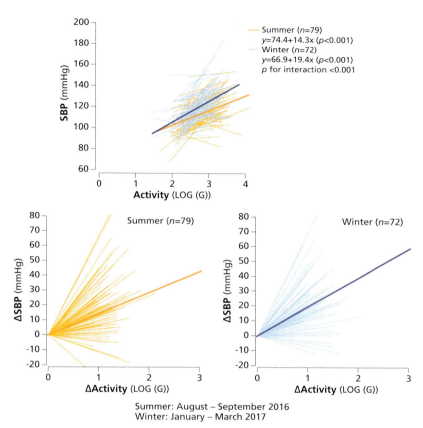

Figure 4.15 Differential actisensitivity between winter and summer in the same hypertensive patients. The actisensitivity is defined as the slope of BP change against the physical activity. Each regression line was calculated from 6 or more ambulatory BP readings with the corresponding 5-minute average of physical activity just before each BP measurement. The thin line represents a regression line calculated from the daytime ambulatory BP measurements in a single patient. The thick line shows the average of all the regression lines of each patient (thin lines). BP, blood pressure; SBP, systolic BP.
Reprinted from *Prog Cardiovasc Dis.*, Kario K. et al., Development of a new ICT-based multisensor blood pressure monitoring system for use in hemodynamic biomarker-initiated anticipation medicine for cardiovascular disease: the national IMPACT program project [9]. Copyright (2017), with permission from Elsevier.

strated that a 10°C decrease in temperature was associated with a 10.4 mmHg increase in SBP (**Figure 4.17**) [9]. For example, based on the analysis, a SBP of 130 mmHg at rest (100 G) in an indoor setting at 25°C will increase to 151 mmHg when the conditions change to walking (1000 G) outdoors at 5°C.

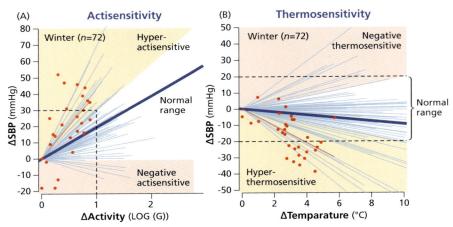

Figure 4.16 Classification of high-risk groups stratified by actisensitivity and thermosensitivity. The blue thick line shows the average of all the regression lines of each patient (thin blue lines). A) Actisensitivity is defined as the slope of BP change against the physical activity. For example, actisensitive hypertension with hyperactisensitivity may be defined as ≥30 mmHg increase in systolic BP by an increase in physical activity from 100 G (resting level) to 1,000 G (walking level). The red plots and the regression line represent 24-h IMS-ABPM data of 77-year-old woman with hypertension, CKD, and hyperuricemia. Her brachial-ankle pulse wave velocity (baPWV) showed high value (right: 2,168 cm/s; left: 2,090 cm/s, corresponding to the vascular age [reference] above 90 years). B) Thermosensitivity is defined as the slope of BP change against change in temperature. For example, cold thermosensitive hypertension with hyperthermosensitivity may be defined as ≥20 mmHg increase in systolic BP by a 10 °C decrease in temperature. The red plots and the regression line represent 24-hour IMS-ABPM data of 69-year-old woman with hypertension, hyperlipidaemia, and insomnia. Her baPWV showed the high value (right: 1,701 cm/s; left: 1,719 cm/s, vascular age: 75 years). BP, blood pressure; CKD, chronic kidney disease; IMS-ABPM, ICT based multi-sensor ambulatory BP monitoring; SBP, systolic BP.
Reprinted from *Prog Cardiovasc Dis.*, Kario K. et al., Development of a new ICT-based multisensor blood pressure monitoring system for use in hemodynamic biomarker-initiated anticipation medicine for cardiovascular disease: the national IMPACT program project [9]. Copyright (2017), with permission from Elsevier.

Multi-sensors and the real-time hybrid Wi-SUN/Wi-Fi transmission system

Our new IMS-ABPM system employs a new ICT/Internet of Things (IoT)-based biological and environmental signal monitoring that can simultaneously monitor the environment (temperature, illumination, humidity) at 5 different locations in a house (the entryway, bedroom, bathing room, toilet, and living room) and activities measured by using wrist-type high-sensitive actigraph to identify the location of patients (**Figure 4.18**) [9]. Using cloud computing with an IoT gate-

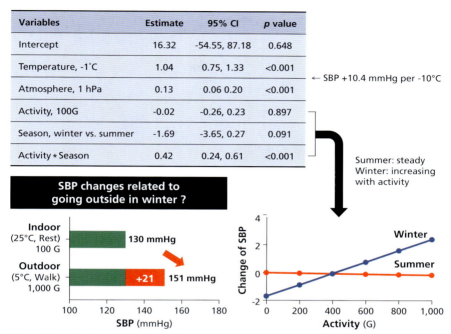

Figure 4.17 Mixed model analysis of the association of daytime ambulatory systolic blood pressure with physical activity, temperature, atmospheric pressure, and season (4,699 data obtained from 79 patients in summer and 72 patients in winter). A 10 °C decrease in temperature was associated with a 10.4 mmHg increase in systolic BP. BP, blood pressure; SBP, systolic BP. Reprinted from *Prog Cardiovasc Dis.*, Kario K. et al., Development of a new ICT-based multisensor blood pressure monitoring system for use in hemodynamic biomarker-initiated anticipation medicine for cardiovascular disease: the national IMPACT program project [9]. Copyright (2017), with permission from Elsevier.

way and bridges based on hybrid Wi-SUN, 92 LTE and Bluetooth Low Energy (BLE) transmission systems, we can collect and store individual time-series home and ambulatory BP data, waveform data, and data on individual physical activity and environmental signals specific to different rooms in the house (**Figure 4.19**) [9]. The IoT bridges collect the data from the IMS-ABPM, wrist-type actigraph and body weight scale via BLE transmission. The data is then converted to Wi-SUN transmission signal format and transmitted to the IoT gateway by a Wi-SUN multi-hop transmission system. The Wi-SUN system is based on IEEE 802.15.4g-based international new IoT standards 92 and certified by the Wi-SUN alliance. In the IoT gateway, the received Wi-SUN signal is also converted to LTE transmission signal format and transmitted to the cloud over a conventional LTE wide-area network. Moreover, each IoT bridge has devices for environmental

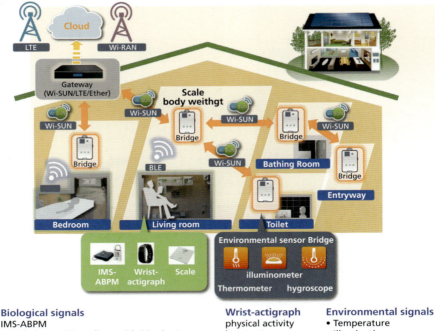

Figure 4.18 Multi-sensors and real-time and hybrid Wi-SUN/Wi-Fi transmission system of individual biological and environmental signals in the living condition. BP, blood pressure; IMS-ABPM, ICT based multi-sensor ambulatory BP monitoring.
Reprinted from *Prog Cardiovasc Dis.*, Kario K. et al., Development of a new ICT-based multisensor blood pressure monitoring system for use in hemodynamic biomarker-initiated anticipation medicine for cardiovascular disease: the national IMPACT program project [9]. Copyright (2017), with permission from Elsevier.

monitoring such as a thermometer, illuminometer and hygroscope. The environment-monitoring data at each IoT bridge is also transmitted to the cloud.

Housing conditions are important for the prevention of cardiovascular disease (CVD) events. The onset of CVD events exhibits significant seasonal variation with a peak in the winter. The death rate, especially the rate of CVD death, increases in the winter. This inverse phenomenon is considered to be partly due to the increasing prevalence of energy-saving homes with good thermal-insulation performance in chilly countries. Our hypothesis is that the heterogeneity of room temperatures within home (i.e., different room temperatures among different rooms, and among the different height even within the same room)

Ambulatory BP monitoring

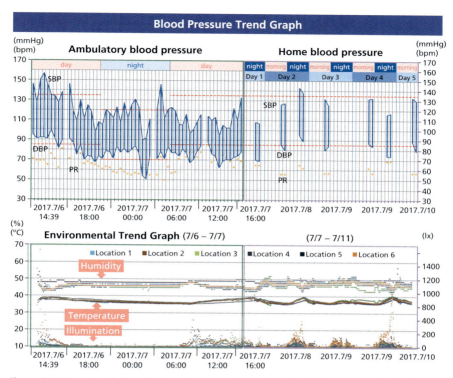

Figure 4.19 Time trend of multi-bioenvironmental signals by the IMS-ABPM and hybrid transmission system in a 78-year-old hypertensive woman who lives in Tatsuno city, Hyogo, Japan. The time-trend data gathered by multisensors in the house are successfully transmitted by the hybrid Wi-SUN/WiFi transmission system. BP, blood pressure; bpm, beats per minute; DBP, diastolic BP; IMS-ABPM, ICT based multi-sensor ambulatory BP monitoring; PR, pulse rate; SBP, systolic BP. Reprinted from *Prog Cardiovasc Dis.*, Kario K. et al., Development of a new ICT-based multisensor blood pressure monitoring system for use in hemodynamic biomarker-initiated anticipation medicine for cardiovascular disease: the national IMPACT program project [9]. Copyright (2017), with permission from Elsevier.

would increase the risk of CVD events through exaggerated BP variability.

HI-JAMP registry

The national general practitioner-based cohort, HI-JAMP registry (Home-Activity ICT-based Japan Ambulatory Blood Pressure Monitoring Prospective study) of patients treated with antihypertensive agents was started in 2017. The aim of the registry is to clarify seasonal and regional differences in trigger-specific sensitivities and their impacts on cardiovascular events (**Figure 4.20**).

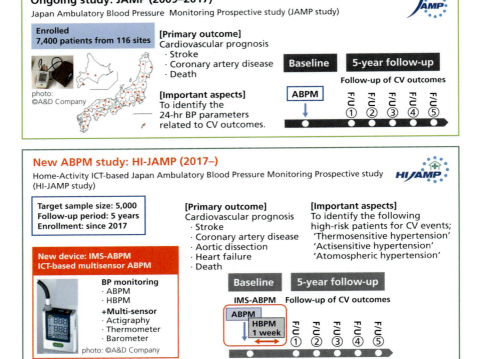

Figure 4.20 Japan Ambulatory Blood Pressure Monitoring Prospective study (JAMP study). Since 2009 the JAMP study has investigated the impact of ambulatory blood pressure control status on cardiovascular prognosis in patients with a history of and/or risk factors for cardiovascular disease. ABPM, ambulatory BP monitoring; BP, blood pressure; CV, cardiovascular; HBPM, home BP monitoring; IMS-ABPM, ICT-based multisensor ABPM. *Source:* Kario K. *Essential Manual on Perfect 24-hour Blood Pressure Management from Morning to Nocturnal Hypertension: Up-to-date for Anticipation Medicine.* Wiley, 2018.

- Studies described under the headings 'Development of ICT-based multisensor-ABPM (IMS-ABPM)', 'New ABPM indices', 'Anticipation of ambulatory BP', and 'Multi-sensors and the real-time hybrid Wi-SUN/Wi-Fi transmission system' in Chapter 4 were supported by the Impulsing Paradigm Change through Disruptive Technologies (ImPACT) Program of the Council for Science, Technology and Innovation (Cabinet Office, Government of Japan).
- A study described under the 'HI-JAMP registry' heading in Chapter 4 was supported by a grant from the Foundation for Development of the Community (Tochigi).

CHAPTER 5

Morning surge in BP

Morning blood pressure surge (MBPS) is one of the components of diurnal BP variability [12, 18, 40-43], and normal MBPS is a physiological phenomenon. However, "exaggerated" MBPS is a pathological form of BP variability, which is significantly associated with other phenotypes of BP variability. In addition to the 24-hour persistent pressure overload, dynamic BP variability from the nadir during sleep to peak early in the morning could contribute to the cardiovascular event continuum, from the early stage of subclinical vascular disease to the final trigger of cardiovascular events [12, 18, 40-43].

Definition of MBPS

There is no consensus on the definition and threshold of pathological MBPS. Use of different definitions and studies of different populations may contribute to the lack of consistency in current findings. MBPS is usually assessed using ambulatory blood pressure monitoring (ABPM); however, there are several definitions of MBPS, such as sleep-trough surge, pre-wakening surge, and rising surge (**Figure 5.1**) [12, 14, 18]. Sleep-trough surge is one of the dynamic diurnal surges during the specific period from sleep to early morning [14], when cardiovascular risk is exaggerated. Thus, it is important to exclude the effects of global diurnal BP variation, such as the dipping status of nighttime BP, in order to establish the clinical implications of sleep-trough morning surge (STMS). As expected, STMS is likely to be associated with extreme dippers with marked nighttime BP fall, and is less likely to be associated with non-dippers with less dipping of nighttime BP or with risers with higher nighttime versus daytime BP [14]. Even after controlling for the nighttime BP dipping status or the mean nighttime BP level, the risk of STMS remains significant [14]. Pre-wakening surge refers to the BP change occurring 4 hours before and after rising [14]. Although the STMS and pre-wakening surges are defined based on the BP difference, theoretically, the speed of the surge (the slope of the increase in morning BP against time) may be a better indicator of the risk of morning surge [44]. The recently proposed measure of the MBPS, derived by the product of the rate of morning surge and the amplitude (day–night difference) giving an effective "power" of the MBPS, may better clarify morning cardiovascular risk [45]. As the rising surge may detect morning risk just after rising [46], it may underscore the BP surge subsequently

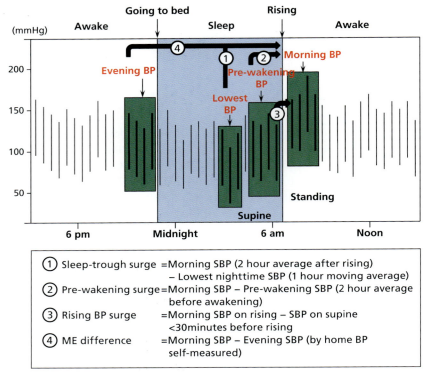

Figure 5.1 Definition of morning BP and morning surge. BP, blood pressure; SBP, systolic BP. *Source:* Kario. 2003 [14] and 2010 [18].

augmented by physical activity in the morning.

Cardiovascular events with MBPS

There are numerous studies indicating that MBPS is a strong predictor for the risk of cardiovascular diseases (stroke, coronary artery disease, total mortality) in both hypertensive outpatients and community-dwelling subjects. Although some studies showed that this predictive ability was independent of average of 24-hour BP, others did not.

The Jichi Medical School (JMS)-ABPM study wave 1 enrolled 519 unmedicated elderly hypertensive Japanese patients with a mean age of 72 years [14]. We first identified two MBPS: a STMS which we defined as morning BP (2-hour average of four 30-minute BP readings just after waking up) minus the lowest nighttime BP (1-hour average of the three BP readings centered on the lowest

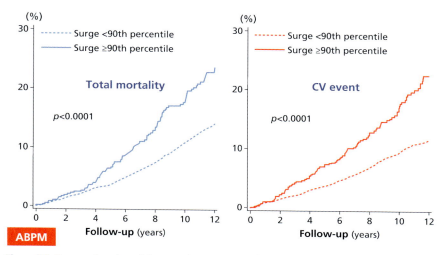

Figure 5.2 Prognostic value of the morning BP surge (Sleep-trough surge) in 5,645 subjects from eight populations (IDACO). CV, cardiovascular. *Source:* Li et al. 2010 [17]

nighttime reading); and a pre-wakening surge defined as the morning BP minus the pre-wakening BP (2-hour average of four BP readings just before waking up). The exaggerated morning surge group was defined as the top 10th percentile of patients with STMS (>55 mmHg), and these patients had a higher stroke incidence than the non-surge group (19% vs. 7.3%, $p=0.004$). After matching for age and 24-hour BP, the relative risk of stroke in the surge group versus the non-surge group was 2.7 ($p=0.04$) (**Figure 2.2**) [14]. This association remained significant after adjusting for nighttime BP dipping status. The pre-wakening surge tended to be associated with stroke risk, although the association was not statistically significant ($p=0.07$). In another Japanese population study, MBPS was associated with cerebral haemorrhage [47].

The International Database on Ambulatory Blood Pressure in Relation to Cardiovascular Outcome (IDACO), including 5,645 subjects from 8 populations, provided definitive data showing that both morning surges (STMS and pre-wakening surges) are independent risk factors for total mortality and cardiovascular events [17]. Like our JMS-ABPM study, this study also found that only individuals with MBPS values in the top 10th percentile were at risk of mortality or cardiovascular events (**Figure 5.2**) [17], even after controlling for covariates including age and 24-hour BP.

Recent meta-analysis demonstrated that a 10 mmHg increase in MBPS was associated with an 11% increase in the risk of stroke [48]. In addition, a population-based prospective study demonstrated that STMS was positively associated with the risk of cardiovascular and all-cause death, and was directly related to indices of 24-hour systolic BP (SBP) variability [43]. In a prospective study of patients with hypertension, blunted MBPS was an independent predictor of cardiovascular events [49]. Similarly, a study of patients referred for ABPM showed that an increased MBPS was significantly associated with decreased mortality, especially in non-dippers [50]. Thus, both extremes, that is, the absence (or a negative value) of MBPS and exaggerated MBPS may be pathological, resulting in non-linear J-shaped (or U-shaped) associations between MBPS and cardiovascular events with specific thresholds [18]. Thus, the identification of pathological thresholds of MBPS is clinically important. In the JMS-ABPM study, the top 10th percentile of SBP was 55 mmHg for elderly hypertensive patients [14], and 37 mmHg for community-dwelling IDACO data [17]. Thus, the threshold of pathological MBPS should be identified for clinical practice in the future.

Recent prospective studies in elderly patients with treated hypertension demonstrated that high morning surge (MS) of SBP predicted coronary events in dippers but not non-dippers [51]. In the same group of patients, even those with normal achieved ambulatory BP, dippers with high MS and non-dippers were at increased cardiovascular risk [52].

In a recent meta-analysis of seven prospective studies evaluating MS in a total of 14,133 patients with a mean follow-up period of 7.1 years, excess STMS was a strong predictor for future all-cause mortality (relative risk: 1.29; $p=0.001$; 4 studies) [53]. Another meta-analysis of 17 studies did not find any clear evidence for the impact of pre-wakening MBPS on prognosis. However, using a continuous scale, which has more power to detect an association, there was evidence that a 10 mmHg increase in MBPS was related to an increased risk of stroke ($n=3$ studies; hazard ratio 1.11, 95% CI 1.03–1.20) [48].

In a recent long-term prospective study of 2,020 participants with 24-hour ambulatory BP data and a median 20-year follow-up, the STMS rate was an independent predictor of cardiovascular death. The amplitude of STMS was derived from the difference between morning SBP and lowest nighttime SBP. The rate of STMS was derived as the slope of linear regression of sequential SBP measures on time intervals within the STMS period. Thresholds for high STMS amplitude and rate were determined by the 95th percentiles (43.7 mm Hg and 11.3 mm Hg/h, respectively). A high STMS rate (hazard ratio, 2.61), but not STMS amplitude, was significantly associated with the risk of cardiovascular mortality [54].

Organ damage with MBPS

MBPS is positively correlated with inflammatory biomarkers, and other types of BP variability, such as orthostatic hypertension (orthostatic increase in BP) and

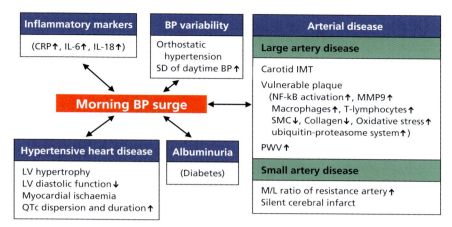

Figure 5.3 Morning BP surge and target organ damage. BP, blood pressure; CRP, C-reactive protein; IL-6, interleukin 6; IL-18, interleukin 18; SD, standard deviation; LV, left ventricular; IMT, intima-media thickness; NF-kB, nuclear factor kappa B; MMP-9, matrix metalloproteinase-9; SMC, smooth muscle cell; PWV, pulse wave velocity, M/L ratio, media thickness to lumen diameter ratio. *Source:* Kario. 2010 [18]

increased daytime ambulatory BP variability [18]. MBPS is associated with target organ damage, including left ventricular hypertrophy (LVH), albuminuria, and large and small artery diseases such as carotid atherosclerosis, arterial stiffness, and silent cerebrovascular disease, independent of the 24-hour BP level (**Figure 5.3**) [18].

Hypertensive heart disease

Many previous studies have demonstrated that an exaggerated MBPS is associated with echocardiographic measures of hypertensive heart disease. MBPS increases cardiac afterload and arterial stiffness, contributing to the progression of LVH.

In elderly hypertensive patients, Kuwajima et al. first reported that the rising surge (change in SBP after rising from bed) was significantly correlated with the left ventricular mass index (LVMI) and the A/E ratio (a measure of diastolic function) [55]. In the Bordeaux study on unmedicated hypertensive patients, rising surge was a significant determinant of LVMI [46]. In addition, hypertensive patients with an exaggerated MBPS had a prolonged QTc duration and QTc dispersion in the morning period (detected by Holter ECG recording) compared with those without MBPS [56]. Given that increased QTc dispersion has been reported to be associated with LVH and cardiac arrhythmia, an exaggerated MBPS could be associated with an increased risk of cardiac arrhythmia and sud-

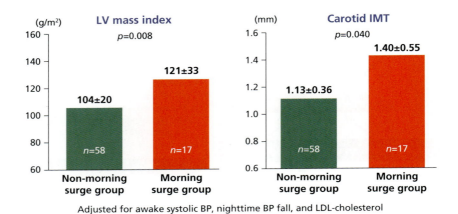

Figure 5.4 Morning BP surge and cardiovascular remodelling in well-controlled hypertensive patients with 24-hour BP <130/80 mmHg (n=75). LV, left ventricular; IMT, intima-media thickness. *Source:* Yano et al. 2009 [58]

den death in the morning in hypertensive patients.

The association between MBPS and LVH is also found in normotensive patients and well-controlled hypertensive patients. In a community-dwelling sample, exaggerated morning BP reactivity (highest quartile of the slope of MBPS against morning physical activity) was associated with LVH [57]. In well-controlled hypertensive patients with 24-hour BP values <130/80 mmHg, MBPS (sleep-trough surge) was significantly associated with increases in LVMI and carotid intima-media thickness (IMT) (**Figure 5.4**) [58]. The association found in both studies was not linear but rather non-linear with a threshold of morning surge. Even in normotensives with clinic BP <140/90 mmHg and 24-hour BP <130/80 mmHg, sleep-trough MBPS was significantly correlated with LVMI [59].

In a recent study on coronary flow reserve in patients with prehypertension or Stage 1 hypertension, increased change in MBPS was associated with microvascular dysfunction in the absence of obstructive coronary artery disease [60].

Vascular disease and inflammation

The morning surge in BP and increased time rate of BP variation in the morning have been associated with carotid atherosclerosis in untreated hypertensive patients [61-64]. This association may be accompanied by increased vascular inflammation that can induce plaque instability.

Hypertensive patients with MBPS (n=128) had greater carotid IMT and higher urinary catecholamine excretion (p<0.001), and higher levels of inflammatory markers such as C-reactive protein (CRP), interleukin-6, and interleukin-18

($p<0.001$), versus those without MBPS ($n=196$) [62]. In our JMS-ABPM study on hypertensive patients, MBPS was significantly correlated with the high-sensitivity CRP (hsCRP) level in patients with the highest quartile of MBPS (sleep-trough surge), but not in the other quartiles [64].

In addition, a histological study on carotid endarterectomy specimens demonstrated that carotid plaques in those with exaggerated MBPS were associated with characteristics of vulnerable plaques (higher numbers of macrophages and T-lymphocytes, increased expression of HLA-DR antigen, reduced numbers of smooth muscle cells and lower collagen content), increased levels of markers of oxidative stress and activation of the ubiquitin–proteasome system [63]. In that study, the finding that subjects with exaggerated MBPS had higher levels of activated subunits (p50, p65) of nuclear factor kappa B (NF-kB: a central transcription factor regulating inflammatory genes), and matrix metalloproteinase-9 (MMP-9: an important enzyme in plaque rupture) suggests that exaggerated MBPS is associated with vascular inflammation and plaque instability. These factors were significantly associated with increased oxidative stress and activation of the ubiquitin–proteasome system. Together, these findings suggest that exaggerated MBPS accelerates both atherosclerotic plaque formation and plaque instability in relation to vascular inflammation. Clinically, hypertensive patients with carotid plaques, which are likely to be vulnerable, may receive potential benefit from anti-inflammatory treatment using statins, renin–angiotensin system (RAS) inhibitors, and thiazolidinediones, as well as from treatment to suppress MBPS [65].

In Asian patients with hypertension, consecutive 3-hourly mean SBP readings during the day were significantly associated with intracranial arterial stenosis (ICAS) (odds ratio [OR] 1.28–1.38 for each 10 mmHg increase; $p \leq 0.001$). However, only mean SBP obtained between 5:00 am and 7:59 am was significantly associated with ICAS after adjusting for all consecutive 3-hourly mean SBP readings (OR 1.30; $p=0.019$). This highlights a significant association between early morning SBP and asymptomatic intracranial stenosis (**Figure 5.5**) [66].

In 743 patients with hypertension or diabetes and healthy normotensives, sleep-trough rising surges were significantly correlated with pulse wave velocity (PWV) (hypertensives: $r=0.126$, $p<0.001$; diabetics: $r=0.434$, $p<0.0001$) and LVMI (hypertensives: $r=0.307$, $p<0.001$; diabetics: $r=0.447$, $p<0.0001$) [67].

In 602 consecutive patients with untreated hypertension (mean age 48 years), STMS ($r=0.16$, $p<0.001$) and rising MBPS ($r=0.12$, $p=0.003$) showed a direct correlation with cf-PWV, and only STMS was independently associated with cf-PWV ($t=1.96$, $p=0.04$) after adjustment for age, sex, height, clinic mean arterial pressure, heart rate, and renal function. ARV, a measure of BP variability (See Chapter 9) was a significant mediator of the relationship between STMS and cf-PWV ($p=0.003$). In untreated hypertension, STMS has a direct relationship with aortic stiffness, which is mediated by increased ARV [68].

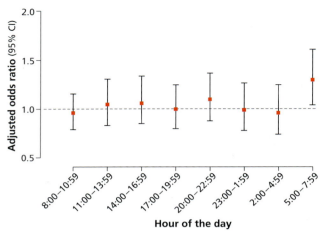

*Computed for a 10 mmHg increase in the consecutive 3-hourly means of SBP during the day.

Figure 5.5 Association between ambulatory systolic blood pressure during the day and asymptomatic intracranial arterial stenosis. SBP, systolic blood pressure. *Source:* Chen et al. 2014 [66]

In the 241 younger adult patients (mean age 36.6 years), those with higher STMS were older ($p=0.003$), had higher carotid IMT ($p=0.05$) and lower E/A ratio ($p=0.01$) than those with lower MBPS. A relationship between MBPS and cardiovascular alterations was observed both in dippers and non-dippers, although in non-dippers, it was less pronounced [69].

In a recent study in 170 patients with prehypertension, independent predictors of greater carotid IMT were greater MBPS (odds ratio [OR] 8.47; $p<0.001$), male sex (OR 2.27; $p=0.047$), and elevated mean platelet volume levels (OR 3.36, $p<0.001$ [70]). Thus, even in relatively younger adults before developing hypertension, MBPS seems partly to be associated with vascular disease.

Silent cerebrovascular disease

Silent cerebral infarcts (SCIs) are the strongest surrogate markers of clinical stroke, particularly in those with an increased CRP level [34]. In the JMS-ABPM study, SCIs (particularly multiple SCIs) were detected more frequently by brain magnetic resonance imaging in the morning surge group than in the non-surge group. The odds ratio for SCI was significantly higher only in patients in the highest quartile of MBPS with higher (above median) hsCRP compared with those in other quartiles of MBPS and with lower hsCRP (below median) (**Figure 5.6**) [64]. This indicates that the relationship between exaggerated MBPS and

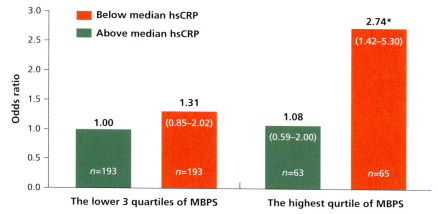

Figure 5.6 Morning BP surge and silent cerebral infarcts in relation to inflammation in elderly hypertensive patients (Jichi Medical University ABPM study wave 1, adjusted for age, gender, body mass index, smoking status, the presence of a glycemic abnormality, dipping status, and 24-h SBP by logistic regression analysis. *$p<0.01$ vs. the patients with the lower 3 quartiles of MBPS and below the median hsCRP level. hsCRP, high-sensitivity C-reactive protein; MBPS, morning blood pressure surge; SBP, systolic blood pressure.
Reprinted from Publication *Atherosclerosis*, vol. 219, Shimizu M, Ishikawa J, Yano Y, Hoshide S, Shimada K, Kario K. The relationship between the morning blood pressure surge and low-grade inflammation on silent cerebral infarct and clinical stroke events, p316-321[64]. Copyright (2011), with permission from Elsevier. Ref. [64]

the presence of SCI is slightly affected by low-grade inflammation.

While it is well known that sympathetic activity, particularly alpha-adrenergic activity, is increased in the morning, SCI has been shown to be more closely associated with the exaggerated MBPS related to alpha-adrenergic activity (defined as the reduction of MBPS by an alpha-adrenergic blocker [doxazosin]) than the overall MBPS (**Figure 5.7**) [71].

Chronic kidney disease

Despite the aforementioned associations between MBPS and cardiac and vascular complications, there have been few studies demonstrating positive associations between MBPS and renal disease. Chronic kidney disease (CKD) is likely to exhibit a non-dipping pattern of nighttime BP falls [72, 73], and this non-dipping pattern might precede microalbuminuria [74]. One cross-sectional study in newly diagnosed type 2 diabetic normotensive patients demonstrated that morning BP levels and MBPS were significantly higher in patients with microalbuminuria than in patients without microalbuminuria [75]. This indicates that

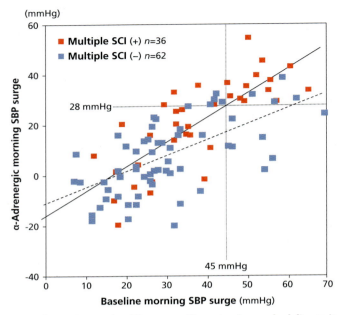

Figure 5.7 Alpha-adrenergic morning BP surge and hypertensive cerebral disease in elderly hypertensive patients. SBP, systolic blood pressure; SCI, silent cerebral infarcts detected by brain MRI. *Source:* Kario et al. 2004 [71].

a systemic BP surge might directly induce MBPS in intraglomerular pressure under the diabetic condition of disrupted autoregulation of the afferent arteriole of the glomerulus. Another study on normotensive subjects and patients with hypertension or diabetes demonstrated only a weak correlation between rising BP surge and albuminuria ($r=0.126$, $p<0.05$) [67].

The resistive index (RI) in renal Doppler ultrasonography is thought to be a good indicator of renal vascular resistance caused by atherosclerosis. It has been shown that MBPS (sleep-trough surge) was significantly associated with higher RI in patients with risks of atherosclerosis [76].

In a prospective study of 622 hypertensive patients (mean age: 57.6 years) with a median of 3.33 years' follow-up, higher MBPS, analysed both as a continuous and categorical variable, was associated with incident CKD in all models [77].

Environmental factors	Risk factor
Winter (cold temperature)	Aging
Monday	Hypertension (high-normal normotension)
Behavioural factors	Diabetes
Alcohol	Orthostatic hypertension
Smoking	Inflammation
Physical stress	
Psychological stress	**Vascular disease**
Poor sleep quality	
Insomnia	**Short-acting**
Obstructive sleep apnoea	**antihypertensive drug**

Figure 5.8 Determinants of morning hypertension and morning surge. *Source:* Kario. 2015 [10]

Determinants of MBPS

Figure 5.8 shows the factors associated with MBPS and morning hypertension [10]. MBPS is increased by various factors, including aging, hypertension, high-normal normotension, diabetes (**Figure 5.9**) [78], inflammation, alcohol intake (**Figure 5.10**) [79], smoking, physical stress, psychological stress, and poor sleep quality [18, 78, 80]. As the underlying mechanism of diurnal BP variation and MBPS, diurnal variation and activation of neurohumoral factors that regulate the vascular tonus and cardiac output, such as RAS and sympathetic nervous activity, potentially in relation to central and peripheral clock genes, may be involved. Orthostatic hypertension, that was found to be associated with extreme dippers, was also associated with an increase only in morning BP level, suggesting that orthostatic hypertension partly contributes to MBPS.

There are weekly and seasonal variations in the MBPS. MBPS is augmented on Mondays (**Figure 5.11**) [81] and over the winter, particularly in elderly subjects [82]. Pre-wakening MBPS was significantly associated with lower outdoor temperature [83]. These BP variations may partly account for the Monday peak and winter peak of cardiovascular events in the elderly [84]. In addition, nocturnal hypoxia or poor sleep quality may augment MBPS, probably through an increase in sympathetic activation and in endothelial dysfunction. Even in children with sleep apnoea without any early vascular damage, MBPS has been shown to be augmented [85].

"Thermosensitive hypertension" and MBPS

Using the data generated by the HEM-7252G-HP, which includes a thermosensor within the device, we first use the "thermosensitive hypertension" to define

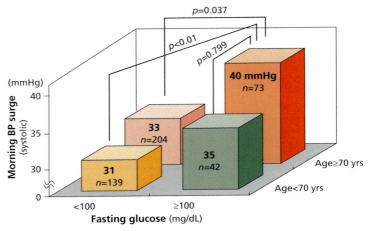

Figure 5.9 Glucose abnormality and morning BP surge in elderly hypertensive patients. JMS ABPM study wave 1 (*n*=458). *Source:* Shimizu et al. 2009 [78]

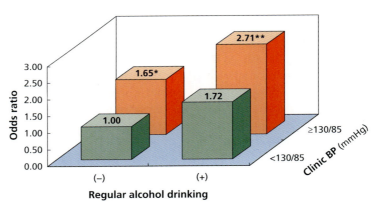

Logistic regression analysis: adjusted by age, sex, BMI, smoking, number of antihypertensive drug classes, and calcium channel blocker use. Odds ratio: vs regular alcohol drinking (–) and clinic BP <130/85 mmHg group, *$p<0.05$, **$p<0.01$

Figure 5.10 Odds ratio of masked morning hypertension. *Source:* Ishikawa et al. 2006 [79]

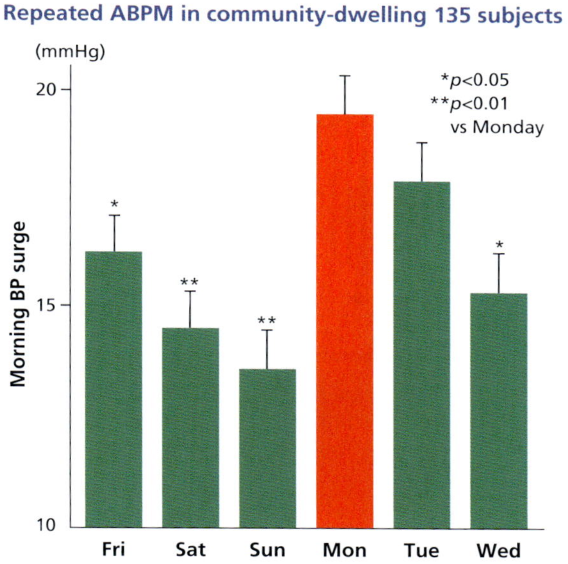

Morning surge in BP

Figure 5.11 Weekly variation of morning BP surge (red bar: Monday morning surge). ABPM, ambulatory BP monitoring; BP, blood pressure. *Source:* Murakami et al. 2004 [81]

the hypertension status in which home BP is closely determined by seasonal changes in temperature (e.g. $R^2>0.3$, change of morning SBP >10 mmHg/10°C) [10]. Morning BP is more closely associated with cold temperature than evening BP. (**Figure 5.12**).

MBPS is augmented in the winter (**Figure 5.13**) [82], especially in the elderly (**Figure 5.14**) [86]. Patients with "thermosensitive hypertension" may exhibit "winter morning surge in BP", which may contribute to increase in cardiovascular events in the winter (**Figure 5.15**). In addition, colder temperature and lower prevalence of well-insulated housing may partly account for regional differences in the winter increase in cardiovascular events. In Hokkaido, located in north area in Japan, the temperature is the coldest but the prevalence of well-insulated housing is higher than other regions, resulting in the lower winter-increase in the cardiovascular events (**Figure 5.16**).

Mechanism of morning risk

The various risk factors related to an increase in cardiovascular risk in the morning are MBPS, imbalance between thrombotic and fibrin lytic activities,

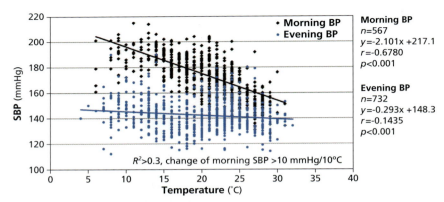

Figure 5.12 A case of thermosensitive hypertension. Measured from March 7, 2015 to December 18, 2015. BP, blood pressure; SBP, systolic BP. *Source:* Kario K. *Essential Manual on Perfect 24-hour Blood Pressure Management from Morning to Nocturnal Hypertension: Up-to-date for Anticipation Medicine.* Wiley, 2018.

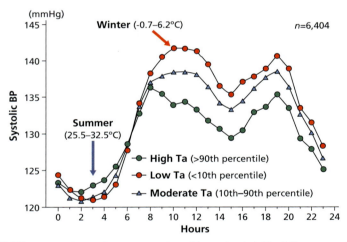

Figure 5.13 Winter morning and summer nocturnal hypertension. Ta, daily mean outdoor air temperature. *Source:* Modesti et al. 2006 [82]

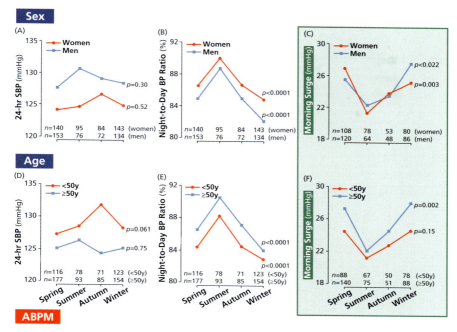

Figure 5.14 Seasonality of the 24-hour systolic blood pressure (SBP) level (A and D), the night-to-day SBP ratio (B and E), and the morning surge in SBP (C and F) stratified by sex and age group. Spring ranged from March 1 to May 31, summer from June 1 to August 31, autumn from September 1 to November 30, and winter from December 1 to the last day of next year's February. Plotted values are means. The number of participants contributing to each data point is given along the horizontal axis. Analysis of variance (ANOVA) p values indicate the significance of the overall differences across seasons. The season-by-sex ($p \geq 0.35$) and season-by-age group ($p \geq 0.13$) interactions were all nonsignificant. ABPM, ambulatory BP monitoring; BP, blood pressure; SBP, systolic BP. *Source:* Sheng et al. 2017 [86]

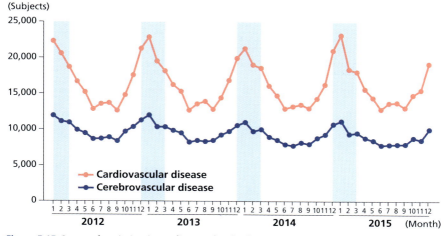

Figure 5.15 Seasonal variation in cardiovascular death in Japan. *Source:* Monthly vital statistics report in japan (approx.). Ministry of health, labour and welfare.

- In Europe, the increment in the death rate in winter is 10% in cold regions (e.g., Finland), whereas in warm regions such as Portugal, UK and Italy, it is around 20%. It suggests that in warm areas there is a lack of energy-saving houses with sufficient insulation and in many residences the indoor room temperature remains low.
- In England, it is thought that blood pressure and circulatory disease may increase at below 18 °C and resistance to respiratory disease declines at below 16 °C. Thus the minimum healthy room temperature in a home has been determined to be 18 °C in winter.*
- The same tendency is found in Japan, and increments in winter death rates are smaller in Hokkaido, a cold part of Japan that contains many well-insulated houses.

*Public Health England, Department of Health 'Cold Weather Plan for England. 2015.10'

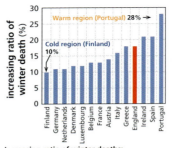

Increasing ratio of winter deaths:
A comparison by European countries.
Annual report of Department of Health U.K. (2010. 3)

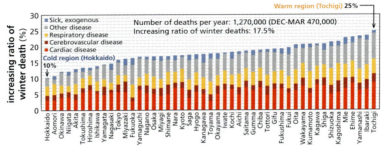

Increasing ratio of winter death: A comparison by prefectures (cause of death)
Drawn using data from 'Demographic statistics (2014), Ministry of Health, Labor and Welfare'.

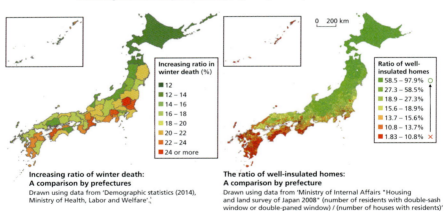

Increasing ratio of winter death:
A comparison by prefectures
Drawn using data from 'Demographic statistics (2014), Ministry of Health, Labor and Welfare'.

The ratio of well-insulated homes:
A comparison by prefecture
Drawn using data from 'Ministry of Internal Affairs "Housing and land survey of Japan 2008" (number of residents with double-sash window or double-paned window) / (number of houses with residents)'

Figure 5.16 A tendency toward low winter mortality rates has been shown in areas (Europe, Japan) where residents are more likely to have sufficient thermal insulation. *Source:* Ikaga. 2017

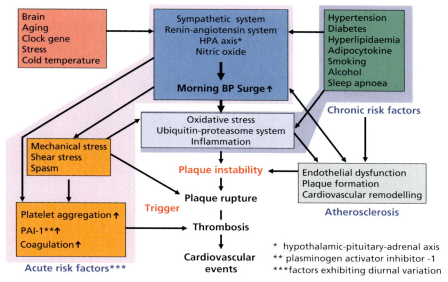

Figure 5.17 Morning BP surge-related cardiovascular risk. *Source:* Kario. 2007 [87]

and endothelial dysfunction (**Figures 5.17** and **5.18**) [87, 88]. There is a circadian rhythm in neurohumoral factors. Sympathetic nervous activity gradually increases before awakening, and overshooting is found after rising. Plasma norepinephrine level has been shown to surge just after awakening (**Figure 5.19-left**) [89]. In a study of muscle sympathetic nerve activity in younger subjects, the ability of the baroreflex to buffer increases in BP via reflexive changes in muscle sympathetic nerve activity may play a role in determining the magnitude of the MBPS [90]. The RAS also exhibits similar variations, with the surge beginning earlier than the sympathetic nervous system. From midnight to early in the morning, RAS is activated, resulting in a peak early in the morning (**Figure 5.19-right**) [91]. The circadian variation of these factors is related partly to circadian variation of haemodynamics, including BP, pulse rate, and circulating volume.

The risk of MBPS triggering cardiovascular events is partly due to increased haemodynamic stress such as vertical pressor stress and increased shear stress generated by exaggerated blood flow on the plaques of the vessel wall. In addition, instability of the plaque may be caused by exaggerated haemodynamic stress as described previously [63].

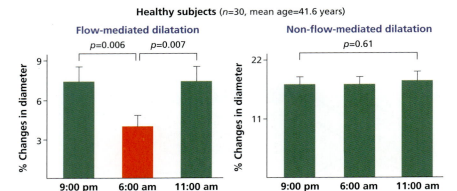

Figure 5.18 Morning endothelial dysfunction in healthy subjects. *Source:* Otto et al. 2004 [88]

Haemostatic abnormality and MBPS

Thrombotic tendency augments the morning risk of cardiovascular events. Thrombus formation results in acute thrombosis at the site of plaque rupture, and haemostatic imbalance in the morning is due to hypercoagulability and hypofibrinolytic activity (increase in plasma level of tissue-type plasminogen activator inhibitor-1 [PAI-1]), and increased platelet aggregation contributes to accelerating thrombus formation at the site of plaque rupture.

In the JMS-ABPM study, an additive increase in stroke risk was found for MBPS and increased plasma level of prothrombin fragment 1+2 (F1+2) and PAI-1 in hypertensive patients (**Figure 5.20**) [92]. F1+2 is the biomarker of activated coagulation factor Xa, and PAI-1 is a well-known inhibitor of fibrinolysis. These biomarkers are known to exhibit circadian variation, with increases in the morning. However, the degree of MBPS per se was not significantly correlated with plasma levels of these biomarkers measured in the morning in our study. These results indicate that exaggerated MBPS additively increases the cardiovascular risk when accompanied by haemostatic abnormalities.

In addition, MBPS has been shown to be significantly associated with increased platelet aggregation assessed by the newly-developed laser scattering intensity method to assess platelet aggregation in different sizes [93]. Spontaneous platelet aggregation in small size particles was significantly correlated with the degree of MBPS (**Figure 5.21**) [93]. The association between morning surge and platelet aggregation was found both in the morning and in the afternoon, but was stronger in the morning. This indicates a very important aspect of BP variability. High shear-stress-induced platelet activation per se due to increased

Morning surge in BP

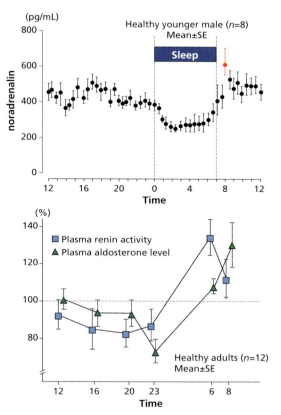

Figure 5.19 Diurnal variation of plasma noradrenalin level, plasma renin activity and aldosterone levels. *Source:* Upper panel, Linsell et al. 1985 [89], Reprinted by permission of Oxford University Press; lower panel, Kawasaki et al. 1990 [91]

BP variability in the morning may partly account for this result. Practically it is important because when hypertensive patients with cardiovascular disease or paroxysmal atrial fibrillation are treated with antithrombotic therapy using antiplatelet or anticoagulation, they are at risk for both thrombotic and haemorrhagic episodes. The Ohasama study demonstrated that MBPS is also a risk for cerebral haemorrhage [47]. Antiplatelet and/or anticoagulation therapy without sufficient reduction of exaggerated MBPS may increase the risk of haemorrhagic events. The strict reduction of exaggerated MBPS in hypertensive patients receiving antithrombotic treatment with antiplatelets or anticoagulants would be critically important to achieve the maximum net clinical benefit [6].

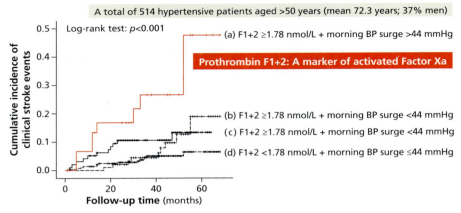

Figure 5.20 Additional impact of morning haemostatic risk factors and morning BP surge on stroke risk in older Japanese hypertensive patients. F1+2, prothrombin fragment 1+2. *Source:* Kario et al. 2011 [92]

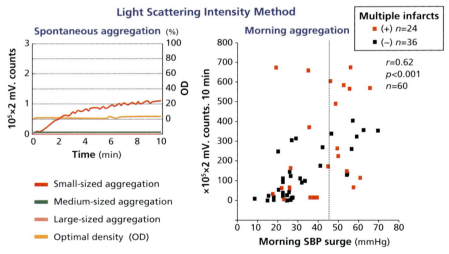

Figure 5.21 Morning BP surge and platelet aggregation in hypertensive patients. Kario et al. 2011 [93]

Morning surge in BP

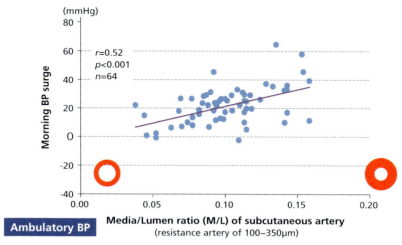

Figure 5.22 Morning BP surge and remodelling of small resistance artery in hypertension. *Source:* Rizzoni et al. 2007 [95]

Vascular mechanism of exaggerated MBPS

Vascular diseases of both the small and large arteries are considered not only to be consequences, but also the leading cause, of exaggerated MBPS, a circumstance giving rise to a vicious cycle in the cardiovascular continuum [18, 87, 94].

An interesting study that directly assessed small artery remodelling by the examination of biopsy specimens demonstrated that the sleep-trough surge was significantly and positively correlated with increased media thickness to lumen diameter ratio (M/L ratio, a measure of remodelling) of the subcutaneous small arteries in patients with essential hypertension (**Figure 5.22**) [95]. The association between contraction of the resistance arteries and vascular resistance is not linear but rather curvilinear in keeping with Folkow's principle [96] that explains the acceleration of hypertension (**Figure 5.23**). Narrowing of the small arterioles has been hypothesised to contribute to the pathogenesis of hypertension [97], but there is little prospective clinical data on this association. Structural narrowing of the small resistance arteries shifts this association curve to the left, compared to the curve for normal arteries. Compared to during sleep when vascular tonus is decreased, the difference in vascular resistance between the small artery with remodelling and that without remodelling is augmented in the morning when vascular tonus is increased.

The activation of various pressor neurohumoral factors including the sympa-

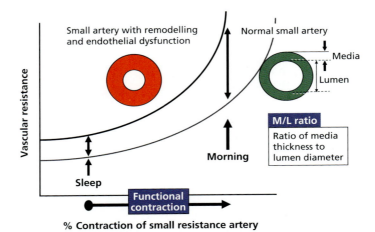

Figure 5.23 Folkow's principle-based mechanism of exaggerated morning BP surge in patients with small artery disease. *Source:* Kario. 2012 [40]

thetic nervous system and the RAS occurs early in the morning. Increased sympathetic activity, particularly of the alpha-adrenergic component [98], increases vascular tone in the small resistance arteries and may contribute to MBPS. In fact, bedtime dosing of an alpha-adrenergic blocker was shown to preferentially reduce morning BP levels and MBPS, particularly in those with small artery diseases (SCIs) [71]. The RAS is activated in the morning and could contribute to MBPS and morning increase in cardiovascular risk. Plasma renin activity, angiotensin II, and aldosterone levels are all increased before awakening and then further increased after awakening [99]. In addition, a previous experimental study demonstrated that the mRNA levels of RAS components in the tissue levels of the cardiovascular system exhibit diurnal variation, particularly in the hypertensive model, with increases occurring during the awakening period [100]. A report demonstrated that a vaccine targeting angiotensin II significantly reduced ambulatory BP throughout a 24-hour period [101]. However, the reduction in BP was most prominent in the morning hours. The fact that the BP reduction by complete 24-hour RAS inhibition was most prominent in the morning period indicates that both the RAS and the related pressor effect are highly activated in the morning. In addition, endothelial dysfunction is found in the morning, even in healthy subjects, and reduces the capacity for vasodilatation [88]. Thus, the threshold of augmentation of BP surge by pressor stimulation may be the lowest in the morning; in other words, the morning is a sensitive period for detecting

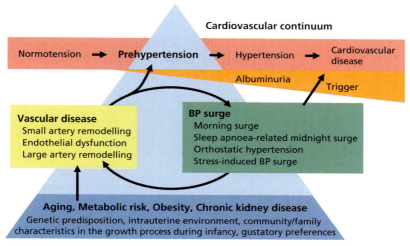

Figure 5.24 Clinical relevance of BP surge on cardiovascular continuum. *Source:* Kario. 2007 [94].

pathological surge and variability in the BP, which reflects vascular status. Using BP surge, the morning may be the best time window to detect the early stage of vascular damage, such as small artery remodelling and endothelial dysfunction.

Considering these data, even when mean clinic BP is within the normal range, masked morning hypertension (isolated morning hypertension) could be considered as "prehypertension" in patients in the early stage of vascular disease (the morning hypertension–prehypertension hypothesis) (**Figure 5.24**) [94]. Other ambulatory BP surges such as sleep apnoea-related nighttime BP surge, orthostatic hypertension, and stress hypertension at the workplace, all of which consist of ambulatory BP variability, could also be considered as forms of "prehypertension," which may precede "true" hypertension with high clinic and 24-hour BP levels. When the duration of pressor conditions persists longer and increase mean 24-hr ambulatory BP to ≥125/75 mmHg, these conditions could be considered as masked hypertension before the clinic BP level increases.

In addition to being a consequence of morning surge, increased arterial stiffness in large artery itself is important as a leading cause of exaggerated BP variability, and MBPS is correlated with vascular disease [67-70]. Baroreceptor sensitivity (BRS) decreases with an increase in large arterial stiffness, and exhibits diurnal variation with a decrease early in the morning [102]. Thus, the reduced BRS in patients with large artery disease may be insufficient to suppress the BP surge (**Figure 5.24**) [94], particularly in the morning. In fact, in hypertensive

Type	Cardiac reactive type	Vascular stiffness type
Age	Younger adult	Elderly
Clinical implication	Prehypertension	Advanced vascular disease
BP characteristics hypertension	Increased heart rate	Systolic
Response to treatment	Easy to treat	Difficult to treat
Day-by-day variability	Stable	Variable
Morning BP surge reactivity	Lower	Higher

Figure 5.25 Age-related characteristics of morning BP surge. BP, blood pressure. *Source:* Kario. 2015 [104]

patients, the impaired dynamic Valsalva-BRS has been significantly correlated with an increase in morning BP [103].

The MBPS can be characterised into 2 types (**Figure 5.25**) [104]: cardiac reactive type and vascular stiffness type. Clinical implications of the former may be the phonotypes of prehypertension before an increase in average BP in younger adults, while the latter may be a direct trigger of cardiovascular events in those with advanced vascular disease. The latter seems difficult to treat.

CHAPTER 6

Nocturnal hypertension

Population-based and clinical studies using ambulatory blood pressure monitoring (ABPM) demonstrated that nighttime BP is a better predictor of cardiovascular diseases than daytime BP [105, 106]. Nocturnal hypertension with higher nighttime BP, and a non-dipper/riser pattern with higher nighttime BP than daytime BP (even if they are normotensive for clinic and 24-hour BP readings) are reported to constitute risks for organ damage and subsequent cardiovascular events [35, 36, 107, 108].

Circadian rhythm of BP

The circadian rhythm of BP is determined partly by the intrinsic rhythm of central and peripheral clock genes, which regulate the neurohumoral factor and cardiovascular systems, and partly by the sleep-wake behavioural pattern.

The pattern of circadian rhythm of BP could be evaluated by ABPM. In healthy subjects, nighttime BP decreases by 10–20% from daytime BP (normal dipper pattern). Hypertensive patients without organ damage also exhibit the dipper pattern; however, those with organ damage tend to exhibit non-dipper patterns with diminished nighttime BP fall. Recent guidelines on the management of hypertension classified dipping patterns of nighttime BP into four groups: dipper, non-dipper, riser, and extreme dippers (**Figure 6.1**) [35, 36]. The definitions of these groups are based on nighttime BP dipping.

Short-term BP variability such as morning BP surge (MBPS), physical or psychological stress-induced daytime BP, and nighttime BP surge triggered by hypoxic episodes in obstructive sleep apnoea modulates this circadian rhythm of BP, resulting in the different individual circadian variation of 24-hour ambulatory BP readings.

Non-dipper/risers of nighttime BP

Non-dippers with diminished nighttime BP fall of 0–10%, and risers with higher nighttime BP than daytime BP are known to have advanced organ damage of the brain, heart, and kidneys, and worse prognosis of cardiovascular events and deaths, compared with normal dippers.

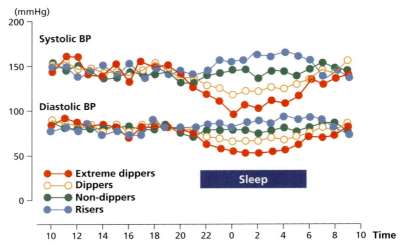

Figure 6.1 Four different dipping status of nighttime BP in hypertensive patients. *Source:* Kario et al. 2001 [36].

Cardiovascular risk

O'Brien et al. first demonstrated that the abnormal non-dipping pattern is associated with advanced organ damage [109]. Nighttime BP fall tends to diminish with advancing age. Shimada et al. first demonstrated that in elderly hypertensive patients, a non-dipper pattern of nighttime BP is associated with advanced silent cerebral disease such as silent cerebral infarcts and deep white matter lesions, both of which were detected by brain magnetic resonance imaging (MRI) [110]. The term "risers" is used to describe patients with a disrupted circadian BP rhythm of higher nighttime BP than daytime BP [111], and "extreme dippers" for patients with an exaggerated nighttime BP fall of 20% or more in the daytime BP reading [35]. Some authors use "reverse dipper" and "inverted dipper" for "risers." In a previous study on elderly hypertensive patients, it was first demonstrated that both extreme abnormal edges of circadian variation, such as risers and extreme dippers with extensive nighttime BP fall by ≥20%, had advanced silent cerebral disease evaluated by brain MRI (**Figure 6.2**) [36], and poor stroke prognosis (**Figure 6.3**) [36]. In particular, risers exhibited a poor prognosis for stroke and cardiac events (**Figure 6.4**) [112].

Shorter sleep duration may increase the cardiovascular risk of non-dippers. In the prospective study, riser pattern and shorter sleep duration synergistically increased cardiovascular risk in hypertensive patients. Non-dippers with a shorter sleep duration exhibited the worst cardiovascular prognosis (**Figure 6.5**) [113].

In addition, the non-dipper pulse rate pattern is also associated with poor car-

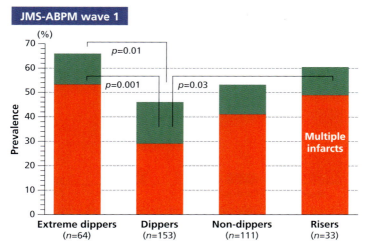

Figure 6.2 Silent cerebral infarcts detected by brain MRI and nighttime BP dipping in elderly hypertensive patients (JMS-ABPM study wave 1). *Source:* Kario et al. 2001 [36]

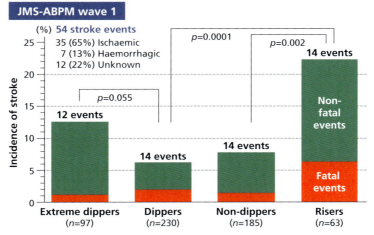

Figure 6.3 Nighttime BP dipping status and stroke prognosis in older sustained hypertensive patients. *Source:* Kario et al. 2001 [36]

diovascular prognosis, especially when it synergistically increases the risk with the non-dipper pattern of nighttime BP fall. In a prospective study on elderly hypertensive patients, non-dippers of nighttime pulse rate showed a 2.4-fold increase in cardiovascular events independent of BP. In addition, non-dippers, of both nighttime BP and nighttime pulse rate, exhibited the worst cardiovascular

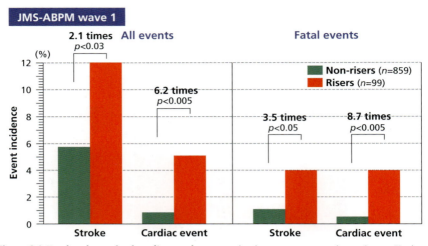

Figure 6.4 Fatal and non-fatal cardiovascular events in risers versus non-risers. *Source:* Kario and Shimada. 2004 [112]

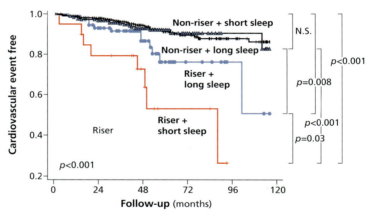

Figure 6.5 Synergistic effect of riser and short sleep on cardiovascular prognosis (*n*=1,255, 70 years, 50 months). *Source:* Eguchi et al. 2008 [113]

prognosis, and a synergistic 8.9-fold increase in cardiovascular events (**Figure 6.6**) [114].

In the patients with heart failure, the riser pattern was more closely associated with the risk of heart failure with preserved ejection fraction (HFpEF) than that of heart failure with reduced ejection fraction (HFrEF) (**Figure 6.7**) [115]. During follow-up, non-dippers and risers with HFpEF had a higher risk of cardiovascular events, while this was not found in HFrEF patients (**Figure 6.8**) [116].

Nocturnal hypertension

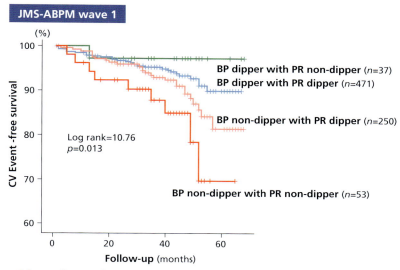

Figure 6.6 Non-dippers of BP and pulse rate and cardiovascular prognosis (JMS-ABPM study wave 1). CV, cardiovascular; PR, pulse rate. *Source:* Kabutoya et al. 2010 [114]. Reprinted by permission of Oxford University Press.

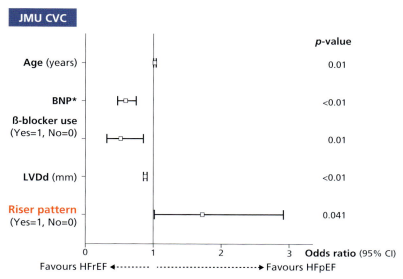

Figure 6.7 Predicting HFpEF or HFrEF in heart failure patients (Jichi Medical University Cardiovascular Center, *n*=508). *Geometric mean. BNP, brain-type natriuretic peptide; HFpEF, heart failure with preserved ejection fraction; HFrEF, heart failure with reduced ejection fraction; LVDd, left ventricular diastolic diameter. *Source:* Komori et al. 2016 [115]

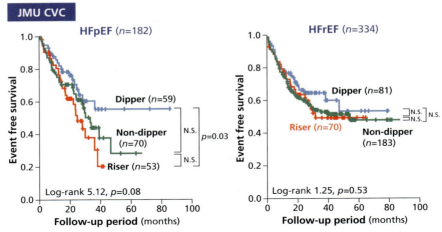

Figure 6.8 Cardiovascular events and disrupted circadian BP rhythm in patients with heart failure (Jichi Medical University Cardiovascular Center, $n=516$). HFpEF, heart failure with preserved ejection fraction; HFrEF, heart failure with reduced ejection fraction.
Source: Komori et al. 2017 [116]

	Dipper $n=49$	Non-dipper + Riser $n=25$	p
Clinic SBP (mmHg)	122±14	123±10	NS
24-hr SBP (mmHg)	112±7.1	111±6.1	NS
LV mass index (g/m^2)	103±26	118±34	<0.05
LV relative wall thickness	0.38±0.07	0.43±0.09	<0.01
Concentric hypertrophy (%)	10	28	<0.05
ANP (pg/ml)	14±10	36±63	<0.01
BNP (pg/ml)	16±12	62±153	<0.05

Figure 6.9 Cardiac overload in normotensive non-dippers (clinic BP <140/90 mmHg, 24-hour BP <125/80 mmHg). Community-dwelling population ($n=74$). ANP, atrial natriuretic peptide; BNP, B-type natriuretic peptide; BP, blood pressure; LV, left ventricular; SBP, systolic BP.
Source: Hoshide et al. 2003 [107]

Organ damage and frailty

Even in normotensive community-dwelling populations with 24-hour BP readings of <125/80 mmHg, normotensive non-dippers and risers showed an increased frequency of concentric cardiac hypertrophy and increased plasma levels of atrial and B-type natriuretic peptides (BNP) (**Figure 6.9**) [107]. In addition, a pulse rate non-dipper pattern was significantly associated with higher plasma BNP level, especially in non-dippers of both BP and pulse rate (**Figure 6.10**) [117].

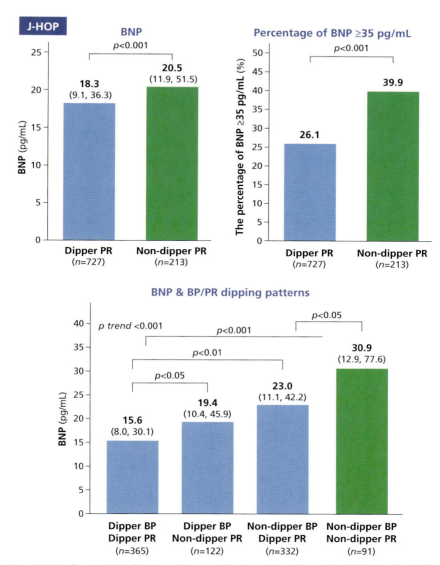

Figure 6.10 Pulse rate (PR) dipping patterns and brain natriuretic peptide (BNP) levels and the percentage of BNP ≥35 pg/mL. Data are presented as median values (25%, 75%) (the J-HOP study, $n=940$) . ABPM was conducted in 940 high-risk Japanese patients enrolled in the J-HOP study. ABPM, ambulatory blood pressure; BP, blood pressure. *Source:* Oba et al. 2017 [117]

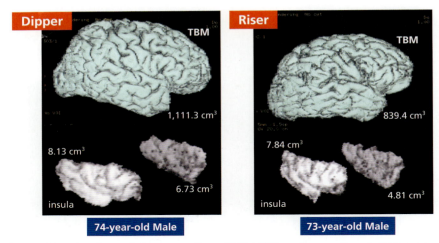

Figure 6.11 Brain volume of riser versus dipper (JMS ABPM study, wave 2 core). TBM, total brain matter. *Source:* Nagai et al. 2008 [118].

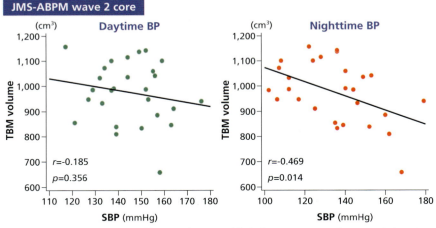

Figure 6.12 Ambulatory BP and brain volume in elderly hypertensive patients (JMS ABPM study, wave 2 core). BP, blood pressure; SBP, systolic BP; TBM, total brain matter. *Source:* Nagai et al. 2008 [118]

Elderly hypertensive non-dippers and risers have been shown to have atrophy of brain and insular cortex (**Figures 6.11** and **6.12**) [118, 119]. The non-dipper pattern and nocturnal hypertension are significantly associated with cognitive dysfunction and slow walking speed in elderly subjects (**Figure 6.13**) [120].

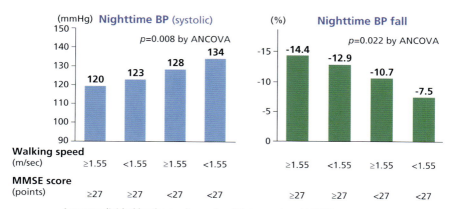

Figure 6.13 Non-dipping and frail elderly (*n*=148, mean 75 years). MMSE, mini-mental state examination. *Source:* Yano et al. 2011 [120]

In patients with heart failure, a riser pattern was significantly associated with mild cognitive impairments [121].

These results indicate that the disrupted circadian rhythm of BP and pulse rate are directly associated with advancing organ damage and subsequent cardiovascular disease.

Definition and risk of nocturnal hypertension

Definition: The definition of nocturnal hypertension is shown in **Figure 2.6**. Nocturnal hypertension is diagnosed by the average of nighttime BP measurements ≥110/65 mmHg. Non-dippers and risers are likely to exhibit nocturnal hypertension.

Cardiovascular risk: In prospective studies, nocturnal hypertension was associated with an increased risk of cardiovascular events, both stroke and coronary. The risk of cardiovascular events is increased along with an increase both in daytime and nighttime BP readings. Only an increase in nighttime BP was associated with increased cardiovascular risk, particularly in medicated patients (**Figure 6.14**) [106]. These BP levels were assessed only at the baseline. Thus, any change in medication would be based on the clinic BP, more closely related to daytime BP levels than nighttime BP levels. Thus, during long-term follow-up, only the risk of nighttime BP remains. This indicates that clinic BP-guided antihypertensive medication does not reduce the risk of nocturnal hypertension.

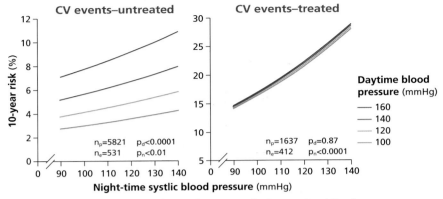

Figure 6.14 Nighttime BP and cardiovascular events. The International Database on Ambulatory blood pressure monitoring in relation to Cardiovascular Outcomes (IDACO); n=7,458, 9.6-year follow-up. n_p and n_e indicate the number of participants at risk and the number of events. p_d and p_n denote the significance of the independent contributions of the daytime and nighttime blood pressures. Reprinted from the *Lancet*, Vol. 370 (9594), Boggia J, Li Y, Thijs L, Hansen TW, Kikuya M, Björklund-Bodegård K, Richart T, Ohkubo T, Kuznetsova T, Torp-Pedersen C, Lind L, Ibsen H, Imai Y, Wang J, Sandoya E, O'Brien E, Staessen JA. Prognostic accuracy of day versus night ambulatory blood pressure: a cohort study, pp.1219-29, Copyright (2007), with permission from Elsevier. Ref. [106]

The risk of cardiovascular events was synergistically associated with higher nighttime pulse rate in the ABP-International study (**Figure 6.15**) [122]. Well-medicated patients with congestive heart failure and uncontrolled nocturnal hypertension with nighttime (sleep) systolic BP (SBP) >120 mmHg, experienced an increase in stroke risk during the follow-up period (**Figure 6.16**) [123].

The impact of nocturnal hypertension is greater in patients with diabetes than that in hypertensive patients without diabetes (**Figure 6.17**) [124]. In a prospective study of hypertensive patients with or without diabetes, the cardiovascular risk associated with nocturnal hypertension (nighttime SBP ≥135 mmHg) versus nocturnal normotension (nighttime SBP <120 mmHg) was increased 2.7 times in the non-diabetic group, but by 10.8 times in the diabetic group (**Figure 6.17**) [124].

In medicated hypertensive patients with well-controlled home BP levels, those with uncontrolled nocturnal hypertension (nighttime SBP ≥120 mmHg by ABPM) exhibited limited reduction of urinary albumin/creatinine ratio (UACR) and increased levels of plasma BNP when compared with those with well-controlled nocturnal hypertension (nighttime SBP <120 mmHg by ABPM) (**Figure 6.18**) [125]. These results indicate that controlling nighttime BP during sleep as well as morning and evening home BP levels is essentially important for reduc-

Nocturnal hypertension

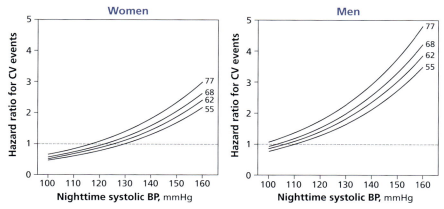

Figure 6.15 Synergistic increase in cardiovascular risk by nighttime blood pressure and pulse rate (ABP-International registry; $n=7,600$; Italy, USA, Australia, Japan). The nighttime pulse rate is represented by four functions corresponding to levels of 55, 62, 68, and 77 beats/min (midpoints within each pulse rate quartile). Risk estimates were adjusted to 52 years of age, non-smoking, lack of diabetes, 206 mg/dl total cholesterol, and 0.9 mg/dl serum creatinine. BP, blood pressure; CV, cardiovascular. Reprinted from *Int J Cardiol.*, Vol. 168, Palatini P, Reboldi G, Beilin LJ, Eguchi K, Imai Y, Kario K, Ohkubo T, Pierdomenico SD, Saladini F, Schwartz JE, Wing L, Verdecchia P, Predictive value of night-time heart rate for cardiovascular events in hypertension. The ABP-International study, pp.1490-5, Copyright (2013), with permission from Elsevier. Ref. [122]

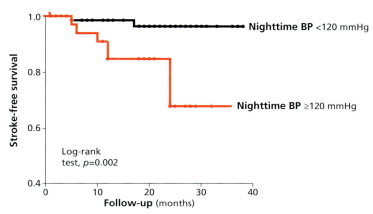

Figure 6.16 Nighttime BP and stroke prognosis in patients with ischaemic/hypertensive heart failure (Jichi Medical University Cardiovascular Center, $n=111$). *Source:* Komori et al. 2008 [123]

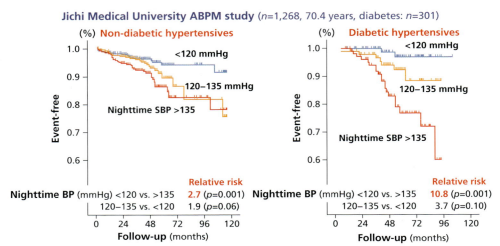

Figure 6.17 Interaction of diabetes on association between nighttime BP (systolic) and cardiovascular prognosis. BP, blood pressure; SBP, systolic BP. *Source:* Eguchi et al. 2008 [124]

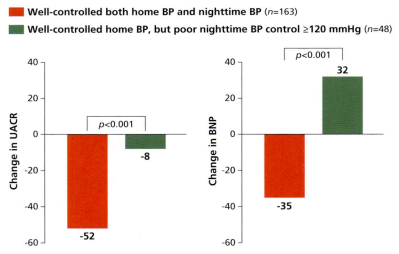

Figure 6.18 Clinical implication of nighttime BP control in addition to controlling home BP in hypertension. BNP, brain natriuretic peptide; BP, blood pressure; UACR, urine albumin/creatinine ratio. Created based on data from Yano et al. 2012 [125].

Nocturnal hypertension

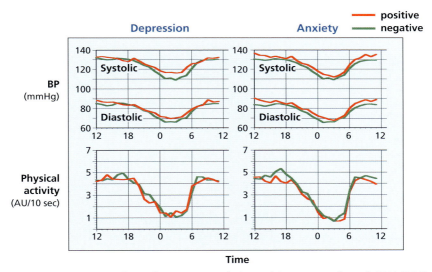

Figure 6.19 Mechanism of non-dipper/riser type nocturnal hypertension. CKD, chronic kidney disease; CHF, congestive heart failure. *Source:* Kario. 2004 [12].

Figure 6.20 Depression and non-dipping (NY work site study). *Source:* Kario et al. 2001 [126]

ing organ damage during antihypertensive treatment.

To minimise the risk of nocturnal hypertension, a staged home-BP guided approach first targeting morning BP to achieve <130/80 mmHg and finally targeting nighttime BP to achieve <110/65 mmHg is recommended (**Figure 2.8**) [10].

Mechanism of nocturnal hypertension

Increased circulating volume, autonomic nervous dysfunction, and poor sleep quality are the three major mechanisms of nocturnal hypertension exhibiting non-dipper and riser patterns (**Figure 6.19**) [12]. Increased circulating volume may have a compensatory effect and increase nighttime BP in addition to day-

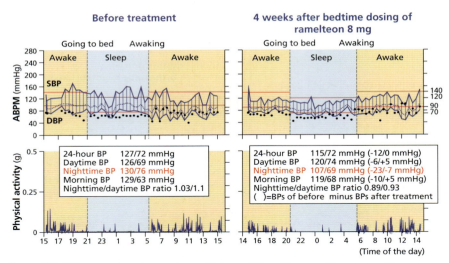

Figure 6.21 Effect of melatonin agonist on 24-hour BP in a 59-year-old woman with uncontrolled nocturnal hypertension and insomnia (treated by Candesartan 8 mg, HCTZ 6.25 mg, and amlodipine 10 mg). ABPM, Ambulatory BP monitoring; BP, blood pressure. *Source:* Kario 2011 [127].

time BP by excreting sodium from the kidney based on Guyton's theory of pressure–natriuresis relationship, resulting in nocturnal hypertension of non-dipper/riser type [72]. Thus, conditions with increased sympathetic nervous activity and renin–angiotensin–aldosterone system associated increases in circulating volume due to reduced sodium excretion, result in non-dipper/riser type of nocturnal hypertension. The effect of the activation of neurohumoral factors due to orthostatic hypotension during the daytime, may persist in the supine position during sleep. Poor sleep quality such as sleep apnoea syndrome (SAS), insomnia in the elderly, depression (**Figure 6.20**) [126], shift-working, etc. contribute to nocturnal hypertension.

Clock gene abnormality and inappropriate secretion of melatonin may contribute to nocturnal hypertension. The administration of ramelteon, a selective MT1/MT2 melatonin-receptor agonist used for insomnia treatment, reduces nighttime BP and restores the circadian rhythm of BP in insomnia patients with isolated uncontrolled nocturnal hypertension (**Figure 6.21**) [127]. In addition, administration of ramelteon shifts the dipping of nighttime BP from the non-dippers/riser type to the dipper type. The orexin receptor antagonist, suvorexant, also decreases 24-hour ambulatory BP levels, especially the nighttime BP level and variability in patients with uncontrolled nocturnal hypertension and insom-

Nocturnal hypertension

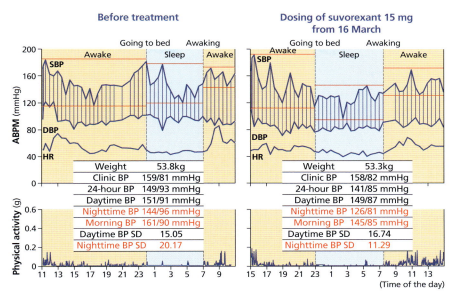

Figure 6.22 Effect of Suvorexant on 24-hour BP in a 71-year-old male with uncontrolled nocturnal hypertension and insomnia. ABPM, ambulatory BP monitoring; BP, blood pressure; HR, heart rate. *Source:* Kario K. *Essential Manual on Perfect 24-hour Blood Pressure Management from Morning to Nocturnal Hypertension: Up-to-date for Anticipation Medicine.* Wiley, 2018.

nia (**Figure 6.22**).

Associated conditions of nocturnal hypertension

Figure 6.23 shows the various determinants and associated conditions of nocturnal hypertension [10]. Diabetes, along with autonomic nervous dysfunction, chronic kidney disease (CKD), and SAS, are common diseases which are frequently associated with nocturnal hypertension. Secondary hypertension and diseases with an increase in sympathetic nervous activity or renin-angiotensin system activity increase the circulating volume, resulting in nocturnal hypertension.

Diabetes

Diabetic patients are likely to have nocturnal hypertension, especially when accompanied with orthostatic hypotension due to autonomic nervous dysfunction. In addition, the CV risk of nocturnal hypertension is augmented in diabetic hypertensive patients compared with non-diabetic patients (**Figure 6.17**) [124]. Thus, the presence of diabetes augments the cardiovascular risk of nocturnal hypertension.

Environmental factors
  Summer (hot temperature)
Behavioural factors
  High salt intake
  Reduced physical activity
  Poor sleep quality
  Nocturia
  Shift-working
Risk factors
  Aging
  Hypertension
  Orthostatic hypotension
  Diabetes
  Asian ethnicity
	Salt sensitivity
	Secondary hypertension
	  Endocrine disease
	    (primary aldosteronism,
	    renovascular hypertension,
	    Cushing syndrome,
	    pheochromocytoma)
	  Chronic kidney disease (CKD)
	  Obstructive sleep apnoea syndrome
	    (OSAS)
	Disease
	  Heart failure
	  Stroke
	  Cognitive dysfunction

Figure 6.23 Determinants of nocturnal hypertension. *Source:* Kario. 2015 [10]

A recent study, in which ABPM and continuous glucose monitoring are performed simultaneously in diabetic patients, demonstrated that the most important determinant of all organ damage (such as left ventricular hypertrophy [LVH], microalbuminuria, carotid intima-media thickness [IMT], and brachial-ankle pulse wave velocity [baPWV]) was the nighttime BP over and above the various other measures of BP and glucose taken during the 24-hour period [128].

In another study, higher fasting glucose increased MBPS in elderly hypertensive patients (**Figure 5.9**) [78], suggesting that the dawn phenomenon may activate sympathetic activity to augment MBPS, especially in those with increased arterial stiffness. In addition, morning hypertension was closely associated with advanced organ damage in diabetic patients [129]. Morning hypertension in patients with diabetes is associated with the non-dipper/riser pattern and nocturnal hypertension.

For diabetic patients it is essential that they achieve "perfect 24-hour BP control."

Chronic kidney disease

CKD is likely to be associated with nocturnal hypertension and the non-dipper/riser pattern. Nighttime BP fall is diminished along with the reduction of glomerular filtration rate and an increase in urinary albumin excretion. In both dippers and non-dippers/risers, CKD is associated with future cardiovascular events. Non-dippers with CKD have the worst cardiovascular risk (**Figure 6.24**) [130].

Sleep apnoea syndrome

See "Trigger nighttime BP monitoring (TNP)" in Chapter 7.

Nocturnal hypertension

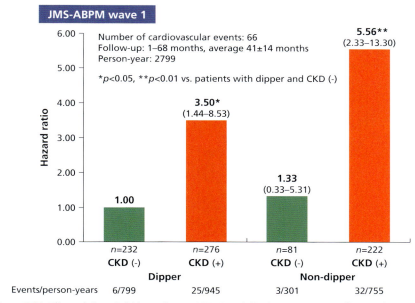

Figure 6.24 Effect of chronic kidney disease (CKD) and dipping status on cardiovascular events (Jichi Medical University ABPM study). *Source:* Ishikawa et al. 2008 [130]

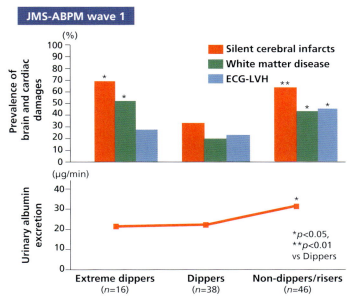

Figure 6.25 Nighttime BP dipping status and organ damage in older sustained hypertensive patients. LVH, left ventricular hypertrophy. *Source:* Kario et al. 1996 [35].

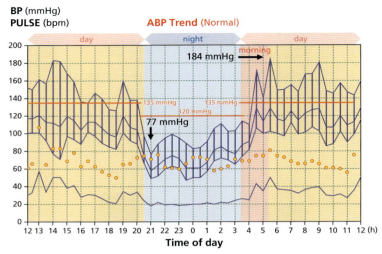

Figure 6.26 24-hour ambulatory BP monitoring of a case of extreme dipper of nighttime BP. A 70-year-old man with a 6-year history of hypertension medicated by 5 mg of amlodipine and 25 mg of losartan. 24-hour BP=135/85 mmHg, daytime BP=154/96 mmHg, nighttime BP=96/62 mmHg, sleep-trough morning surge=68 mmHg, pre-wakening morning surge=44 mmHg. ABP, ambulatory blood pressure; BP, blood pressure. *Source:* Kario. 2017 [8]

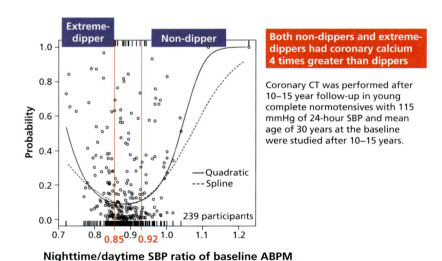

Figure 6.27 U-curve association between nighttime BP dipping and coronary calcium: CARDIA study. ABPM, ambulatory BP monitoring; BP, blood pressure; SBP, systolic BP. *Source:* Viera et al. 2012 [134]

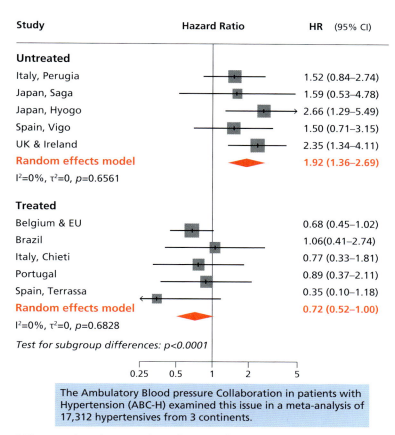

Figure 6.28 Forest plots of meta-analysis of extreme dipping pattern for total cardiovascular events. Adjustment for average 24-hour systolic blood pressure. *Source:* Salles et al. 2016 [135]

Extreme dipper

We first demonstrated that extreme dippers with an extensive nighttime BP fall of >20% had advanced silent cerebral disease detected by brain MRI (**Figure 6.25**) [35]. **Figure 6.26** demonstrates the typical case of an extreme-dipper [8]. In addition, in the prospective JMS-ABPM study wave 1, it was shown that elderly hypertensive patients exhibiting an extreme dipper pattern had an increased risk of future clinical stroke events (**Figure 6.3**) [36]. Another brain MRI study demonstrated that deep white matter lesion was advanced in extreme dippers [131]. Some studies also demonstrated that extreme dippers had reduced cerebral blood flow [132], and increased pulse wave velocity (PWV) [133].

In the CARDIA study on young normotensive subjects, extreme dippers,

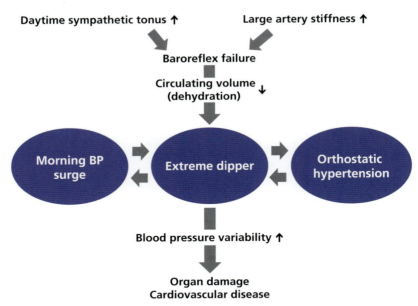

Figure 6.29 Mechanism of extreme dippers and related phenotypes of blood pressure variability. BP, blood pressure. *Source:* Kario. 2017 [8]

non-dippers and risers, defined by the baseline ABPM, developed more advanced coronary calcification which was detected by coronary CT performed in middle-aged adults 10 years or more after the baseline ABPM. Even after controlling for baseline covariates, the risk of having coronary calcium was four or more times greater in both extreme dippers and non-dippers/risers compared with normal dippers (**Figure 6.27**) [134].

In a recent meta-analysis of data from 17,312 hypertensive patients from three continents, the ABC-H (the Ambulatory Blood pressure Collaboration in patients with Hypertension) found that an extreme-dipper pattern was significantly associated with cardiovascular events only in unmedicated patients (**Figure 6.28**) [135].

The pathophysiology of extreme-dippers is not well-known. Baroreflex failure caused by increased daytime sympathetic activity in patients with increased arterial stiffness may be one of the pathophysiology (**Figure 6.29**) [8]. Increased plasma vasopressin level, following head-up tilting, has been shown to be significantly higher in extreme-dippers than in dippers. This might counteract reduced circulating blood volume in extreme-dippers [136]. Extreme-dippers are associated with other phenotypes of BP variability, resulting in the risk of organ damage and cardiovascular events.

CHAPTER 7
Development of nighttime home BP monitoring

Studies have demonstrated that sleep disturbance is closely associated with hypertension, metabolic disease, and various types of cardiovascular disease (**Figure 7.1**) [4, 5, 10, 137-139]. Sleep disturbance includes sleep deprivation, shift-working, insomnia, obstructive sleep apnoea syndrome (OSAS), restless leg syndrome and narcolepsy. Nighttime blood pressure (BP) and its variability could be the new haemodynamic cardiovascular risk indicator of these sleep-related disorders.

Cutting-edge of home BP monitoring

Ambulatory BP monitoring (ABPM) has historically been the gold standard for measuring nighttime BP. However, self-measured home BP monitoring (HBPM) could be used to evaluate nighttime BP, with results that are comparable to those of ABPM. The Jichi Medical University and Omron Healthcare Co., Ltd. (Kyoto, Japan) have been conducting cutting-edge collaboration programme projects in the SURGE (SUper ciRculation monitoriNG with high tEchnology) research and development centre to develop new home BP variability monitoring systems and clarifying a new clinically relevant index of BP variability (**Figure 7.2**) [4, 140].

Recommendation for nighttime home BP measurement

There is no consensus of the standard measurement of nighttime home BP. **Figure 7.3** is a demonstration of how to take a nighttime home BP measurement. A validated home BP monitor should be used, and patients should be shown how to put the cuff of the BP monitor on the upper arm or wrist. Automatic BP measurements should be set for 1–3 times during sleep at either of the following time intervals: 1) fixed o'clock time (2:00 am, 3:00 am, 4:00 am), 2) individual behaviour time (2–4 hours after going to bed) for two or more nights. The average of at least six measures is required to be considered as the nighttime home BP. Nocturnal hypertension is diagnosed when nighttime home BP is ≥110/65 mmHg.

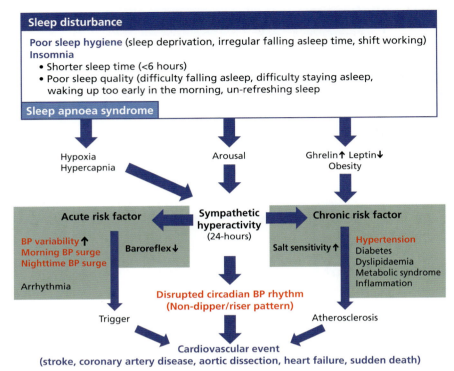

Figure 7.1 Sleep disturbance and related mechanism of cardiovascular disease. BP, blood pressure. Reprinted from *Encyclopedia of Cardiovascular Research and Medicine*, 1st Edition, Kario K, Sleep and Circadian Cardiovascular Medicine, pp 424-437, Copyright (2018), with permission from Elsevier. Ref. [139]

1. Basic home nighttime BP monitoring (Medinote)

2. Trigger nighttime BP monitoring (TNP)
   → IT-based TNP (ITNP)

3. Wearable Beat-by-beat surge BP monitoring (WSP)

Figure 7.2 Cutting-edge nighttime BP monitoring at home (Jichi Medical University - Omron Healthcare Co., Ltd.). *Source:* Kario K. *Essential Manual on Perfect 24-hour Blood Pressure Management from Morning to Nocturnal Hypertension: Up-to-date for Anticipation Medicine*. Wiley, 2018.

Development of nighttime home BP monitoring

Nighttime home BP measurement is performed as follows
Set the cuff of BP monitoring on the upper arm or wrist
Set automatic BP measurements 2–3 times during sleep
Timing of measurements (at least twice)
1) 2:00 AM, 3:00 AM, 4:00 AM
2) 2–4 hours after going to bed
Days
2 or more nights
Calculation
Average of ≥6 measures

Figure 7.3 Nighttime home BP measurement. BP, blood pressure. *Source:* Kario K. *Essential Manual on Perfect 24-hour Blood Pressure Management from Morning to Nocturnal Hypertension: Up-to-date for Anticipation Medicine.* Wiley, 2018.

Basic nighttime home BP monitoring (Medinote)

Medinote, a semi-automatic HBPM device was developed, with the function of allowing automatic fixed-interval BP measurement during sleep (**Figure 7.4**) [141]. The BP data are stored in the memory file in this device. The development of Medinote was the first step in detecting basic nighttime BP information using at-home, self-measured BP monitoring as opposed to ABPM. The Medinote device has now advanced to an IT-based new nighttime home BP monitoring device, HEM-7252G-HP.

In the Japan Morning Surge Home Blood Pressure (J-HOP) study [142], the largest nationwide home BP cohort, used the Medinote monitoring device with data memory to successfully measure nighttime home BP three times during sleep (2:00 AM, 3:00 AM, 4:00 AM), as well as three times each in the morning and evening for 14 days. Data from 2,562 participants indicated that self-measurement of nighttime BP at home was feasible (**Figure 7.5**) [143]. There was no difference between the nighttime home systolic BP (SBP) at 2:00 AM and 3:00 AM, whilst that at 4:00 AM was slightly higher by 1.5 mmHg ($p<0.0001$). Thus, we defined nighttime home BP as the average of three nighttime BP readings measured at 2:00 AM, 3:00 AM, and 4:00 AM. Nighttime home SBP was significantly correlated with the urinary albumin/creatinine ratio (UACR), left ventricular mass index (LVMI), brachial-ankle pulse wave velocity (baPWV), maximum carotid intima-media thickness (IMT), and plasma levels of N-terminal pro-brain natriuretic peptide (NT-proBNP) and high-sensitive cardiac troponin T level (**Figure 7.6**) [143]. In addition, nighttime home BP was significantly correlated with organ damage independently of clinic, morning, and evening

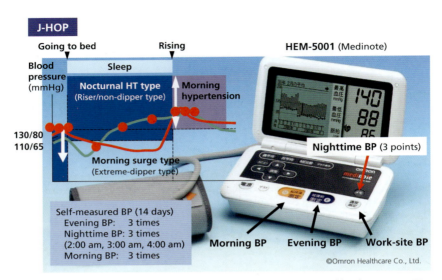

Figure 7.4 Semi-automatic home BP monitoring device (Medinote). BP, blood pressure; HT, hypertension.

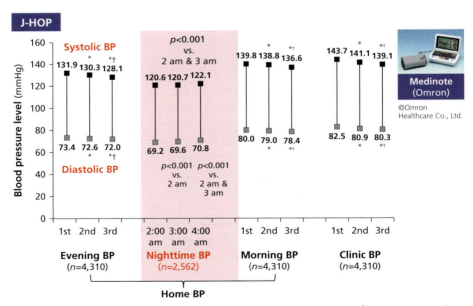

Figure 7.5 Home BP levels in J-HOP study. *$p<0.001$ vs first measurement. †$p<0.001$ vs second measurement by paired t test. BP, blood pressure. *Source:* Kario. 2015 [143]

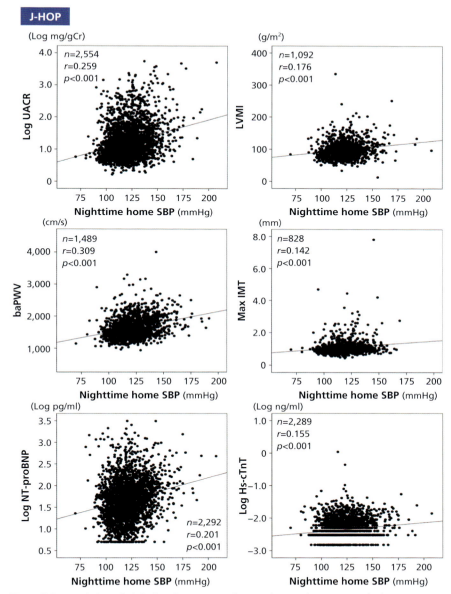

Figure 7.6 Association of nighttime home BP and organ damage in J-HOP study. baPWV, brachial-ankle pulse wave velocity; hs-cTnT, high-sensitivity cardiac troponin T; IMT, intima media thickness; LVMI, left ventricular mass index; NT-proBNP, N-terminal pro-brain natriuretic peptide; UACR, urine albumin-to-creatinine ratio. *Source:* Kario. 2015 [143]

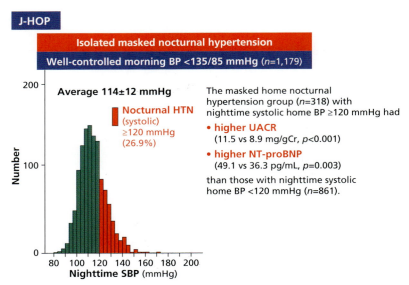

Figure 7.7 Distribution of nighttime home BP levels in J-HOP study BP, blood pressure; HTN, hypertension; NT-proBNP, N-terminal pro-brain natriuretic peptide; UACR, urinary albumin/creatinine ratio. *Source:* Kario. 2015 [143]

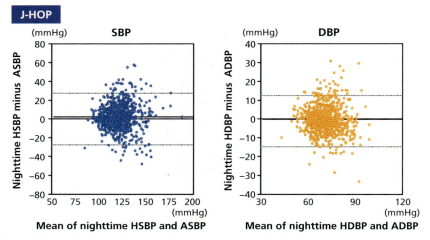

Figure 7.8 Bland–Altman plots of nighttime BP measured by home BP monitoring and ABPM (J-HOP study) (n=854). ADBP, ambulatory DBP; ASBP, ambulatory SBP; DBP, diastolic blood pressure; HDBP, home DBP; HSBP, home SBP; SBP, systolic blood pressure. *Source:* Ishikawa et al. 2012 [141]

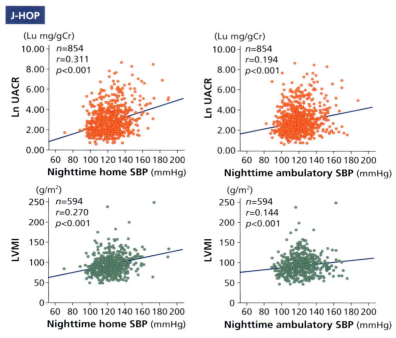

Figure 7.9 Nighttime BP and organ damage. LVMI, left ventricular mass index; SBP, systolic blood pressure; UACR, urinary albumin/creatinine ratio. *Source:* Ishikawa et al. 2012 [141]

BP readings. Even in those with well-controlled morning home SBP <135/85 mmHg, 27% exhibited "masked home nocturnal hypertension" with nighttime home SBP ≥120 mmHg (**Figure 7.7**) [143]. These patients had higher UACR and NT-proBNP, indicating that masked home nocturnal hypertension, which is associated with advanced organ damage, remains unrecognised by conventional HBPM.

In a J-HOP subanalysis, the nighttime home BP measured was almost comparable to nighttime BP defined by ABPM (**Figure 7.8**) [141], and the association with organ damage (LVH and microalbuminuria) was greater for nighttime home SBP than nighttime SBP detected by ABPM (**Figure 7.9**) [141]. Nighttime home BP was also a better indicator of BP control during antihypertensive treatment. In the Japan Morning Surge-Target Organ Protection (J-TOP) study, the reduction of nighttime home BP was more closely associated with the regression of LVH evaluated by cardiac echography and electrocardiography (**Figure 7.10**) [144].

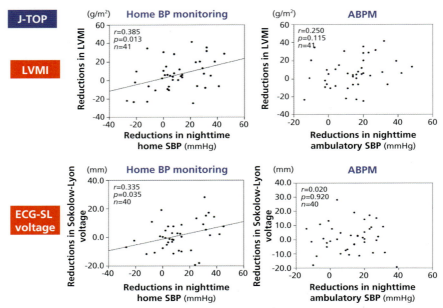

Figure 7.10 Association of reduction of nighttime BP and cardiac hypertrophy by antihypertensive treatment. ABPM, ambulatory blood pressure monitoring; LVMI, left ventricular mass index; SBP, systolic blood pressure. *Source:* Ishikawa et al. 2014 [144]

Trigger nighttime BP monitoring (TNP)

The second advance was the development of trigger nighttime BP monitoring (TNP), which was based on the automated fixed interval-measurement technique of Medinote with an added trigger function that initiates BP measurement when oxygen desaturation falls below the variable threshold continuously monitored by pulse oximetry (**Figure 7.11**) [140]. OSAS is characterised by uncontrolled nocturnal hypertension with increased BP variability (both morning and nighttime BP surges) (**Figure 7.12**) [145]. TNP can detect the specific nighttime BP surges triggered by hypoxic episodes in patients with sleep apnoea syndrome (SAS) [146, 147]. However, neither previous HBPM nor ABPM with fixed time-interval measurement could detect the nighttime BP surge specific to each sleep apnoea episode.

In addition, the pulse rate-trigger function was added to TNP to detect the "basal nighttime BP," which is determined by the circulating volume and structural cardiovascular system without any increase in sympathetic tonus. This double TNP is a brand-new concept for evaluating the pathogenic pressor mecha-

Development of nighttime home BP monitoring

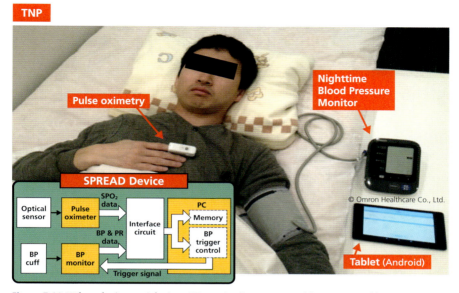

Figure 7.11 IT-based trigger nighttime BP monitoring system with oxygen and heat rate triggers and Cloud system (ITNP1, 2015) (Jichi Medical University, Omron Healthcare Co., Ltd. Kyoto, Japan). BP, blood pressure; PR, pulse rate. *Source:* modified from Kario et al. 2015 [145]

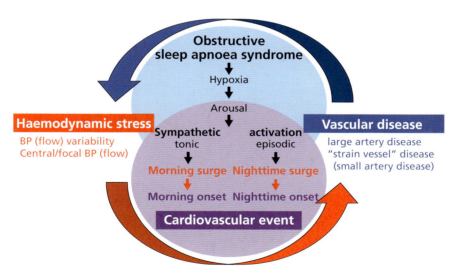

Figure 7.12 Obstructive sleep apnoea-triggered systemic haemodynamic atherothrombotic syndrome (SHATS) - acceleration of the risk of cardiovascular events and organ damage via a vicious cycle of haemodynamic stress and vascular disease. BP, blood pressure. *Source:* Kario et al. 2015 [145]

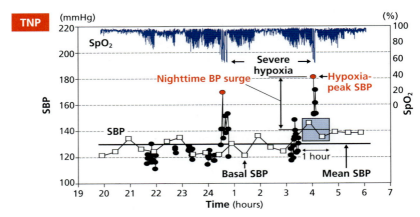

Figure 7.13 Definition of nighttime BP parameters by trigger nighttime BP monitoring (TNP). SBP, systolic blood pressure. *Source:* Kario et al. 2014 [148].

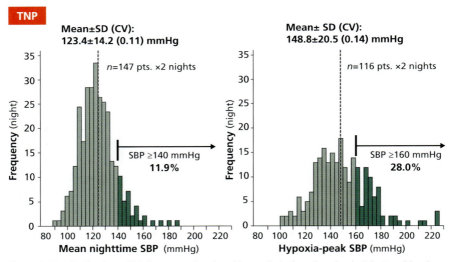

Figure 7.14 Distribution of higher mean level and hypoxia-induced peak of nighttime blood pressure in patients with suspected sleep apnoea. SBP, systolic blood pressure. *Source:* Kuwabara et al. 2017 [149].

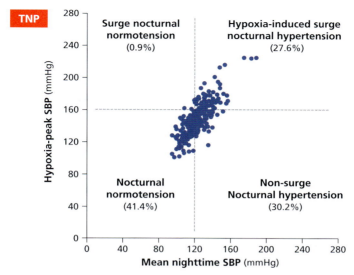

Figure 7.15 Prevalence of hypoxia-induced surge nocturnal hypertension in patients with suspected sleep apnoea . SBP, systolic blood pressure. *Source:* Kuwabara et al. 2017 [149]

nism of nighttime BP.

Figure 7.13 shows the nighttime BP parameters obtained from TNP [148]. The distribution and reproducibility of hypoxia-triggered nighttime BP parameters were evaluated and compared with those of fixed-interval nighttime BP parameters for two consecutive nights in 147 OSA patients. The mean and distribution (standard deviation [SD]) of the hypoxia-peak SBP were significantly greater than that of the mean nighttime SBP (148.8±20.5 vs 123.4±14.2 mm Hg, $p<0.001$) (**Figure 7.14**) [149]. The repeatability coefficient (expressed as % MV) of hypoxia-peak SBP between night one and night two was comparable to that of mean nighttime SBP (43% vs 32%). In conclusion, hypoxia-peak nighttime BP was much higher than mean nighttime BP, and it was as reproducible as mean nighttime BP. In the patients with nocturnal hypertension (mean nighttime SBP ≥120 mmHg), approximately 50% had increased hypoxia-induced nighttime BP surge ≥160 mmHg (**Figure 7.15**) [149]

Figure 7.16 demonstrates the nighttime BP readings detected by TNP in the two cases with drug-resistant hypertension and SAS [140]. Although patients had comparable SAS severity (as measured by the apnoea-hypopnoea index [AHI]), the trigger function of TNP revealed quite different nighttime BP surges between these patients. It is well known that cardiovascular events occurred

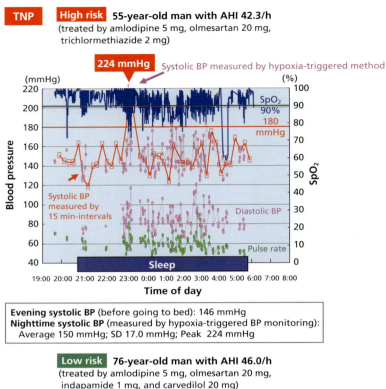

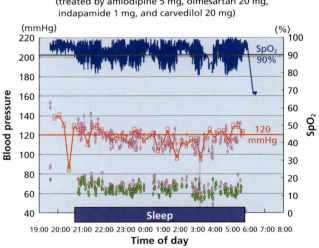

Figure 7.16 Different nighttime BP surges in two patients with resistant hypertension and sleep apnoea syndrome. AHI, apnoea hypopnoea index. *Source:* Kario. 2013 [140]

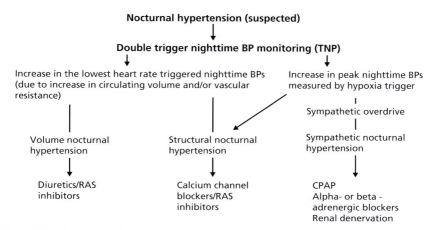

Figure 7.17 Three types of nocturnal hypertension and selective drugs based on the double-trigger nighttime BP monitoring (TNP). CPAP, continuous positive airway pressure; RAS, renin angiotensin system. *Source:* Kario. 2015 [10]

more frequently during sleep periods in patients with OSAS. The hypoxia-induced nighttime BP surge could trigger the sleep-onset cardiovascular events in SAS patients. Using this TNP device, it is possible to specifically identify the SAS patients at high risk for sleep-onset cardiovascular events.

Although nocturnal hypertension exhibits similar average nighttime BP readings; there may be a different mechanism: peak nighttime BP levels measured by hypoxia trigger may be attributed to sympathetic overdrive, whilst basal nighttime BP levels measured by lowest heart rate trigger may be due to circulating volume and vascular structure (**Figure 7.17**) [10]. The former BP component of nocturnal hypertension may be suppressed by nighttime dosing of sympatholytic drugs, while the latter BP component may be suppressed by diuretics, calcium channel blocker, and/or RAS inhibitors.

IT-based trigger nighttime BP monitoring system

Finally, an IT-based nighttime BP monitoring system (ITNP) with oxygen and heart rate triggers and a 3G web system has been developed with our colleagues at Omron Healthcare Co., Ltd. (Toshikazu Shiga, Takahide Tanaka, Mitsuo Kuwabara, Osamu Shirasaki, Yutaka Kobayashi). The ITNP system is a cloud-computing-based composite management and analysis system for data sent from the BP device in the patient's home. The most important benefit of this system is to detect the day-by-day variabilities in nighttime BP as well as

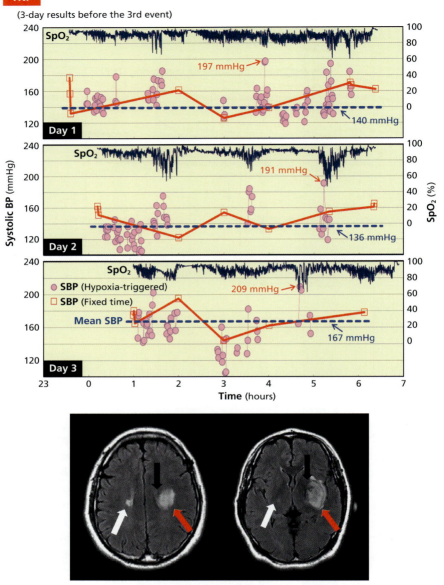

Figure 7.18 36-year-old hypertensive man developed three haemorrhagic strokes. Upper figure: Closed circles represent SBP measured by an oxygen-triggered function; Open boxes represent SBPs measured by the fixed-point function. The hypoxia-related nighttime SBP surges were observed on all three days. Lower figure: Brain MRI at the time of the 3ed event. All the 3 events occurred during sleep. Red arrows represent the sites of acute left putaminal haemorrhage. Black arrows represent the sites of an earlier left putaminal haemorrhage. White arrows represent an old lacunar infarction. SBP, systolic blood pressure; SpO_2, oxygen saturation monitored by pulse oximetry. Reprinted from *J Am Soc Hypertens.*, vol. 10, Yoshida T, Kuwabara M, Hoshide S, Kario K., Recurrence of stroke caused by nocturnal hypoxia-induced blood pressure surge in a young adult male with severe obstructive sleep apnea syndrome., p201-4, Copyright (2016), with permission from Elsevier. Ref. [150]

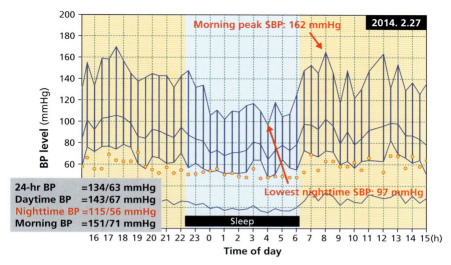

Figure 7.19 Exaggerated morning blood pressure surge detected by ambulatory blood pressure monitoring in a 76-year-old woman with obstructive sleep apnoea syndrome. Nighttime blood pressure was <120/70 mmHg. BP, blood pressure; SBP, systolic BP. *Source:* Kario et al. 2015 [145]

morning BP, and nighttime BP surges associated with sleep apnoea episodes, the degree of which can be affected by daily environmental changes. Using this ITNP, the prospective study of Sleep Pressure and disordered breathing in REsistant hypertension And cardiovascular Disease (SPREAD) has been started. It is a registry to evaluate the clinical implications of nighttime BP and nighttime BP surges in high-risk patients with resistant hypertension and/or cardiovascular disease.

In the SPREAD study, ITNP detected the exaggerated nighttime BP surges triggered by sleep apnoea-related hypoxia in a 36-year-old man. The patient developed the sleep-onset of ischaemic and haemorrhagic stroke three times (**Figure 7.18**) [150]. In a 74-year-old woman with OSAS, even when the average of nighttime BP levels measured by ABPM with fixed 30-minute intervals was <120/70 mmHg (**Figure 7.19**) [145], ITNP detected repetitive exaggerated nighttime BP surges (**Figure 7.20**) [145].

The assessment of SAS was repeated using ITNP in a real-life setting and increased the sensitivity of the diagnosis of SAS and related nighttime BP surge. Using polysomnography in alcohol-prohibited conditions in hospitals may underestimate the severity of SAS and may miss diagnosing patients with moderate SAS. The SPREAD study participants with mild-to-moderate SAS exhibited significant night-by-night variability of the degree of apnoea/hypopnoea episodes.

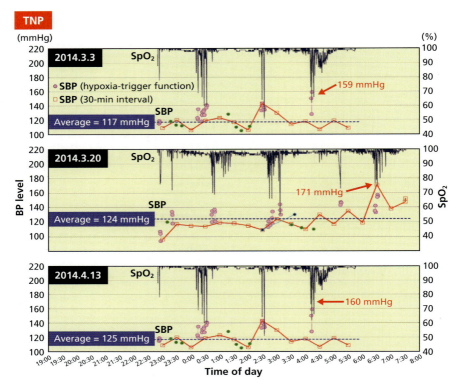

Figure 7.20 Nighttime BP surge detected by trigger nighttime BP monitoring (TNP). BP, blood pressure; SBP, systolic BP. *Source:* Kario et al. 2015 [145]

These patients exhibited apnoea/hypopnoea more frequently, and nighttime BP and surge increased on the day of alcohol intake (**Figure 7.21**).

ITNP will help to detect high-risk SAS patients with nocturnal hypertension and/or nighttime BP surge, and assess the quality of BP control during continuous positive airway pressure (CPAP) and/or antihypertensive treatment (**Figure 7.22**) [10]. Strict BP control throughout a 24-hour period, including nighttime BP and hypoxia-induced peak, could effectively suppress the development of organ damage and cardiovascular events in OSAS patients. The ITNP system would contribute to achieving this goal.

CPAP adherence and nighttime BP surge

CPAP treatment almost eliminates nighttime BP surge in patients with OSAS (**Figure 7.23**) [147, 151]. However, cardiovascular protection and the BP-low-

Development of nighttime home BP monitoring

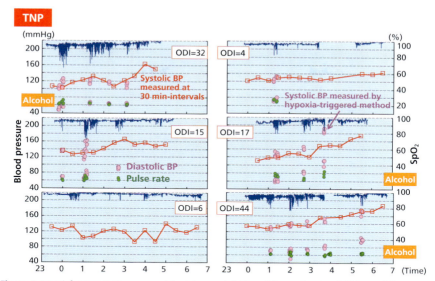

Figure 7.21 Nighttime BPs measured by trigger nighttime BP monitoring (TNP) on different days in a patient registered in the SPREAD registry. ODI, oxygen desaturation index. *Source:* Kario. 2015 [10]

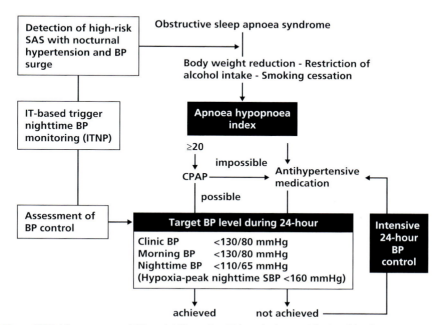

Figure 7.22 Management of BP variability using IT-based trigger nighttime blood pressure monitoring (ITNP) in sleep apnoea. BP, blood pressure; CPAP, continuous positive airway pressure; SAS, sleep apnoea syndrome; SBP, systolic BP. *Source:* Kario. 2015 [10]

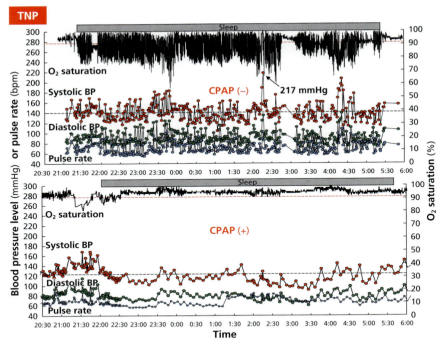

Figure 7.23 Effect of continuous positive airway pressure (CPAP), on nighttime BP measured by trigger nighttime BP monitoring (TNP). in a hypertensive patient with sleep apnoea syndrome. *Source:* Kario. 2009 [147]

ering effect of CPAP are not perfect, and OSAS patients may still develop cardiovascular events [152, 153]. The 2017 AHA/ACC guidelines state that the effectiveness of CPAP to reduce BP in adults with hypertension and OSAS is not well established, and recommended CPAP only as having Class IIb evidence [1]. It is possible that good adherence to CPAP therapy may be the key for this treatment approach to be effective.

The ITNP could evaluate the adherence and efficacy of CPAP on a day-by-day basis. Even in SAS patients receiving CPAP every night, the CPAP mask may be off the face (**Figure 7.24**), and the pressure of CPAP may be insufficient in the presence of other conditions such as upper tract infection and allergic rhinitis (**Figures 7.24** and **7.25**). Effective CPAP can reduce mean nighttime SBP by 8 mmHg (**Figure 7.26**), and by up to 42 mmHg when evaluated by hypoxia peak nighttime SBP (**Figure 7.27**). These results suggest that ITNP could be a useful tool for assessing the therapeutic efficacy of CPAP therapy.

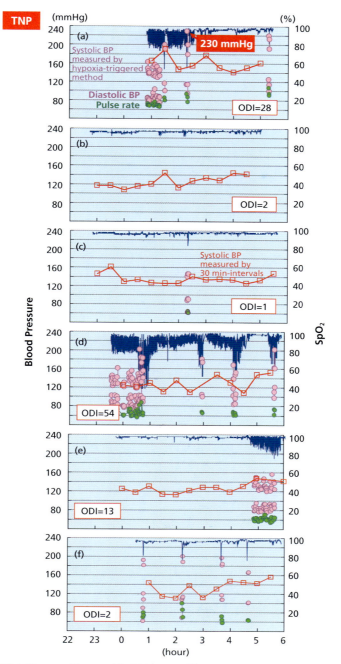

Figure 7.24 A 58-year-old man with OSAS treated by continuous positive airway pressure (CPAP), who developed cardiopulmonary arrest during sleep period at home. Figures (a) to (f) are BP data from six different days during IT-based trigger nighttime BP monitoring (ITNP). (a) Short sleep-triggered marked nighttime BP surge that reached 230 mmHg. After rising with this episode, he initiated CPAP. (b), (c) Well treated with CPAP. (d) The CPAP mask was not worn for the total duration of the sleep period. Marked nighttime BP surges were detected with severe hypoxic clusters. (e) CPAP mask was no longer in place 1.5 hours before rising in the morning. (f) Spike hypoxic episodes triggered marked nighttime BP surges even when well treated with CPAP. This is the day the patient developed severe rhinorrhoea. ODI, oxygen desaturation index. *Source:* Kario. 2015 [10]

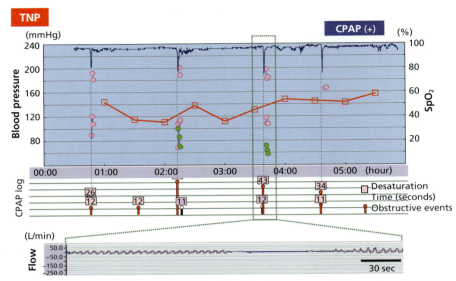

Figure 7.25 A 58-year-old man who developed cardiopulmonary arrest during sleep at home. On the day of Figure 7.24 (f), continuous positive airway pressure (CPAP) log data were measured concurrently with triggered BP monitoring. In harmony with nighttime BP surges during desaturation episodes, the flags of obstructive apnoea events and decreased nasal air flow are clearly observed in CPAP log data. *Source:* Kario. 2015 [10]

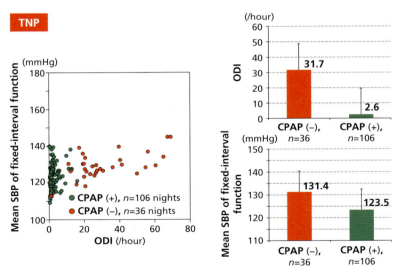

Figure 7.26 Mean nighttime BP measured by trigger nighttime BP monitoring (TNP) in a patient registered in the SPREAD registry. BP, blood pressure; CPAP, continuous positive airway pressure; ODI, oxygen desaturation index; SBP, systolic BP. *Source:* Kario. 2015 [10]

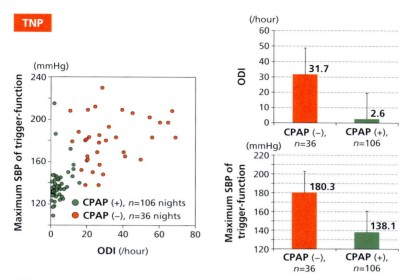

Figure 7.27 Hypoxia-peak nighttime BP measured by trigger nighttime BP monitoring (TNP) in a patient registered in the SPREAD registry. CPAP, continuous positive airway pressure; ODI, oxygen desaturation index. *Source:* Kario. 2015 [10]

Antihypertensive medication on nighttime BP surge

Only a small dose of doxazosin reduced nighttime BP surge and basal nighttime BP in patients with OSAS, while the cluster of hypoxic episodes was similar at baseline and during treatment (**Figure 7.28**) [147], indicating that OSAS-induced nocturnal hypertension and nighttime BP surge at least partly attribute to sympathetic overdrive caused by nocturnal hypoxia. In a recent study of TNP, bedtime dosing of nifedipine and carvedilol, significantly reduced all nighttime BP measures (**Figure 7.29**) [148], while the nighttime BP-lowering property was different between the two drugs. Carvedilol reduced peak nighttime BP to a similar extent as nifedipine, but had less effect in reducing basal BP, resulting in significant suppression of hypoxia-induced nighttime BP surge (**Figure 7.30**) [148]. Even in a SAS patient with well-controlled mean nighttime SBP, 55% of hypoxia-triggered peak nighttime SBP values were above 140 mmHg (**Figure 7.31**) [148]; bedtime dosing of nifedipine reduced both mean and hypoxia-peak SBP.

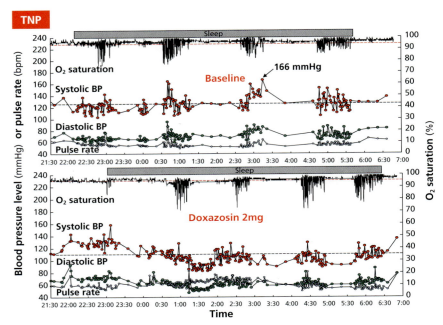

Figure 7.28 Effect of evening dose of doxazosin on nighttime BP measured by trigger nighttime BP monitoring (TNP) in a hypertensive patient. *Source:* Kario. 2009 [147]

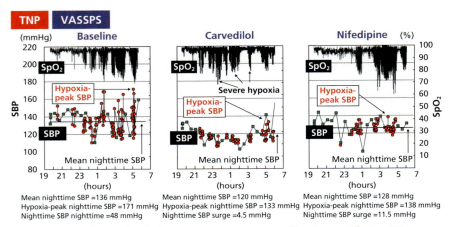

Figure 7.29 Typical case of nighttime BP parameters measured by tirgger nighttime BP monitoring (TNP) at baseline and carvedilol or nifedipine-administered nights. The red circles indicate SBPs measured by an oxygen-triggered function, and green boxes indicate SBPs measured by the fixed-interval (30 minutes) function. VASSPS (Effects of Vasodilating vs Sympatholytic Antihypertensives on Sleep Blood Pressure in Hypertensive Patients with Sleep Apnea Syndrome) study. BP, blood pressure; SBP, systolic BP. *Source:* Kario et al. 2014 [148]

Development of nighttime home BP monitoring

VASSPS

	Baseline	Carvedilol	Nifedipine
Morning SBP	150.8	137.4**	118.2***†††
Morning heart rate	61.8	57.0**	64.7†††
Nighttime SBP	137.3	121.8***	112.8***†
Nighttime heart rate	59.8	57.2*	62.4†††
Nighttime heart rate	164.7	143.0**	138.0**
Minimum nighttime SBP	113.6	99.6***	88.6***††
Nighttime SBP surge (mmHg)	30.8	18.6*	22.1

Figure 7.30 Morning and nighttime BPs at baseline and carvedilol or nifedipine-administered days. Data are shown as mean (mmHg). *$p<0.05$, **$p<0.01$, ***$p<0.001$ versus baseline, by paired t-test; †$p<0.05$, ††$p<0.01$, †††$p<0.001$ versus carvedilol-added phase, by paired t-test; SBP, systolic blood pressure. *Source:* Kario et al. 2014 [148]

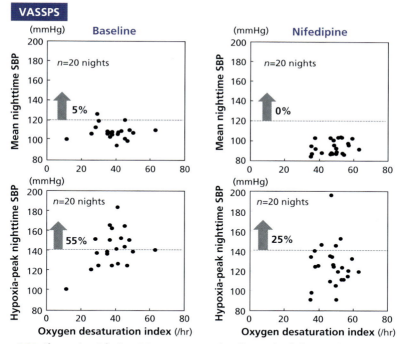

Figure 7.31 Change in nighttime BP parameters at baseline and nifedipine-administered nights in a hypertensive patient with sleep apnoea. SBP, systolic blood pressure. *Source:* Kario et al. 2014 [148]

Studies described in Chapter 7 were partly supported by JSPS KAKENHI, Grant-in-Aid for Scientific Research B (Grant Number JP26293192) from Japan Society for the Promotion of Science.

CHAPTER 8

Development of wearable beat-by-beat (surge) BP monitoring

There are marked individual differences in the short-term dynamic blood pressure (BP) change caused by various triggers (**Figure 8.1**) [154]. Wearable non-invasive beat-by-beat BP monitoring has been the dream of doctors who manage hypertension. Omron Healthcare Co., Ltd. recently publicised the prototype of a wearable surge BP monitoring (WSP) that uses recent advances in automatically-controlled technology and measures absolute values of the maximum peaks of beat-by-beat pressure (**Figure 8.2**) [4]. The first prototype (WSP-1) has two tonometry sensor plates and the angle of the arrayed sensor plate to cover the radial artery is automatically adjusted in order to obtain effective applanation. This device is being tested and improved in collaboration with Omron, with the goal of developing more accurate beat-by-beat WSP (**Figure 8.2**) [4].

Using the WSP device, continuous beat-by-beat BP during sleep was monitored simultaneously with polysomnography (**Figure 8.3**) [139]. The nighttime BP level and variability were significantly lower in the stage 2 and stage 3 sleep, but were higher in stage 1 sleep as well as in REM (rapid-eye-movement) sleep and during waking hours (**Figure 8.4**) [139]. Three nighttime BP surges were

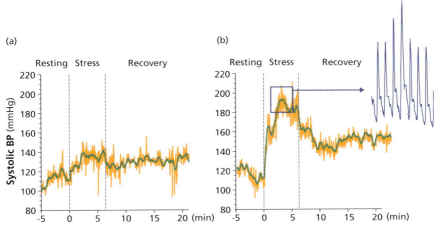

Figure 8.1 A typical hyperreactive case triggered psychological stress (anger recall) (a) normal control. (b) hyperreactive case. BP, blood pressure. *Source:* Kario et al. 2002 [154]

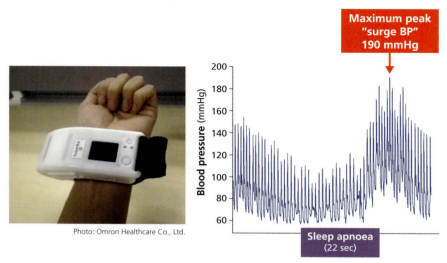

Figure 8.2 Beat-by-beat tonometry-type wearable surge BP monitoring-1 (WSP-1) device and nighttime surge triggered by sleep apnoea. Nighttime BP surges detected by WSP-1 in a hypertensive patient with sleep apnoea. BP, blood pressure. *Source:* Kario. 2016 [4]

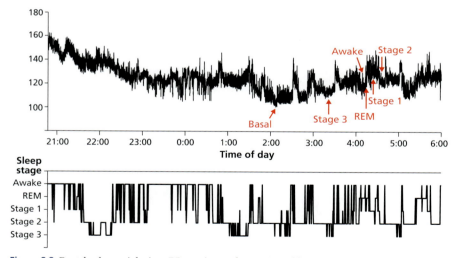

Figure 8.3 Beat-by-beat nighttime BP continuously monitored by the newly developed tonometry-type wearable surge BP monitoring-1 (WSP-1) in different sleep stages defined by the simultaneous polysomnography. Data were obtained from a 43-year-old healthy woman. REM, rapid-eye movement. *Source:* Kario. 2018 [139]. Reprinted from *Encyclopedia of Cardiovascular Research and Medicine*, 1st edition, Kario K., Sleep and circadian cardiovascular medicine, pp.424-437, Copyright (2018), with permission from Elsevier.

Development of wearable beat-by-beat (surge) BP monitoring

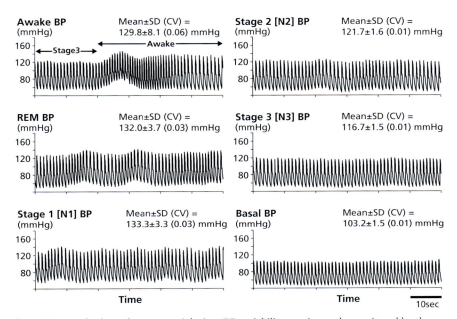

Figure 8.4 Beat-by-beat short-term nighttime BP variability continuously monitored by the newly developed tonometry-type wearable surge BP monitoring-1 (WSP-1) in different sleep stages shown in Figure 8.3. The BP surges during awake or REM sleep are more pronounced than those during slow wave sleep (N3). The basal BP, the lowest BP, is usually found during N3 sleep. REM, rapid-eye movement. *Source:* Kario. 2018 [139]. Reprinted from *Encyclopedia of Cardiovascular Research and Medicine*, 1st edition, Kario K., Sleep and circadian cardiovascular medicine, pp.424-437, Copyright (2018), with permission from Elsevier.

detected, associated with REM sleep, arousal (unconscious microarousal) (**Figure 8.5 upper Fig.**), and a sleep apnoea episode (**Figure 8.5 lower Fig.**) [139].

The peak of sleep apnoea-triggered nighttime BP surge was successfully detected by analysing data from a newly developed tonometry-type WSP-1 device together with data obtained from a hypoxia-triggered nighttime BP monitoring. The peak systolic BP (SBP) surge was detected by the beat-by-beat WSP-1 was 242 mmHg and was higher than the hypoxia-triggered BP surge detected by trigger nighttime BP monitoring (TNP) using the oscillometric method (208 mmHg) (**Figure 8.6**) [139]. In a 50-year-old normotensive woman with obstructive sleep apnoea (OSA), WSP-2 (equipped with a calibration function based on BP values obtained using the oscillometric method) detected the highest peak of nighttime BP surge one day before (Day 1: baseline) and on the day of nighttime dosing of carvedilol 20 mg (Day 2: carvedilol-added). Carvedilol was associated with a reduction in the Surge Index (frequency of surge per hour) from

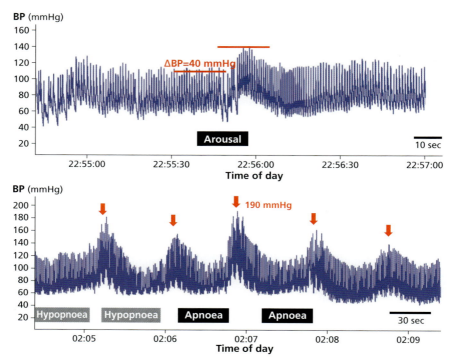

Figure 8.5 Nighttime BP surges triggered by arousal (upper panel: data from a 36-year-old healthy man) and apnoea/hypopnoeas (lower panel: data from a 50-year-old man with severe obstructive sleep apnoea). Beat-by-beat nighttime BP was continuously monitored by the newly developed tonometry-type wearable surge BP monitoring-1 (WSP-1).
Reprinted from *Encyclopedia of Cardiovascular Research and Medicine*, 1st edition, Kario K., Sleep and circadian cardiovascular medicine, pp.424-437, Copyright (2018), with permission from Elsevier. Ref. [139]

17.2/hour to 7.4/hour. The peak of surge was also decreased from 178 mmHg to 133 mmHg by the oscillometric method (**Figure 8.7 upper Fig.**), and from 184 mmHg to 137 mmHg by the continuous beat-by-beat method (**Figure 8.7 lower Fig.**) [139]. There are limitations of WSP-1, because the weaknesses of a tonometry BP monitoring device are that (1) the sensor must be strictly positioned to cover the artery, and (2) artifacts caused by movement of the wrist, which disturb effective applanation, are frequent.

Teams at Omron Healthcare Co., Ltd. (Mitsuo Kuwabara, Noboru Shinomiya, Shingo Yamashita, Toshikazu Shiga, Takahide Tanaka), Jichi Medical University, (Kazuomi Kario, Naoko Tomitani, Satoshi Hoshide, Tomoyuki Kabutoya, Yuri Matsumoto) and Kyusyu University are now collaborating on research and

Development of wearable beat-by-beat (surge) BP monitoring

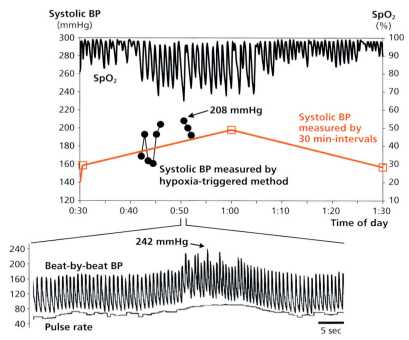

Figure 8.6 The peak of sleep apnoea-triggered nighttime BP surge detected by the newly developed tonometry-type wearable surge BP monitoring-1 device. Data were obtained from a 53-year-old man with obstructive sleep apnoea. *Source:* Kario. 2018 [139]. Reprinted from *Encyclopedia of Cardiovascular Research and Medicine*, 1st edition, Kario K., Sleep and circadian cardiovascular medicine, pp.424-437, Copyright (2018), with permission from Elsevier. Ref. [139]

development of new BP monitoring systems utilising haemodynamic indices, such as "Surge Index" and "baroreflex index (BRI)" (**Figure 8.8**) [155].

> Studies described in this chapter was partly supported by Japan Agency for Medical Research and Development (AMED) under Grant Number JP17he1102002h0003.

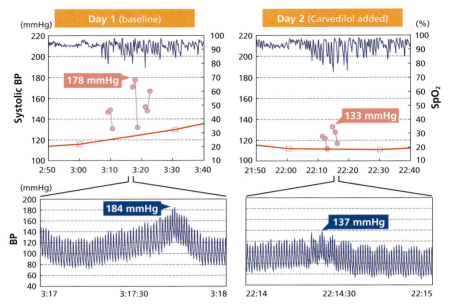

Figure 8.7 Nighttime surges in BP monitoring at the time of apnoea episode in a 50-year-old normotensive woman with obstructive sleep apnoea syndrome (upper: BPs detected by trigger nighttime BP monitoring [TNP]; closed circles represent SBP measured by an oxygen-triggered function, lower: BPs monitored by wearable surge BP monitoring [WSP]-2). BP, blood pressure. *Source:* Kario K. *Essential Manual on Perfect 24-hour Blood Pressure Management from Morning to Nocturnal Hypertension: Up-to-date for Anticipation Medicine.* Wiley, 2018.

Figure 8.8 Innovation of BP monitoring device and new haemodynamic indices. BP, blood pressure; CV, cardiovascular. *Source:* Kario K. *Essential Manual on Perfect 24-hour Blood Pressure Management from Morning to Nocturnal Hypertension: Up-to-date for Anticipation Medicine.* Wiley, 2018.

CHAPTER 9

BP surge

BP variability with different time phase

There are various types of blood pressure (BP) variability with different time phases, from short-term to long-term [104, 156]. These include beat-by-beat, orthostatic, physical- or psychological stress-induced, diurnal, day-by-day, visit-to-visit, seasonal, and yearly BP variability, and clinically these are detected by different clinic, home, and ambulatory BP monitoring (ABPM) methods (**Figure 9.1**) [104, 156].

BP variability is considered the master biomarker of human healthcare, since it is not only a modifiable risk factor of organ damage and cardiovascular disease but also a sensor of cardiovascular dysregulation that is affected by individual characteristics and stressors of daily psychobehavioural factors and environmental conditions, as well as medication status [157-161]. Almost all of the BP variability phenotypes are partly correlated with each other and are reported to be cardiovascular risk factors [42, 162-164].

The components of BP variability may have different clinical impacts on cardiovascular disease. A long-term increase in the average of BP values would be considered a chronic risk factor for advancing endothelial dysfunction and subsequent atherosclerosis, whereas relatively short-term exaggerated BP variability (e.g. the BP surge) would be considered an acute risk factor which triggers an atherothrombotic cardiovascular disease event by a mechanical stress-induced plaque rupture.

These different roles of the risks presented by BP variability are similar to the risks of heart failure: chronically advancing left ventricular hypertrophy, and the triggering of acute heart failure by afterload mismatch due to an abrupt increase in systolic BP.

The resonance hypothesis of BP surge

We are now proposing the 'resonance hypothesis' of BP surge [155, 157]. On the basis of reduced baroreceptor sensitivity and small-artery remodelling associated with aging, each type of BP variability has different time phase increases. The degree of increase in each type of BP variability may be different in different

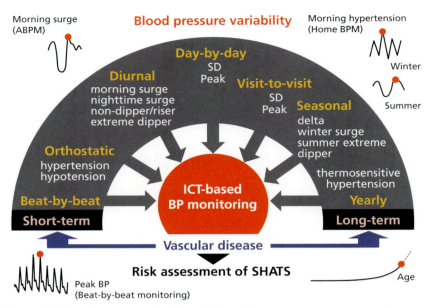

Figure 9.1 ICT-based assessment of different BP variability parameters and vascular damage in systemic haemodynamic atherothrombotic syndrome (SHATS); see Chapter 10. BP, blood pressure; ICT, information and communication technology; SD, standard deviation. *Source:* Modified from Kario. 2015 [104]

individuals. There are a number of triggers of BP surge in the real world, such as physical and mental stress, and environmental factors, especially cold temperature, diet, and sleep (**Figure 9.2**) [155]. When the timing of each type of BP surge wave is unsynchronised, the total summation of BP surge at each time is small. However, when the timing of all of the BP surge waves with different time phases is synchronised and resonance of the pulse wave occurs, this could result in the generation of a critically large dynamic BP surge that would trigger a cardiovascular disease (CVD) event (**Figure 9.2**).

For example, the morning BP surge is one of the typical surges [104] which can be potentiated synergistically by a resonance of various components of BP surges, resulting in morning-onset CVD [155]. In ABPM studies, the morning BP surge was exaggerated in the winter, especially in elderly patients (the winter morning surge in BP) [84]. On the top of basic morning BP surge, the coexistence of exposure of airborne PM2.5 [161] and smoking, with high salt and alcohol intake at the last dinner and poor sleep the previous night, may occur at the same timing in the morning in the cold winter. This cluster of triggers results

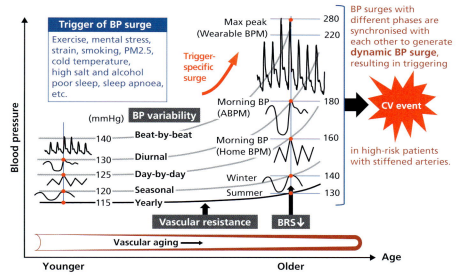

Figure 9.2 Synergistic resonance hypothesis of BP variability. ABPM, ambulatory blood pressure monitoring; BP, blood pressure; BPM, blood pressure monitoring; BRS, baroreceptor sensitivity; CV, cardiovascular. *Source:* Modified from Kario. 2016 [155]. Reprinted by permission of Oxford University Press.

in a marked dynamic morning BP surge, and could precipitate a cardiovascular event, especially in high-risk patients with vascular disease.

Evidence and mechanism of BP variability

An increase in various phenotypes of BP variability is associated with advanced organ damage, finally resulting in cardiovascular disease (**Figure 9.3**) [165]. Recent evidence that increased BP variability constitutes a risk factor for organ damage and cardiovascular events (independent of average BP) is accumulating [104, 156, 166-178] (**Figure 9.4**).

There are a number of determinants of BP variability with different time phases. Short-term BP variability is mainly determined by physiological regulation of the neural network, and disruption of short-term BP variability is determined by the impaired baroreflex caused by increased central sympathetic tonus and/or vascular stiffness. On the other hand, other factors can contribute to long-term BP variability, including patient behaviour.

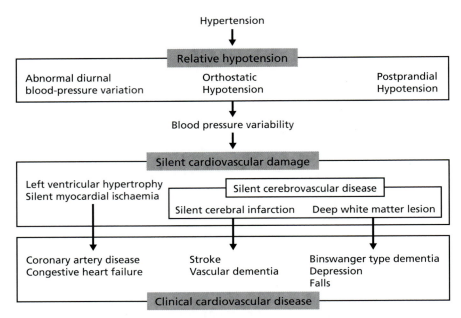

Figure 9.3 Clinical significance of BP variability in elderly people with hypertension. Reprinted from the *Lancet*, Vol. 355(9215), Kario K, Pickering TG. Blood pressure variability in elderly patients., pp. 1645-1646., Copyright (2000), with permission from Elsevier. Ref. [165]

Visit-to-visit variability in clinic BP

There is a lot of evidence on the association between visit-to-visit variability of clinic BP and organ damage and cardiovascular events.

Rothwell et al. demonstrated the prognostic importance of visit-to-visit variability of clinic BP and maximum systolic BP (SBP) for stroke and coronary events in the ASCOT-BPLA database (**Figure 9.5**) [168]. We have previously shown that delta SBP (peak minus the lowest reading of clinic BP over 12 months, a measure of visit-to-visit variability of clinic BP readings) was significantly correlated with measures of vascular disease (intima-media thickness [IMT] and stiffness of the common carotid artery) in elderly patients at high risk of cardiovascular disease (mean age 80 years; $n=201$) (**Figure 9.6**) [179]. Insomnia augments the impact of vascular disease on an increase in delta SBP (**Figure 9.7**) [180]. In addition, delta SBP was a significant determinant of cognitive dysfunction (Mini Mental State Examination [MMSE] <24 points), independent of the average of clinic BP readings over a 12-month period (**Figure 9.8** [170]). The impact of increased delta SBP on cognitive impairment was augmented by the presence of advanced vascular disease (**Figure 9.9**) [175].

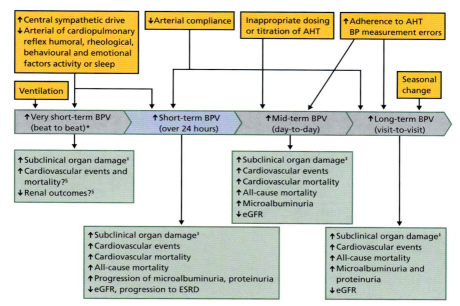

Figure 9.4 Various types of BP variability, their determinants, and prognostic relevance for cardiovascular and renal outcomes. *Assessed in laboratory conditions; ‡cardiac, vascular, and renal subclinical organ damage; §BPV on a beat-to-beat basis has not been routinely measured in population studies. AHT, antihypertensive treatment; BP, blood pressure; BPV, blood pressure variability; ESRD, end-stage renal disease; eGFR, estimated glomerular filtration rate. Reprinted by permission from Macmillan Publishers Ltd: *Nat Rev Cardiol* (vol.10, pp.143-155), copyright (2013). Ref. [156]

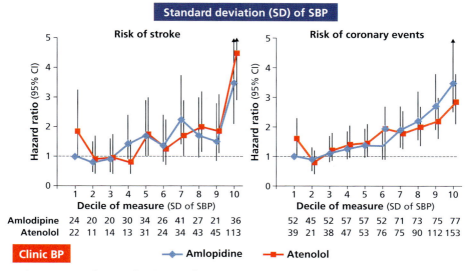

Figure 9.5 Distribution of patients in the two treatment groups in ASCOT-BPLA according to deciles of mean standard deviation of systolic blood pressure and the associations of each of the variables with risk of stroke and risk of coronary events.
Reprinted from the *Lancet*, Vol. 375 (9718), Rothwell et al., Prognostic significance of visit-to-visit variability, maximum systolic blood pressure, and episodic hypertension, pp. 895-905, Copyright (2010), with permission from Elsevier. Ref. [168]

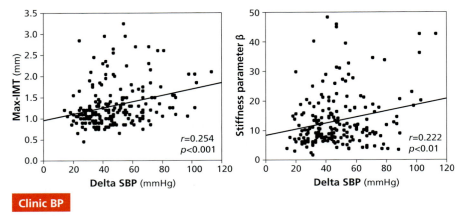

Figure 9.6 The relationship of visit-to-visit BP measures with common carotid artery intima-media thickness in elderly patients at high risk of cardiovascular disease (mean age 80 years; $n=201$). BP, blood pressure; IMT, intima-media thickness; SBP, systolic BP.
Reprinted from *J Am Soc Hypertens.*, Vol. 5, Nagai M et al., Visit-to-visit blood pressure variations: New independent determinants for carotid artery measures in the elderly at high risk of cardiovascular disease, pp.184-192. (2011), with permission from Elsevier. Ref. [179]

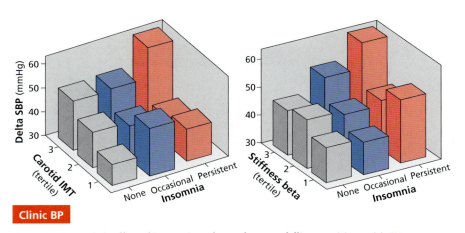

Figure 9.7 Synergistic effect of insomnia and vascular remodelling on visit-to-visit BP variability. BP, blood pressure; IMT, intima-media thickness; SBP, systolic BP. *Source:* Nagai et al. 2013 [180]. Reprinted by permission of Oxford University Press.

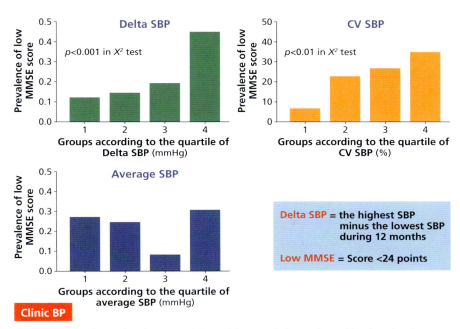

Figure 9.8 The relationships between visit-to-visit BP variation and cognitive function (mean age 80 years; $n=201$). CV, coefficient of variation; MMSE, mini mental state examination; SBP, systolic blood pressure. Created based on data from Nagai et al. 2012 [170]

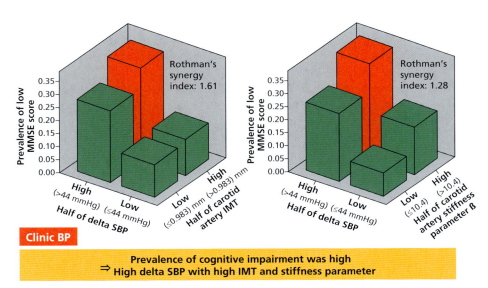

Figure 9.9 Visit-to-visit BP variability and cognitive impairment interacted by carotid artery remodelling ($n=205$). IMT, intima media thickness; MMSE, mini mental state examination; SBP, systolic blood pressure. *Source:* Nagai et al. 2014 [175].

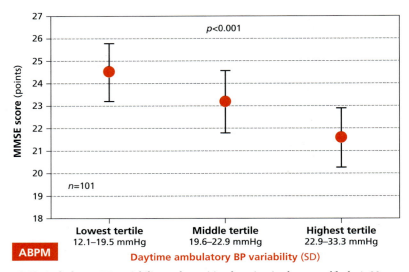

Figure 9.10 Ambulatory BP variability and cognitive function in the very elderly (>80 years; mean age 84 years). BP, blood pressure; MMSE, mini mental state examination; SD, standard deviation. Created based on data from Sakakura et al. 2007 [181]

Ambulatory BP variability

There is also significant evidence of the association between ambulatory BP variability and organ damage and cardiovascular events. An increase in ambulatory BP variability has been shown to be significantly associated with cognitive dysfunction assessed by the MMSE in the very elderly (age >80 [mean 84] years) (**Figure 9.10**) [181]. In addition, even in the 232 elderly patients (mean age 77.7 years) with well-controlled ambulatory BP, increased ambulatory BP variability (weighted standard deviation of ambulatory SBP), but not the average ambulatory BP level, was significantly associated with cognitive dysfunction (reduction of Japanese version of the Montreal Cognitive Assessment [MoCA-J] score) (**Figure 9.11**) [182].

Home BP variability

Home BP monitoring (HBPM) is the best practical method to detect the wide range of BP variability with different time phases, from relatively short-term (diurnal) to long-term (seasonal, and yearly) variability. HBPM could exclude the white-coat effect to detect pathological BP variability which is reproducible.

There are several promising measures of home BP variability, which might

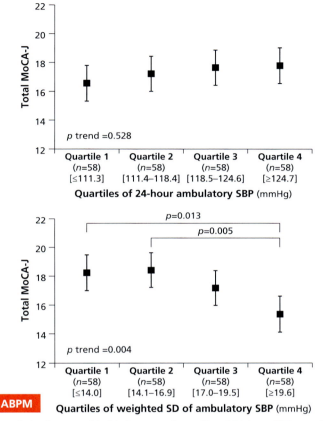

Figure 9.11 Association between MoCA-J score and quartiles of 24-hour SBP or weighted SD of SBP in the population with well-controlled BP (n=232, mean age 77.7 years, antihypertensive treatment 85%, 24 hour BP 118/68 mmHg). BP, blood pressure; SBP, systolic BP. *Source:* Cho et al. 2017 [182]. Reprinted by permission of Oxford University Press.

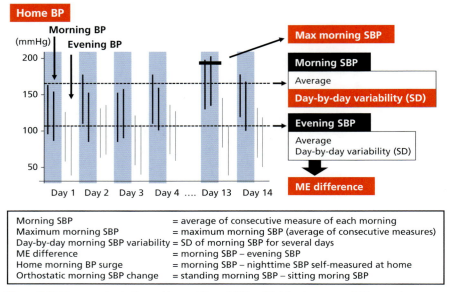

Figure 9.12 Three major indices of home BP variability. BP, blood pressure; ME, morning-evening; SBP, systolic blood pressure. *Source:* Kario. 2012 [40]. Reprinted with permission of Springer.

have clinical relevance (**Figure 9.12**) [40]. These are maximum home SBP (max home SBP) and SD of home SBP by the conventional home BP measurement. Morning–evening difference (ME-dif) is also one of the important measures of home BP variability as described above.

Maximum home SBP

Maximum home SBP was significantly associated with increases in left ventricular mass index (LVMI) and carotid IMT evaluated by echocardiography, and microalbuminuria, independent of BP level in unmedicated hypertensive patients (**Figure 9.13**) [183]. In this study, even in well-controlled hypertensive patients with home BP <135/85 mmHg, the maximum home SBP was significantly correlated with LVMI and carotid IMT. Maximum home SBP was found in the morning BP readings in 67% of all samples.

An increase in maximum morning SBP and/or increased SD of morning SBP readings would reflect the instability of morning BP surge (MBPS). In addition to the reproducible exaggerated morning surge (**Figure 9.14, Patient B**), the exaggerated MBPS with poor reproducibility increases cardiovascular risk (**Figure 9.14, Patient C**) [18]. Given that the degree of MBPS in high-reactive patients

Home BP

Max SBP for 14 days was derived from morning SBP in 240 patients (67%)	Total population (n=356)		Subgroup Analysis			
			Mean home BP <135/85 mmHg (n=135)		Mean home BP ≥135/85 mmHg (n=221)	
Variable	β (SE)	p	β (SE)	p	β (SE)	p
Dependent variable: LVMI* (g/m²)						
Maximum home SBP (mmHg)	0.598 (0.094) Model R^2=0.32	<0.001	0.512 (0.188) Model R^2=0.21	0.007	0.655 (0.145) Model R^2=0.24	<0.001
Dependent variable: Carotid IMT† (mm)						
Maximum home SBP (mmHg)	0.003 (<0.001) Model R^2=0.27	<0.001	0.003 (0.001) Model R^2=0.26	0.006	0.003 (0.001) Model R^2=0.24	<0.001
Dependent variable: UACR‡ (mg/gCr)						
Maximum home SBP (mmHg)	0.004 (0.002) Model R^2=0.20	0.02	0.001 (0.003) Model R^2=0.15	0.68	0.003 (0.002) Model R^2=0.17	0.18

*This model was adjusted by age, sex, habitual drinking, and mean clinic SBP.
†This model was adjusted by age, sex, hypertension duration, smoking, diabetes mellitus, and mean clinic SBP.
‡This model was adjusted by age, sex, diabetes mellitus, and mean clinic SBP.

Figure 9.13 Multivariate regression analyses between maximum home SBP and organ damage in 356 never-treated hypertensive patients. *Source:* Matsui et al. 2011 [183]

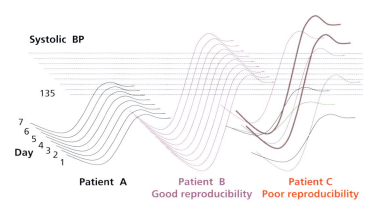

Figure 9.14 Poor reproducibility does not directly imply that morning BP surge is a less important cardiovascular risk. *Source:* Kario. 2010 [18].

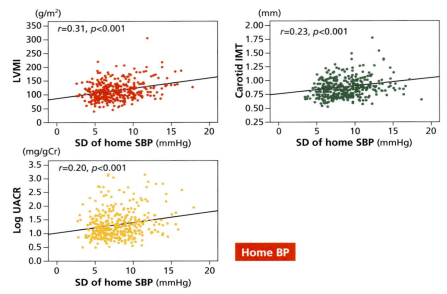

Figure 9.15 Day-by-day variability of home BP and organ damage in never treated hypertensive patients. IMT, intima-media thickness; LVMI, left ventricular mass index; SBP, systolic blood pressure; SD, standard deviation; UACR, urinary albumin/creatinine ratio. *Source:* Matsui et al. [183].

is highly dependent on morning physical activity [18, 37], high-reactive patients would exhibit poorly reproducible exaggerated MBPS with increased day-to-day variability of morning BP (**Figure 9.14, Patient C**). Exaggerated MBPS reactivity may pose the greatest risk, when physical activity is maximised. Thus, the unstable morning BP surge with increased day-by-day variability may be associated with worse phenotypes (**Figure 9.14**) [18].

Standard deviation of morning home BP

The increase in SD of home BP readings is associated with organ damage. In a study of unmedicated hypertensive patients, the SD of home BP level readings measured three times at a single time point in the morning and evening for 14 days was associated with urinary albumin/creatinine ratio (UACR), LVMI, and carotid IMT (**Figure 9.15**) [183]. The Ohasama study on a community-dwelling population also demonstrated that an increase in the SD of home BP self-measured in the morning was an independent risk for cardiovascular mortality (**Figure 9.16**) [166]. In addition, in the recent population-based prospective Finn-Home study, the variability of home BP, defined as the SD values of ME difference, day-by-day, and first minus second measurements, was associated

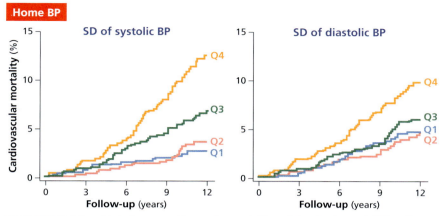

Figure 9.16 Relationship between cardiovascular mortality and day-by-day variability of home BP: the Ohasama study (n=2,455, median follow-up 11.9 years). BP, blood pressure. Q1 to Q4 indicate ascending quartiles; cutoff points were 6.5, 8.2, and 10.3 mmHg for systolic and 4.9, 6.1, and 7.6 mmHg for diastolic. BP, blood pressure. *Source:* Kikuya et al. 2008 [166]

with future cardiovascular events independent of BP [184]. The association with cardiovascular risk was stronger for BP variability of morning SBP than that for evening SBP. Thus, the BP variability assessed by self-measured home BP has clinical relevance independently of average home BP levels.

In the J-HOP study (n=4,231), the impact of three different measures of home BP variability was evaluated (**Figure 9.17**). The incidence of cardiovascular events was significantly higher across quartiles of all measures of home BP variability (**Figure 9.18**) [185].

Morning-evening difference (ME-dif)

In both medicated and non-medicated hypertensive patients, the ME difference of self-measured home BP was associated with LVMI and the risk of concentric hypertrophy, as well as with increased pulse wave velocity (PWV) [186-188]. ME-dif has been significantly associated with left ventricular hypertrophy (LVH), and increased brachial-ankle PWV (baPWV) (**Figure 9.19**) [186], and morning hypertension defined by the ME-dif and the average of morning and evening BP readings (ME-ave) was shown to be a determinant of concentric LVH (**Figure 9.20**) [187]. Even among patients with normal home BP (white-coat hypertensives), patients with ME-dif ≥15 mmHg had a higher percentage of concentric remodelling than those with ME-dif <15 mmHg (32.5% vs 14.7%, p=0.017). Recently, ME-dif assessed either by ABPM or by HBPM was reported to be associated with cardiovascular risk independently of the ME-ave [16, 184]. The ME-dif

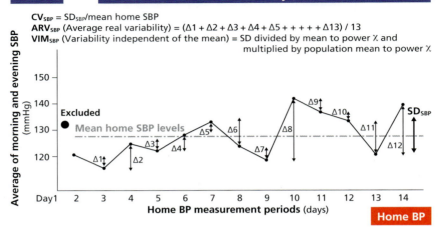

Figure 9.17 SD_{SBP}, CV_{SBP}, and ARV_{SBP} over home BP readings. An example of one patient's home BP readings over 14 days is given. The absolute differences of home systolic BP (SBP) (average of morning and evening SBP) between successive SBP measurements are shown as Δ1 to Δ13. For example, Δ1 represents the absolute difference in SBP between Day 2 and Day 3 SBPs. ARV_{SBP} is calculated as (Δ1 + Δ2 + Δ3 + Δ4 + Δ5 + Δ6 + Δ7 + Δ8 + Δ9 + Δ10 + Δ11 + Δ12 + Δ13)/13. Mean home SBP and SD_{SBP} over the readings was calculated from 13 SBP measurements (Day 2–Day 14 SBPs) for each individual, and CV_{SBP} was calculated as SD_{SBP}/mean home SBP over visits. VIM was calculated as the SD divided by the mean to the power χ and multiplied by the population mean to the power χ. The power χ was obtained by fitting a curve through a plot of SD against mean values using the model SD = a times mean^χ, where χ was derived by a nonlinear regression analysis as implemented in the SAS PROC NLIN procedure. *Source:* Kario K. *Essential Manual on Perfect 24-hour Blood Pressure Management from Morning to Nocturnal Hypertension: Up-to-date for Anticipation Medicine.* Wiley, 2018.

of ABPM is an independent predictor of future stroke events in elderly hypertensive patients [16].

Evening BP measurement in addition to morning measurement is recommended, especially for diabetic hypertensive patients, because the reduction of evening BP as well as morning BP is closely correlated with the reduction of UACR [189].

Morning orthostatic hypertension

In a previous study on the association with orthostatic BP change in disrupted circadian rhythm, a very unique phenomenon was found of not transient, but persistent, orthostatic BP increase in extreme dippers (**Figure 9.21**) [162]. This orthostatic hypertension was also associated with MBPS evaluated by ABPM

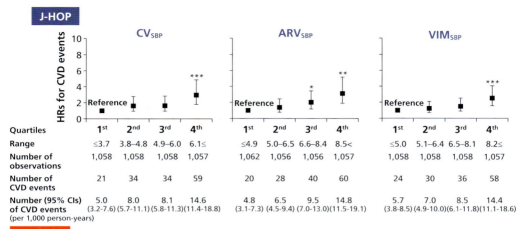

Figure 9.18 Incident CVD risk by quartiles of home BP variability measurements ($n=4{,}231$, 65 years). Bars represent adjusted HR (95% CIs) of incident CVD risk by quartiles of CV_{SBP}, ARV_{SBP}, and VIM_{SBP}. $*p<0.05$, $**p<0.01$, $***p<0.001$ vs. reference group. ARV, average real variability; CVD, cardiovascular disease; VIM, BP variability independent of the mean. Among 4,231 participants (mean±SD age 64.9±10.9 years; 53.3% women) 79.1% taking antihypertensive medication. *Source:* Hoshide et al. 2018 [185]

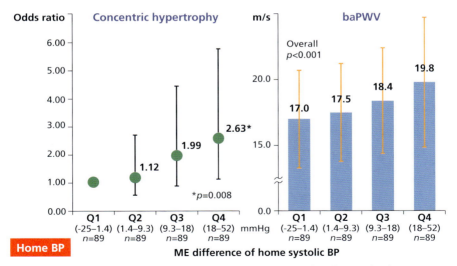

Figure 9.19 Morning–evening difference (ME-dif) of home BP and cardiovascular disease in unmedicated hypertensive patients ($n=356$). baPWV, brachial-ankle pulse wave velocity. *Source:* Matsui et al. 2009 [186]

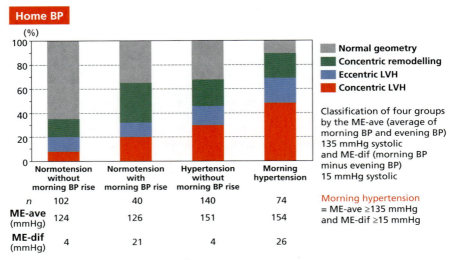

Figure 9.20 Morning hypertension and left ventricular hypertrophy in unmedicated hypertensive patients (n=356). LVH, left ventricular hypertrophy. *Source:* Matsui et al. 2010 [187]

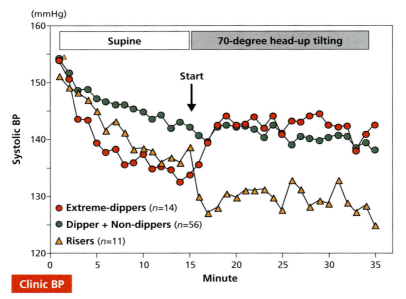

Figure 9.21 Persistent orthostatic hypertension evaluated by head-up tilting test. Persistent orthostatic systolic hypertension was detected in subjects with an extreme dipping pattern of nighttime BP by the head-up tilting test (70 degree). *Source:* Kario et al. 1998 [162]

BP surge

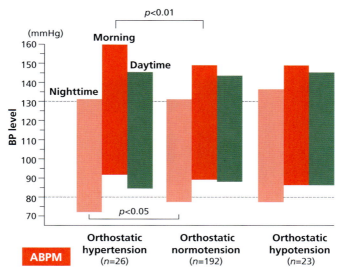

Figure 9.22 Orthostatic hypertension and 24-hour ambulatory BP profile in elderly hypertensive patients. Created based on data from Kario et al. 2002 [163]

(**Figure 9.22**) [163]. Orthostatic hypertension, as well as orthostatic hypotension, is one of the phenotypes of positional BP variability, which is known as a new risk factor for cardiovascular disease. Three phenotypes of BP variability – the morning BP surge, nighttime BP dipping, and orthostatic BP change – are partly associated with each other. Exaggerated morning surge, extreme-dipper, and orthostatic hypertension are associated with each other as hyperreactive BP variability, while blunted or inverse morning surge, riser, and orthostatic hypotension are associated with each other as disrupted BP variability (**Figure 9.23**) [104].

Home BP self-measured conventionally in the morning in a sitting position may underestimate the risk of ambulatory MBPS, which is augmented by standing and morning physical activity. Orthostatic stress may also clarify the reactive BP profile and **Figure 9.24** shows the different diagnostic methods to detect orthostatic hypertension [42]. The head-up tilting test is the standard test to assess the orthostatic BP change; however, the simple home active standing test (HAST) using HBPM (two measures on the active standing after two measures in the sitting position) is clinically useful to exclude the white-coat effect and to identify the reproducible and pathological "home orthostatic hypertension/hypotension" (**Figure 9.25**) [190].

By the HAST, orthostatic hypertension is defined by the orthostatic BP

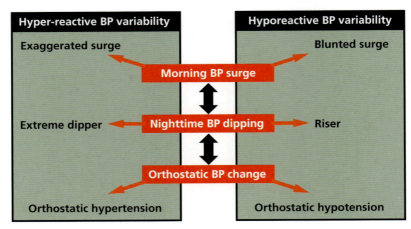

Figure 9.23 U-curve associations among both pathological extremes of differences in blood pressure variability. *Source:* Kario. 2015 [104]

Tests	Method of orthostatic stress	BP measurements	Diagnostic threshold of orthostatic hypertension (orthostatic increase in systolic BP)
Head-up tilting	Supine for 5 minutes or more followed by passive tilting with 60–70° tilt angle for 20 minutes or more	every 1 minute	• 20 mmHg (definitive) • 10 mmHg (probable)
Active standing			
Clinic	Supine for 5 minutes or more followed by active standing for 3 minutes	At least 3 times (one before standing, two during 3-minutes standing)	• 20 mmHg (definitive) • 10 mmHg (probable) • 5 mmHg for predicting masked hypertension and future hypertension
Home	Sitting for 5 minutes or more followed by active standing for 3 minutes	At least 3 times (one before standing, two during 3-minute standing)	• 10 mmHg

Figure 9.24 Recommendation of diagnostic method and definition of orthostatic hypertension. *Source:* Kario. 2013 [42]

BP surge

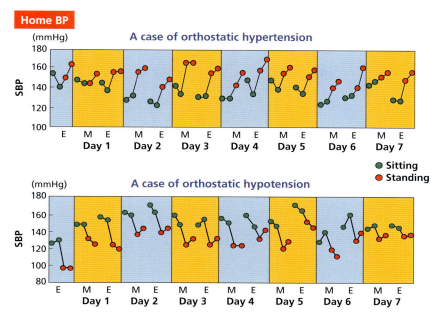

Figure 9.25 Reproducible orthostatic hypertension and hypotension detected by home BP monitoring. E, evening; M, morning. *Source:* Kario. 2009 [190]

increase (SBP measured by HBPM in standing position minus that in the sitting position) ≥10 mmHg (**Figure 9.21**) [104]. Even in normotensive patients defined by sitting home BP, orthostatic hypertension may be a risk for future cardiovascular events.

In recent studies on orthostatic BP changes evaluated by self-measured BP monitoring at home (four BP measures: two in the sitting position followed by two in the standing position), both orthostatic hypertension and orthostatic hypotension (two standing SBP measures minus two sitting SBP measures) were significantly associated with microalbuminuria (**Figure 9.26**) and plasma BNP levels in hypertensive patients [164]. After nighttime dosing of doxazosin, a reduction in the orthostatic BP increase in patients with orthostatic hypertension at home was associated with a reduction of UACR independent of the reduction in sitting home BP (**Figure 9.27**) [191].

Orthostatic hypertension is closely associated with exaggerated ambulatory MBPS, while orthostatic hypotension is closely associated with nocturnal hypertension. The HAST contributes to identifying masked hypertension in those exhibiting exaggerated MBPS and nocturnal hypertension and in those who could not be detected by conventional sitting HBPM.

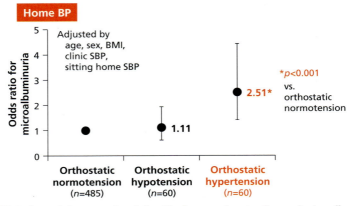

Figure 9.26 Orthostatic hypertension defined by home active standing and microalbuminuria (JMS-1 study). SBP, systolic blood pressure. *Source:* Hoshide et al. 2008 [164].

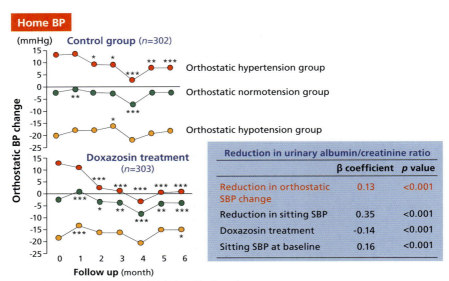

*$p<0.05$, **$p<0.005$, ***$p<0.001$ vs. baseline in each group

Figure 9.27 Reproducible orthostatic hypertension could be restored by alpha-blockade (JMS-1 study). SBP, systolic blood pressure. *Source:* Hoshide et al. 2012 [191].

CHAPTER 10
What is systemic haemodynamic atherothrombotic syndrome?

In 2013, we first proposed a novel disease entity, called systemic haemodynamic atherothrombotic syndrome (SHATS) that is characterised by a vicious cycle between haemodynamic stress and vascular disease and is a risk factor for cardiovascular events and organ damage (**Figure 10.1**) [41, 42, 192]. There are four domains of SHATS biomarkers: 1) pressure biomarkers, 2) haemodynamic regulation biomarkers, 3) vascular biomarkers, 4) cardiorenal brain biomarkers (**Figure 10.1**). The pressure biomarkers of SHATS could be detected by home blood pressure monitoring (HBPM), ambulatory blood pressure monitoring (ABPM), and the active standing test.

A typical case of SHATS

A 72-year-old woman who had been registered and was being followed in the Japan Morning Surge Home Blood Pressure study (J-HOP) [142] developed acute stroke just after rising in the morning to take a walk (**Figure 10.2**) [192]. Her neurological deficits were dizziness and conjugate deviation. The responsible lesion (shown in diffusion MRI) was located in a small artery, the paramedian branch (the perforating artery supplying the posterior circulation) of the posterior cerebral artery. The patient had a past history of hypertension from age 36 years, hyperlipidaemia from age 57 years, and acute myocardial infarction at age 58 years. Before the onset of stroke, she had achieved good control of her clinic BP (<130/80 mmHg), her home BP self-measured in the sitting position (125/75 mmHg), her average 24-hour BP (<120/75 mmHg) (**Figures 10.3** and **10.4**), and other metabolic risk factors by a regimen of aspirin, candesartan, hydrochlorothiazide (HTCZ), bisoprolol, and a statin. However, before the onset of stroke, she already had advanced SHATS with advanced vascular disease and exaggerated haemodynamic stress. The vascular evaluation tests performed before the onset of stroke revealed advanced systemic vascular disease: flow-mediated dilatation of the brachial artery 2.4% (normal range >5%); intima-media thickness (IMT) of the common carotid artery (right 2.2 mm, left 2.2 mm; normal range: <1.0 mm) and brachial-ankle pulse wave velocity (baPWV) (1935 cm/sec, corresponding to 93-year-old healthy reference subjects), and carotid augmentation index (26%) (**Figure 10.5**). In addition, she had advanced haemodynamic risk factors such as exaggerated morning BP surge (MBPS) (SBP >55 mmHg) (**Figure**

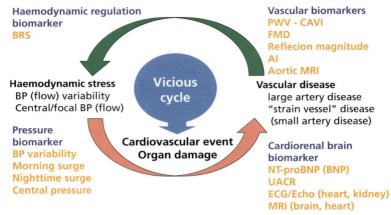

Figure 10.1 Concept and biomarkers of systemic haemodynamic atherothrombotic syndrome (SHATS). BRS, baroreceptor sensitivity; BPV, blood pressure variability; PWV, pulse wave velocity; CAVI, cardio-ankle vascular Index; FMD, Flow-mediated dilation; AI, augmentation index; MRI, magnetic resonance imaging; UACR, urinary albumin/creatinine ratio; BNP, B-type natriuretic peptide; NT-proBNP; N terminal-proBNP; ECG, electrocardiography; Echo, echography. *Source:* Kario. 2013 [42]; Kario. 2016 [4]

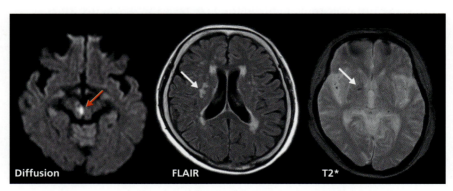

Figure 10.2 A 72-year-old woman who developed morning-onset stroke. The paramedian branch of the posterior cerebral artery exhibited the signs of branch atheromatous disease and this anatomical location corresponded to the site of high intensity of diffusion MRI and her neurological deficit. The red arrow shows the acute infarction in diffusion MR imaging and the white arrows show old deep white matter infarcts (FLAIR) and microbleed (T2*). *Source:* Kario. 2015 [192]

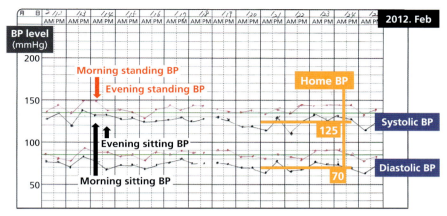

Figure 10.3 The self-measured home active standing BP monitoring four months before the onset of stroke. This home active standing BP monitoring performed in the morning and evening (two occasions per day) for 14 days clearly demonstrated persistent orthostatic hypertension (orthostatic increase in systolic BP >15 mmHg) at home. The black dots and lines represent the second read of the sitting BP measurements and the red ones represent the standing BP readings consecutively measured just after standing. *Source:* Kario. 2015 [192]

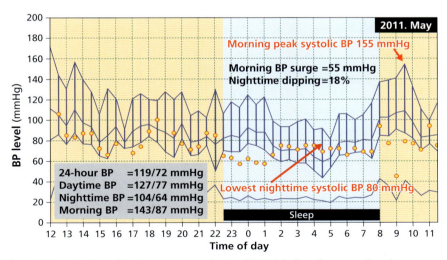

Figure 10.4 Ambulatory blood pressure monitoring (ABPM) before the onset of stroke event. ABPM performed 13 months before the stroke event demonstrated an exaggerated morning BP surge with marked daytime blood pressure variability, even when the average of the 24-hour BP level was well controlled to <130/80 mmHg. *Source:* Kario. 2015 [192]

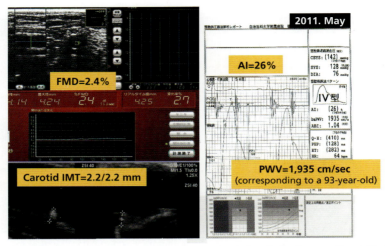

Figure 10.5 Vascular evaluation tests. AI, augmentation index; FMD, flow mediated dilation; IMT, intima-media thickness; PWV, pulse wave velocity. *Source:* Kario. 2015 [10]

10.4) and orthostatic hypertension detected by orthostatic HBPM before stroke (**Figure 10.3**). This case indicates that even if conventional risk factors are well controlled, the cardiovascular risk still remains significant. After the stroke event, her neurological deficit completely recovered. Amlodipine was added to previous medication and the peak of morning BP was markedly diminished, while the lowest BP during sleep was not changed, resulting in the specific suppression of MBPS (**Figure 10.6**).

Current guidelines on the management of hypertension stress the importance of out-of-clinic BP, and that the BP control status is assessed by the average of clinic, home, or 24-hour BP readings. However, even if the average value of one of these BP measures is well below the recommended threshold of target BP level, there is still a blind spot in the disease management: exaggerated BP surge still poses a risk for organ damage and cardiovascular events.

Clinical relevance of SHATS

The novel contribution of SHATS is its synergistic consideration of various types of BP variability and haemodynamic stress in relation to vascular disease [41, 42, 140]. That is, SHATS is defined by both vascular (one or more clinical/subclinical vascular diseases) and BP components (one or more phenotypes of BP variability), although the precise definition and criteria of SHATS are not yet clearly established [41, 42, 140]. Nonetheless, the concept underscores that clinicians should recognise the synergistic risk posed by exaggerated BP variability and

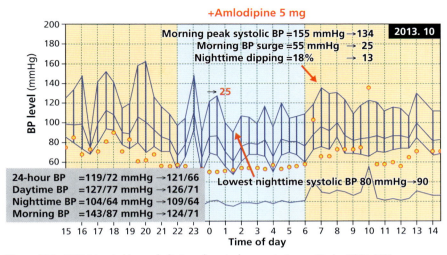

Figure 10.6 ABPM treated by amlodipine after stroke event. *Source:* Kario. 2015 [10]

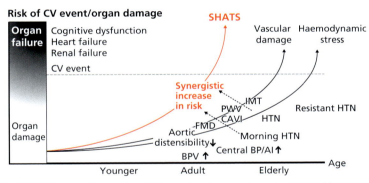

Figure 10.7 SHATS on cardiovascular (CV) event and organ damage worsened by vicious cycle of haemodynamic stress and vascular damage. AI, augmentation index; BPV, blood pressure variability; CAVI, cardio-ankle vascular index; FMD, flow-mediated dilatation of brachial artery; HTN, hypertension; IMT, intima-media thickness of carotid artery; PWV, pulse wave velocity. *Source:* Kario. 2015 [192]

vascular damage in clinical practice (**Figure 10.7**).

The clinical relevance of SHATS is different for younger and older subjects. SHATS is clinically important for predicting future sustained hypertension in younger subjects. Early detection of SHATS may raise the alert for prevention of organ damage in this early stage. In older subjects, SHATS is important as a direct

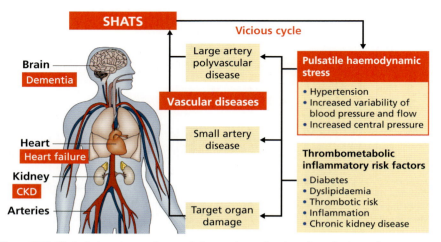

Figure 10.8 Clinical phenotypes of systemic haemodynamic atherothrombotic syndrome (SHATS). CKD, chronic kidney disease. *Source:* Modified from Kario. 2013 [42].

risk for triggering cardiovascular events. The suppression of SHATS leads directly to reduced cardiovascular events.

Pathological target of SHATS

The arteries with different size and microcirculation organ interaction are the target of SHATS (**Figure 10.8**) [42]. In high-risk patients, an advanced vulnerable plaque may be the first target. MBPS triggers plaque rupture by mechanical stress of BP and shear stress from exaggerated variability of blood flow, resulting in the onset of cardiovascular events. The small arteries branching rectangularly from large arteries may be an appropriate second target [41, 42, 140]. These vessels are the so-called "strain vessels" that are anatomically exposed to high pressure and that must maintain strong vascular tone in order to provide large pressure gradients from the parent vessels to the capillaries [193].

Large artery disease will augment the impact of exaggerated MBPS on atherosclerotic and small-artery-related cardiovascular events. An increase in large artery stiffness decreases the attenuation of the pulse to transmit to the peripheral arteries (**Figure 10.9**) [194]. As shown in **Figure 10.9**, soft ascending aorta dilate (11.562% dilatation) to absorb the power of the pulse (**Figure 10.10 left**). However, dilation of a stiffened aorta is limited (2.675% dilatation) (**Figure 10.10 right**). Thus, the pulse is transmitted to the brain without absorption in the ascending aorta (**Figure 10.11**). When plaque exists in the major artery, the pulse reaching a disrupted plaque could trigger cerebral infarction (**Figure 10.11 left**).

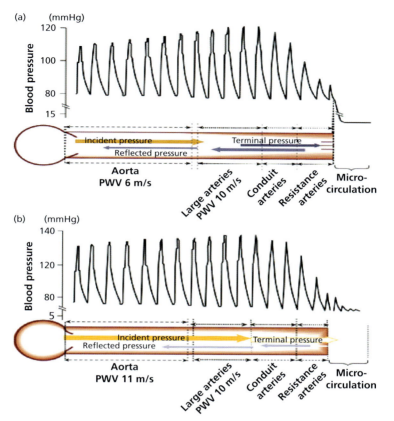

Figure 10.9 Attenuation of transmission of pulsatile pressure energy to microcirculation by arterial stiffness gradient. (a) When an arterial stiffness gradient is present (aortic pulse wave velocity [PWV] < peripheral PWV), partial reflections occur far from the microcirculation and return at low PWV to the aorta in diastole, thereby maintaining central-to-peripheral amplification. Partial reflections limit the transmission of pulsatile pressure energy to the periphery and protect the microcirculation. (b) When the stiffness gradient disappears or is inverted (aortic PWV > peripheral PWV), pulsatile pressure is not sufficiently dampened and is transmitted, damaging the microcirculation. In parallel, the central-to-peripheral pressure amplification is attenuated. *Source:* Briet et al. 2012 [194]

Even when such a plaque does not exist, pulse transmission to small perforating arteries could result in white matter disease (**Figure 10.11 right**). White matter disease predisposes elderly patients to dementia, depression, apathy, and falls.

Cerebral haemorrhage and infarction occur most frequently in the regions of the small perforating arteries. In fact, in elderly hypertensive patients, silent cerebral infarcts (SCIs), particularly when occurring as multiple SCIs, are more

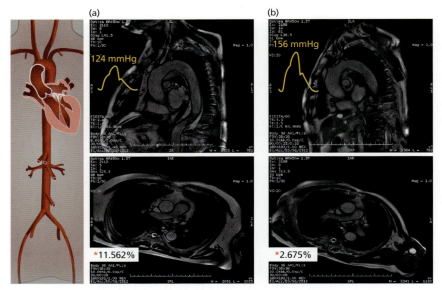

Figure 10.10 Assessment of aortic stiffness using dynamic MRI. (a) soft aorta. (b) stiffened aorta. * % dilation of ascending aorta during systolic phase. *Source:* Kario K. *Essential Manual on Perfect 24-hour Blood Pressure Management from Morning to Nocturnal Hypertension: Up-to-date for Anticipation Medicine.* Wiley, 2018.

frequently detected by brain MRI in the exaggerated MBPS group than in the normal MBPS group (**Figures 2.2** and **2.3**) [14]. In addition, cerebral haemorrhage was observed more frequently in the exaggerated MBPS group than the normal MBPS group [47].

For example, the nearer the large artery (arcuate artery), the greater the pressure overload in the afferent arterioles of the glomeruli (**Figure 10.12**) [193]. The source of microalbuminuria is first the glomeruli in the cortex near the arcuate arteries of the outer medulla. These vascular structures are found in the cerebral perforating arteries, renal juxtamedullary afferent arterioles, and retinal and coronary arteries (**Figure 10.13**) [193].

Mechanism of vicious cycle of SHATS

Exaggerated MBPS, specifically potentiated by neurohumoral activation in the morning, is the BP variability phenotype of SHATS. SHATS is characterised by an increase in BP variability and clinically detected by one of the specific surges, which may partly be associated with each other. In fact, MBPS is associated with other phenotypes such as orthostatic hypertension (a 15–20 mmHg increase in

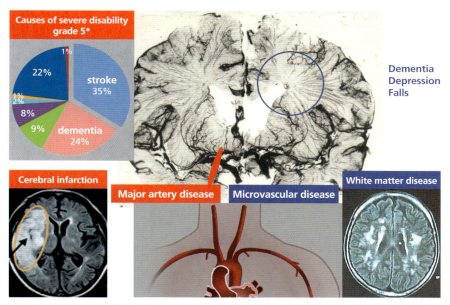

Figure 10.11 Hypertension affects two causes (stroke, dementia) of severe disability. Created based on Dr. Vladimir Hachinski's slide with his permission. *Created based on data from 2013 Comprehensive Survey of Living Conditions (Ministry of Health, Labour and Welfare; http://www.mhlw.go.jp/toukei/saikin/hw/k-tyosa/k-tyosa13/; accessed on December 23, 2017)

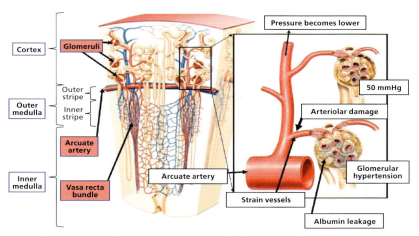

Figure 10.12 Strain vessel hypothesis: a viewpoint for linkage of albuminuria and cerebrocardiovascular risk. *Source:* Ito et al. 2009 [193]

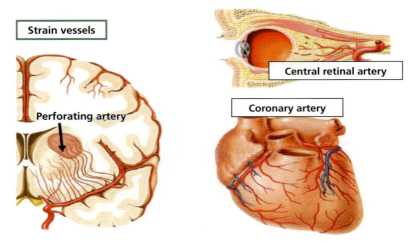

Figure 10.13 Strain vessel hypothesis: a viewpoint for linkage of albuminuria and cerebro-cardiovascular risk. *Source:* Ito et al. 2009 [193]

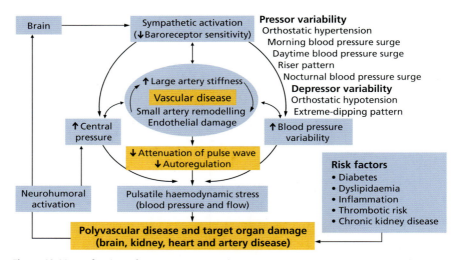

Figure 10.14 Mechanism of SHATS. *Source:* Kario. 2013 [42]

SBP on standing), increase in the SD of daytime ambulatory BP readings, and circadian BP variation, especially with extreme dipping of nighttime BP (a nighttime SBP fall ≥20%) [41, 42, 140, 162, 163].

Increases in BP variability, central pressure, and impaired baroreceptor sensi-

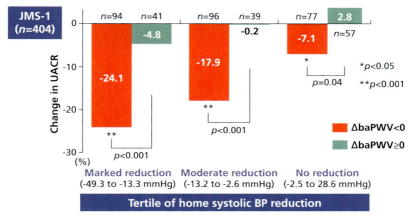

Figure 10.15 Reduction of baPWV (brachial-ankle pulse wave velocity) is important for reduction of UACR in hypertensive patients. UACR, urinary albumin/creatinine ratio. *Source:* Matsui et al. 2010 [195]

tivity are the three BP measures of SHATS, and are closely related (**Figure 10.14**) [42]. The overall underlying mechanism of SHATS may include impaired neural and vascular components of baroreflex due to increased central sympathetic activity and decreased carotid dispensability, respectively. In addition, small artery remodelling as well as large artery disease may contribute to increases in BP variability [42, 140]. Arterial stiffness and pressure wave reflections are two important components of pulsatile haemodynamics. The measurements of ambulatory BP, including MBPS, can reflect pulsatile haemodynamics through the influences of arterial stiffness and wave reflections. The degree of central and peripheral neurohumoral activation and their related cardiovascular reactivity in each specific condition may determine the different phenotypes of BP variability.

Synergistic protection of the end organ was found between the BP and vascular disease. In the titration of doxazosin to target home BP <135/85 mmHg by HBPM, not only the reduction in home BP, but also the reduction in PWV was important for reducing micoalbuminuria (**Figure 10.15**) [195].

Invasive strategies may reduce exaggerated BP variability and pulse wave reflection, resulting in the suppression of the vicious cycle of SHATS. Carotid artery stenting (CAS) significantly reduces the day-by-day variability of home BP levels in patients with carotid artery disease (**Figure 10.16**) [196]. After percutaneous transluminal angioplasty (PTA), reductions in left ventricular hypertrophy (LVH) and microalbuminuria are correlated with the augmentation index of the carotid artery in patients with peripheral artery disease (PAD) (**Figure 10.17**) [197].

Even when conventional risk factors are well-controlled, hypertensive

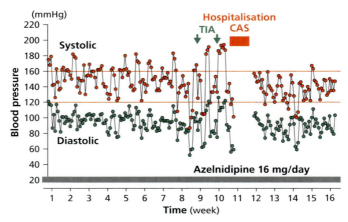

Figure 10.16 Stabilisation of BP variability after CAS (carotid artery stenting) in a 62-year-old hypertensive patient with TIA (transient ischaemic attack). *Source:* Toriumi et al. 2014 [196]

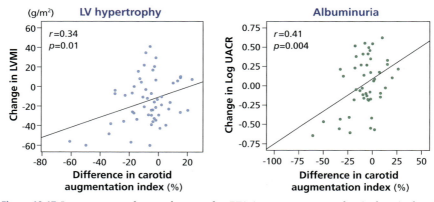

Figure 10.17 Improvement of organ damage after PTA (percutaneous transluminal angioplasty) in PAD (peripheral artery disease) patients (*n*=76, mean 70 years). LVMI, left ventricular mass index; UACR, urinary albumin/creatinine ratio. *Source:* Eguchi et al. 2014 [197]

patients may be at risk of advanced organ damage and cardiovascular events. The detection of phenotypes of BP variability to assess SHATS, especially in high-risk patients with cardiovascular disease and during antihypertensive treatment, can be achieved by considering the time of medication dosing targeting BP peaks, by measures to confer vascular protection, and/or by neuromodulation with renal denervation or baroreceptor sensitisation therapy, resulting in more effective organ protection.

CHAPTER 11

Biomarker of SHATS

There are four classes of biomarkers of systemic haemodynamic atherothrombotic syndrome (SHATS). The two core biomarkers are pressure and vascular biomarkers. Pressure biomarkers include variability of visit-to-visit clinic, home, and ambulatory blood pressure (BP) readings, morning and/or nighttime BP surge, and central pressure. Vascular biomarkers are pulse wave velocity (PWV), cardio-ankle vascular index (CAVI), flow-mediated dilation (FMD), arterial wave form (reflection magnitude, augmentation index), and aortic stiffness evaluated by aortic MRI. The two other biomarkers are haemodynamic regulation (baroreceptor sensitivity) and organ damage (ECG and/or cardiac echo-validated hypertensive heart disease, urinary albumin/creatinine ratio [UACR], eGFR, echo-validated resistive index of kidney, serum levels of N-terminal proBNP [NT-proBNP], high sensitivity troponin T [hs-TnT], growth differentiation factor 15 [GDF-15], and MRI-validated cardiac and brain damage) (**Figure 10.1**) [4].

Vascular biomarkers

1) CAVI/PWV

The cardiac and vascular screening system, VaSera device (Fukuda Denshi Co., Ltd., Tokyo, Japan), is able to measure the following four different measures to evaluate cardiovascular damage: ECG, cardiac sound, brachial and ankle pulse waves (**Figure 11.1**). These measures are useful to evaluate hypertensive heart disease, aortic valvular disease, central pressure, cardiac function, and ankle-brachial index (ABI) to calculate the BP-independent CAVI at one examination. This system stores the intracuff pressure wave form of four different extremities.

In a cross-sectional study of 1,391 patients with moderate to high risk for coronary artery disease (CAD), CAVI is an independent predictor of CAD evaluated by 64-slice multidetector CT coronary angiography, and the addition of CAVI to the traditional risk score significantly improves the diagnostic yield of CAD (**Figure 11.2**) [198].

In the recent meta-analysis of 14,673 participants without history of cardiovascular disease using 6.4-year follow-up data from eight cohort studies in Japan, the brachial-ankle PWV (baPWV) was an independent predictor of future cardiovascular disease. In analysis based on baPWV quintile ranges, the multivariable-adjusted hazard ratio increased significantly in parallel with increasing

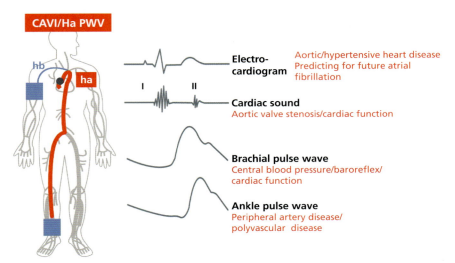

Figure 11.1 Development of a device for predicting future heart failure by analysing wave forms obtained from three modalities. CAVI, cardio-ankle vascular index. *Source:* Kario K. *Essential Manual on Perfect 24-hour Blood Pressure Management from Morning to Nocturnal Hypertension: Up-to-date for Anticipation Medicine.* Wiley, 2018.

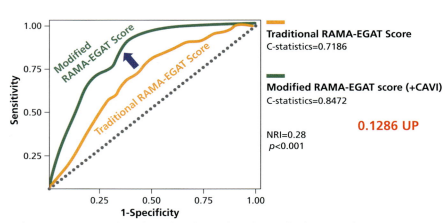

* The RAMA-EGAT score is traditional cardiovascular risk score for diagnosis of coronary artery disease in thailand.

Figure 11.2 Incremental value of CAVI. Comparison of receiver operating characteristic (ROC) curve of modified RAMA-EGAT score (EGAT+ cardio-ankle vascular index [CAVI]) and traditional RAMA-EGAT score (EGAT score). *Source:* Yingchoncharoen et al. 2012 [198]

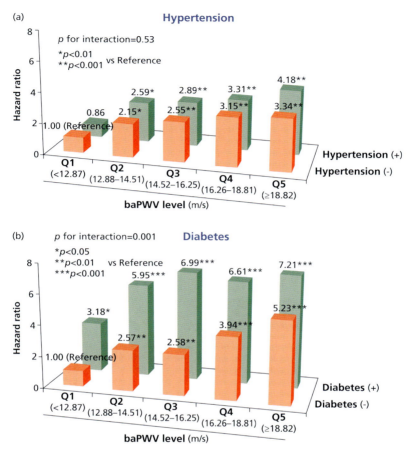

Figure 11.3 Multivariate-adjusted hazard ratios for the development of cardiovascular disease according to baPWV level by presence or absence of hypertension or diabetes. baPWV, brachial-ankle pulse wave velocity. a) Multivariate-adjustment was made for age, sex, diabetes, body mass index, total cholesterol, high-density lipoprotein cholesterol, and current smoking habits. b) Multivariate-adjustment was made for age, sex, brachial systolic blood pressure, use of antihypertensive agents, body mass index, total cholesterol, high-density lipoprotein cholesterol, and current smoking habits. *Source:* Ohkuma et al. 2017 [199]

baPWV quintile (**Figure 11.3**) [199]. The hazard ratio for cardiovascular disease for baPVW values in quintile 5 versus quintile 1 was 3.50 (2.14–5.74, $p<0.001$). Adding baPWV to a model with Framingham risk score significantly increased the c-statistics from 0.8026 to 0.8131 ($p<0.001$) and the category-free net reclassification improvement (0.247, $p<0.001$), suggesting that baPWV could provide

Coupling Japan
CardiOVascUlar Prognostic Coupling Study in Japan

The COUPLING study (since 2015) aimed to clarify the relationship between blood pressure variability and vascular properties in hypertensive patients and to investigate its relationships with the onset of cardiovascular events in patients at high risk of cardiovascular disease.

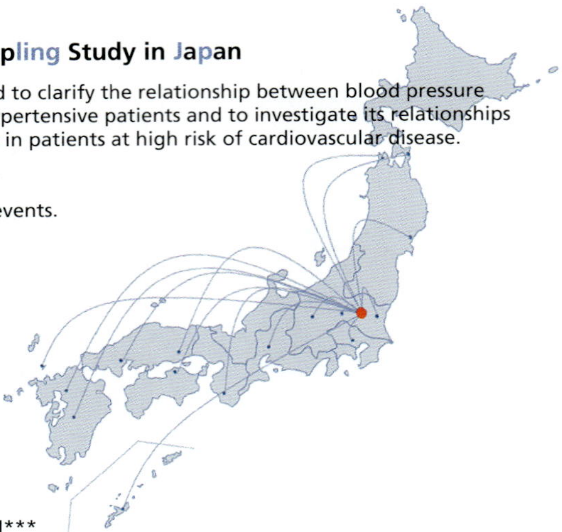

[Primary outcomes]
Time to onset of major cardiovascular events.
1. A composite of cerebral infarction
2. Cerebral haemorrhage
3. Subarachnoid haemorrhage
4. Unknown type of stroke
5. Myocardial infarction
6. Cardiovascular intervention due to angina pectoris
7. Sudden death

[Secondary outcomes]
1. Time to onset of various events*
2. Change in blood pressure (BP)
3. Increase in CAVI** or decrease in ABI***
4. Development of left ventricular hypertrophy
5. Adverse events

Target sample size: 5,000
Follow-up period: 7 years (every 1–2 years)

Figure 11.4 The COUPLING study. *Each fatal and non-fatal cardiovascular event, hospitalisation for angina pectoris or heart failure, aortic dissection, peripheral arterial disease, end-stage renal disease; doubling of serum creatinine level; new onset of atrial fibrillation, dementia, need of nursing care; total death. **CAVI (cardiac-ankle vascular stiffness index) = $a\{(2\rho/\Delta P)\times\ln(Ps/Pd)PWV^2\}+b$. a and b, constants; ρ, blood density; ΔP, Ps–Pd; Ps, systolic BP; Pd, diastolic BP. ***ABI, ankle-brachial index. *Source:* Kario. 2016 [4]

additional predictive information on cardiovascular disease beyond traditional risk factors [199]. Despite a lack of longitudinal studies from the US and Europe, the AHA recommends baPWV measurements or the determination of the CAVI as useful measures for prediction of cardiovascular outcome in Asian populations (*Class I; Level of Evidence B*), as part of recommendations for improving and standardising vascular research on arterial stiffness [200].

The nationwide COUPLING (Cardiovascular Prognostic Coupling) study has been underway since 2015 in collaboration with Fukuda Denshi Co., Ltd. Its aim is to clarify the relationship between the BP variability and vascular properties in hypertensive patients, and to investigate its relationships with the onset of cardiovascular events in high-risk patients (**Figure 11.4**) [4].

Method of waveform recording	Device	Company	Method of calibration	Method of estimation	Clinical applicability[†]
Radial tonometry	Bpro	HealthSTATS	Brachial-radial cuff BP	GTF (radial-aortic)	++
	SphygmoCor	AtCor	Brachial-radial cuff BP	(i) GTF (radial-aortic)	+
				(ii) Late systolic shoulder	+
	HEM9000AI	Omron	Brachial Cuff BP	(i) Algorithm	++
				(ii) Late systolic shoulder	++
Brachial cuff PVP	Mobil-O-Graph (ARCsolver)	IEM	Brachial cuff BP	GTF (radial-aortic)	+++
	Centron cBP301	Centron Diagnostics	Brachial cuff BP	GTF (radial-aortic)	++++
	Vicorder	Skidmore Medical	Brachial cuff BP	GTF (radial-aortic)	+++
	XCEL	AtCor Medical	Brachial cuff BP	GTF (radial-aortic)	+++
Supra-systolic brachial cuff PVP	Arteriograph	TensioMed	Brachial cuff BP	Late systolic wave amplitude	+++
	Cardioscope II	Pulsecor	Brachial cuff BP	Algorithm	++++

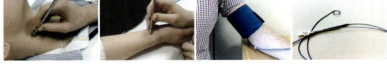

Figure 11.5 Indirect, non-invasive method for estimating central pressure. GTF, generalized transfer function; PVP, pulse volume plethysmography. [†]Personal view based on experience, operator-dependency, need for computer/software interface, with + indicating limited applicability to routine clinical practice and ++++ indicating high applicability.
Source: McEniery et al. 2014 [201]. Reprinted by permission of Oxford University Press.

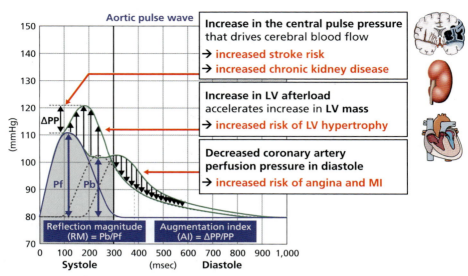

Figure 11.6 Role of increased central aortic and pulse pressures in the increase of cardiovascular events. LV, left ventricular; MI, myocardial infarction. Pf, amplitude of forward pulse wave; Pb, amplitude of backward pulse wave; PP, pulse pressure.
Source: Kario K. *Essential Manual on Perfect 24-hour Blood Pressure Management from Morning to Nocturnal Hypertension: Up-to-date for Anticipation Medicine.* Wiley, 2018.

2) Central pressure

Central pressure could be calculated from the pulse wave form obtained using a variety of non-invasive methods (**Figure 11.5**) [201]. However, there is no standardisation of the measurement. From pathophysiological viewpoints, central pressure is more closely related to organ damage and cardiovascular risk – an increase in central pressure increases the risk of stroke and chronic kidney disease (CKD), an increase in left ventricular load (direct afterload) increases left ventricular hypertrophy, and a decrease in coronary perfusion pressure in diastole increases the myocardial ischaemia (**Figure 11.6**). Aortic central pressure consists of forward wave and reflection wave (**Figure 11.7**). The following two vascular indices of the relative impact of reflection wave versus forward percussion wave could be calculated from the pulse wave form: RM and AI. The RM and AI might be potential indicators of vascular stiffness and vascular tonus of the peripheral artery. Previous evidence demonstrates that central systolic and pulse pressures are better predictors than brachial systolic and pulse pressures, respectively (**Figure 11.8**) [202].

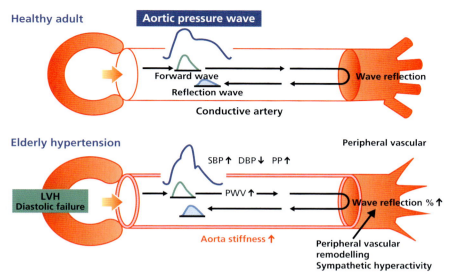

Figure 11.7 Relationship between central blood pressure and wave reflection. DBP, diastolic blood pressure; LVH, left ventricular hypertrophy; PWV, pulse wave velocity; PP, pulse pressure; SBP, systolic BP. *Source:* Kario K. *Essential Manual on Perfect 24-hour Blood Pressure Management from Morning to Nocturnal Hypertension: Up-to-date for Anticipation Medicine.* Wiley, 2018.

3) Flow-mediated dilatation (FMD)

A semiautomatic measurement device to measure FMD of the brachial artery is now available in clinical practice (UNEX corp., Nagoya, Japan). This device provides a new integrated FMD response, the area under the dilation curve during the 120-second dilation period after cuff deflation (FMD-AUC120), which is a more reliable indicator of endothelial dysfunction. FMD-AUC120 is more closely associated with home BP control, Framingham risk score and UACR than ΔFMD. (**Figure 11.9**) [203, 204].

Cardiac biomarkers

Assays for the following cardiac biomarkers are available from F. Hoffmann-La Roche Ltd (Basel, Switzerland).

1) NT-proBNP

The major determinant of serum NT-proBNP level is left ventricular wall stress, especially during systole (**Figure 11.10**). As the wall stress is determined by

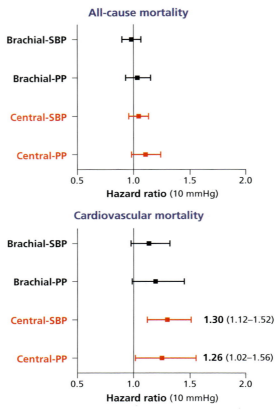

Figure 11.8 Hazards ratios of the individual blood pressure variables per 10 mmHg increment for all-cause and cardiovascular mortality. 10-year all-cause and cardiovascular mortality in 1,272 participants (47% women aged 30–79 years) from a community of homogeneous Chinese. PP, pulse pressure; SBP, systolic blood pressure. *Source:* Wang et al. 2009 [202]

both cavity pressure and left ventricular cavity radius, an increase in serum NT-proBNP level reflects an increase in preload (increased circulating volume) and afterload (systolic BP), and myocardial ischaemia. Even within the normal range (NT-proBNP <125 pg/mL, BNP <28 pg/mL), individual change reflects the quality of BP control (nocturnal hypertension, BP variability and central pressure), circulating volume, systemic hypoxia, and myocardial ischaemia, suggesting that change in NT-proBNP could be a useful biomarker of cardiovascular risk status during antihypertensive treatment (**Figure 11.11**).

In fact, on-treatment serum NT-proBNP level is a predictor of cardiovascular events in high-risk hypertensive patients (ASCOT) (**Figure 11.12**) [205].

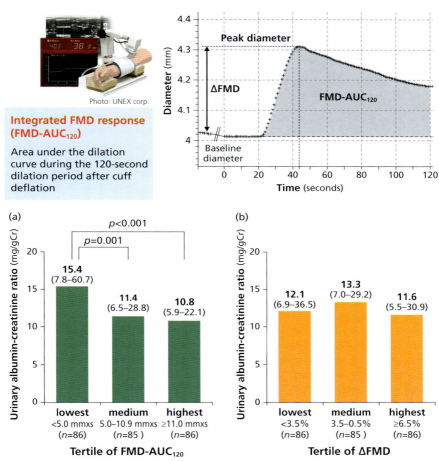

Kabutoya T, Hoshide S, Ogata Y, Eguchi K, Kario K. Relationship between endothelial dysfunction and kidney disease. *J Clin Hypertens* (Greenwich). 2014; 16: 156.

Figure 11.9 FMD-AUC$_{120}$ and urinary albumin-creatinine ratio. FMD, flow mediated dilation. *Source:* Kabutoya et al. 2012 [203]; Kabutoya et al. 2013 [204]

Amlodipine recipients who achieved a 6-month NT-proBNP below the median (61 pg/mL) were at lower risk of CVD compared with those who did not (odds ratio 0.58) after adjustment for confounders including baseline NT-proBNP and achieved BP. Thus, NT-proBNP would be a biomarker for the efficacy of antihypertensive treatment [205].

Levels of NT-proBNP could also be used as a biomarker to assist in achieving perfect 24-hour BP control. An increase in the NT-proBNP level during anti-

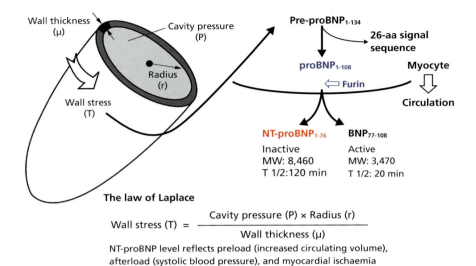

Figure 11.10 Systolic left ventricular wall stress is the major determinant of NT-proBNP level. NT-proBNP, N-terminal pro-brain natriuretic peptide. *Source:* Kario K. *Essential Manual on Perfect 24-hour Blood Pressure Management from Morning to Nocturnal Hypertension: Up-to-date for Anticipation Medicine.* Wiley, 2018.

Threshold (pg/mL)		
NT-proBNP	BNP	Clinical implication
<400	<100	Even within normal range (NT-proBNP <125, BNP <28), individual change reflects quality of BP control (nocturnal hypertension, BP variability, and central pressure), circulating volume, hypoxia, and myocardial ischaemia, suggesting cardiovascular risk status during antihypertensive treatment
≥400	≥100	Suspected heart failure*
≥2,000	≥400	Chronic heart failure likely*

Figure 11.11 NT-proBNP as the sensitive biomarker of perfect 24-hour blood pressure control. *Diagnosis of heart failure in untreated patients with suggestive heart failure. BP, blood pressure; BNP, brain natriuretic peptide; NT-proBNP, N terminal-proBNP. *Source:* Kario K. *Essential Manual on Perfect 24-hour Blood Pressure Management from Morning to Nocturnal Hypertension: Up-to-date for Anticipation Medicine.* Wiley, 2018.

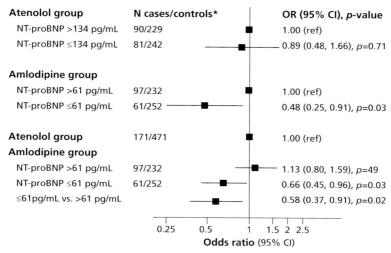

Figure 11.12 On-treatment serum NT-proBNP level as the predictor of cardiovascular events in high-risk hypertensive patients (ASCOT). *Number of cases and controls in corresponding category, they are not the discordant sets for estimating odds ratios. BP, blood pressure; CVD, cardiovascular disease; NT-proBNP, N-terminal pro-brain natriuretic peptide. *Source:* Welsh et al. 2014 [205]

hypertensive treatment suggests an increase in the left ventricular wall stress [125]. Even in medicated hypertensive patients with well-controlled clinic BP, the causes of an increase in wall stress should be examined. Nocturnal hypertension and/or sleep apnoea might be occurring during sleep (**Figure 11.13**).

2) High-sensitivity troponin T (hs-TNT) and growth differentiation factor 15 (GDF-15)

These two biomarkers may be measures of cardiac wall stress and fibrosis [206].

3) Electrocardiography (ECG)

ECG-derived measures are important biomarkers of hypertensive heart disease. ECG-derived left ventricular hypertrophy (LVH) is a powerful predictor of cardiovascular events, especially stroke in the elderly hypertensive patients (**Figure 11.14**) [207]. Data from the general population-based JMS Cohort ($n=10,755$, follow-up 10 years) demonstrated that the Cornell product-defined LVH (Cornell product >244 mV×msec), is a good prognostic predictor of stroke (**Figure 11.15**) [208]. In addition, in this cohort, a prolonged corrected QT interval (>440 msec in males, >460 msec in females) is also predictive of future stroke events even in subjects without ECG-diagnosed LVH (**Figure 11.16**) [209].

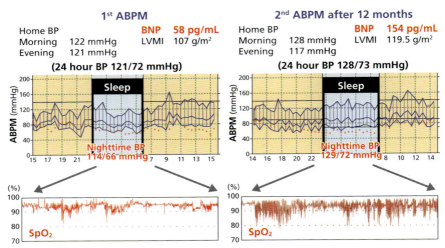

Figure 11.13 How to use BNP as biomarker to achieve perfect 24-hour BP control. A 68-year-old woman with amlodipine 2.5 mg and candesartan 12 mg per day was well-controlled for home and 24-hour ambulatory BP (the first ABPM). However, her BNP level increased (from 58 to 154 pg/mL), even when clinic and home BP levels remained well controlled. The second ABPM and nocturnal pulse oximetry performed on the same day detected nocturnal uncontrolled hypertension with sleep apnoea. ABPM, ambulatory BP monitoring; BNP, B-type natriuretic peptide; BP, blood pressure; LVMI, left ventricular mass index.
Source: Kario K. *Essential Manual on Perfect 24-hour Blood Pressure Management from Morning to Nocturnal Hypertension: Up-to-date for Anticipation Medicine.* Wiley, 2018.

Microalbuminuria

Microalbuminuria, an increase in the UACR, is a renal biomarker. It is also a good biomarker of cardiovascular events [210], because various pathological conditions are associated with microalbuminuria (**Figure 11.17**). The UACR could be used as a biomarker of perfect 24-hour BP control, especially nighttime BP control and BP variability (**Figures 6.18**, **6.25**, **7.7**, **7.9**, **9.13**, **9.15**, **9.26**, **9.27** and **10.15**, see Chapter 13) [35, 125, 141, 143, 164, 183, 191, 195].

Brain

High BP induces profound alterations of cerebral circulation autoregulation that, in combination with structural alterations, compromise blood supply to the brain and increase the risk of stroke and dementia (**Figure 11.18**) [211].

Silent cerebral infarcts (SCI) and white matter lesions are the morphological

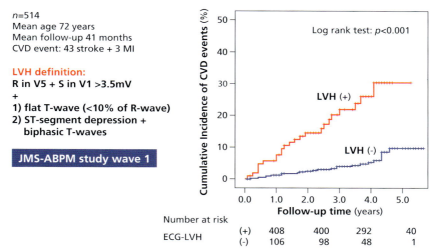

Figure 11.14 ECG-LVH and cardiovascular events in the elderly hypertensive patients: JMS-ABPM study wave 1. CVD, cardiovascular disease; ECG-LVH, electrocardiographic left ventricular hypertrophy. *Source:* Edison et al. 2015 [207]. Reprinted by permission of Oxford University Press.

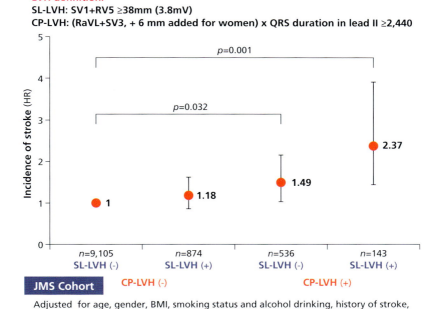

Adjusted for age, gender, BMI, smoking status and alcohol drinking, history of stroke, history of myocardial infarction, status of diabetes mellitus, presence of hyperlipidaemia, systolic blood pressure, and antihypertensive medication use.

Figure 11.15 ECG-LVH and stroke risk in JMS Cohort study (n=10,755, follow-up 10 years). CP, Cornell product; LVH, left ventricular hypertrophy; SL, Sokolow-Lyon. Created based on data from Ishikawa et al. 2009 [208]

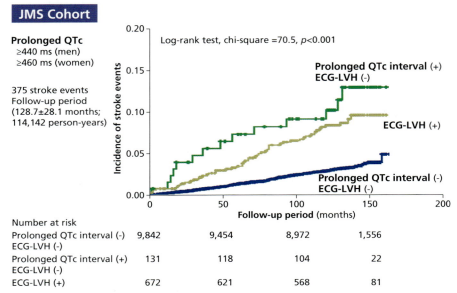

Figure 11.16 QTc and stroke risk in JMS Cohort study (n=10,643, follow-up 10 years). LVH, left ventricular hypertrophy; QTc, corrected QT. Source: Ishikawa et al. 2015 [209]

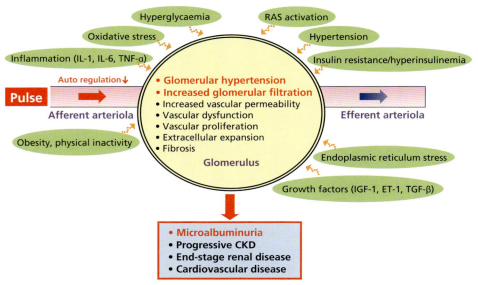

Figure 11.17 Cardiometabolic syndrome and CKD. CKD, Chronic kidney disease; RAS, renin–angiotensin system. Source: Kario K. Essential Manual on Perfect 24-hour Blood Pressure Management from Morning to Nocturnal Hypertension: Up-to-date for Anticipation Medicine. Wiley, 2018.

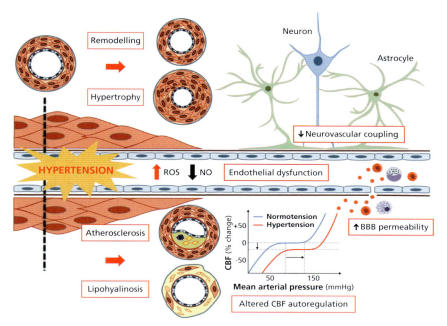

Figure 11.18 Hypertension and cerebral blood vessels. BBB, blood–brain barrier; CBF, cerebral blood flow; ROS, reactive oxygen species. *Source:* Faraco and Iadecola. 2013 [211]

phenotypes of hypertensive cerebral disease. Both predispose to clinical stroke, dementia, apathy, and falls in the elderly. In the JMS-ABPM wave 1 study, SCI, especially multiple SCI, was the strong predictor of future clinical stroke in elderly hypertensive patients (**Figure 11.19**) [34]. Higher 24-hour BP and diabetes are important determinants of multiple SCI; both increase the risk of SCIs (**Figure 11.20**) [212].

Proton (H1)-MR spectroscopy could quantitatively measure cerebral metabolites such as N-acetyl asparate (NAA), which is an indicator of functional neuronal mass, because NAA is located only in neurons (**Figure 11.21**) [213]. NAA in white matter lesions is significantly decreased in diabetic hypertensive patients compared with normotensive and non-diabetic hypertensive patients (**Figure 11.22**) [214].

Clinically, Mini-Mental State Examination (MMSE) and the Japanese version of the Montreal Cognitive Assessment (MoCA-J) are used to evaluate cognitive function.

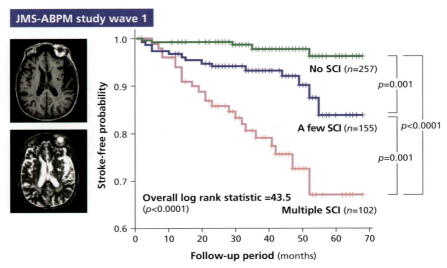

Figure 11.19 Impact of silent cerebral infarct (SCI) on clinical stroke prognosis in Japanese patients. Created based on data from Kario et al. 2001 [34]

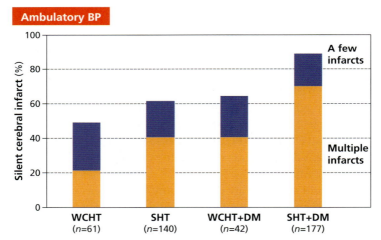

Figure 11.20 Prevalence of silent cerebral infarcts in hypertensive patients with diabetes mellitus. DM, diabetes mellitus; SHT, sustained hypertension; WCHT, white-coat hypertension. *Source:* Eguchi et al. 2003 [212]

Biomarker of SHATS

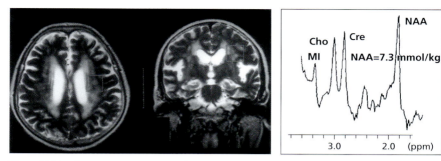

Figure 11.21 H^1-MR spectroscopy in white matter lesion. NAA, N-acetyl-asparate, an indicator of functional neuronal mass (normal range =8.5–10 mmol/kg). *Source:* Kario et al. 1999 [213]

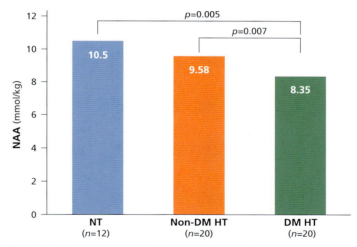

Figure 11.22 Cerebral N-acetyl aspartate (NAA; an indicator of functional neuronal mass) was lower in the diabetic hypertensive patients. DM, diabetes mellitus; HT, hypertensive; NT, normotensive. Created based on data from Kario et al. 2005 [214]

Baroreflex sensitivity

Figure 11.23 shows the Baroreflex, a negative feedback loop in the autonomic nervous system. Baroreflex sensitivity (BRS) could be calculated from the agreement between beat-by-beat BP and heart rate, measured using a tonometry device (**Figure 11.24**). Different calcium antagonists improve BRS to differing extents. Azelnidipine significantly reduced heart rate and increases BRS, while the amlodipine had no effect [215].

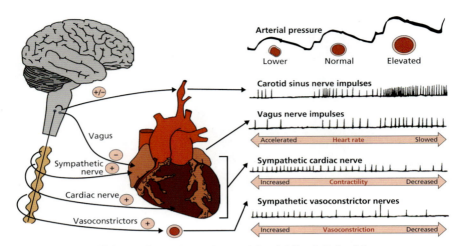

Figure 11.23 Carotid sinus reflexes. *Source:* Amerena J and Julius S. Role of the nervous system in human hypertension. In: Hollenberg NJ, Braunwald E, eds. *Atlas of Hypertension*. 5th ed. Current Medicine, Philadelphia, PA, LLC, 2005, reprinted with permission of Springer Nature.

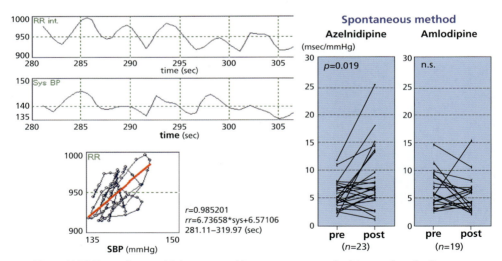

Figure 11.24 Baroreflex sensitivity measured by spontaneous method (spectral method). *Source:* Eguchi et al. 2007 [215]

CHAPTER 12
Antihypertensive strategy

The 2017 AHA/ACC hypertension management guidelines recommended a simple "universal blood pressure (BP) goal" of <130/80 mmHg for all BP measurements including clinic, home, and daytime BP for all hypertensive patients with different specific conditions (**Figure 12.1**) [1].

In clinical practice, morning home BP-guided titration of antihypertensive drugs is the first step to achieving "perfect 24-hour BP control" and consists of three components (**Figure 0.4**) [40]: lowering 24-hour BP; keeping normal circadian rhythm (dipper-type); and suppressing exaggerated BP variability, especially for morning surge. Controlling morning home systolic BP (SBP) to <145 mmHg is the first step in reducing relatively short-term risk, with the goal being morning home BP <130 mmHg, and ideally <125 mmHg for home SBP (**Figure 3.13**) [10].

Chronotherapy

Non-specific medication for perfect 24-hour BP control of morning and nocturnal hypertension includes long-acting drugs (**Figure 12.2**). Longer-acting antihypertensives are better at controlling nighttime and morning BP levels. These drugs are usually administered once daily in the morning, and they provide continuous BP reduction over a 24-hour period to attenuate the exaggerated morning BP surge.

Specific chronologic treatment includes the time of antihypertensive dosing and selecting the class of agents. Specific treatment of the morning BP surge may be achieved using antihypertensive medication that reduces the pressor effect of neurohumoral factors potentiated in the morning (**Figure 5.19**) [89], such as inhibitors of sympathetic activity or the renin-angiotensin-aldosterone system (RAS) (**Figure 12.2**). Practically, bedtime dosing of antihypertensive drugs, especially calcium channel blockers (CCB), alpha-blockers, and RAS inhibitors, suppresses the exaggerated morning BP surge without excessive nocturnal hypotension during sleep. These treatments are also effective for nocturnal hypertension. On the other hand, specific drugs for reducing nighttime BP are diuretics including thiazide-type diuretics, indapamide, and aldosterone blockers.

Clinical Condition (s)	BP Threshold (mmHg)	BP Goal
General		
Clinical CVD or 10-year ASCVD risk ≥10%	≥130/80	<130/80
No clinical CVD and 10-year ASCVD risk <10%	≥140/90	<130/80
Older persons (≥65 years of age; noninstitutionalised, ambulatory, community-living adults)	≥130 (SBP)	<130 (SBP)
Specific comorbidities		
Diabetes mellitus	≥130/80	<130/80
Chronic kidney disease	≥130/80	<130/80
Chronic kidney disease after renal transplantation	≥130/80	<130/80
Heart failure	≥130/80	<130/80
Stable ischaemic heart disease	≥130/80	<130/80
Secondary stroke prevention	≥140/90	<130/80
Secondary stroke prevention (lacunar)	≥130/80	<130/80
Peripheral arterial disease	≥130/80	<130/80

ASCVD indicates atherosclerotic cardiovascular disease; BP, blood pressure; CVD, cardiovascular disease; and SBP, systolic blood pressure.

Figure 12.1 BP thresholds for and goals of pharmacological therapy in patients with hypertension according to clinical conditions. Reprinted from Whelton et al. 2017 [1]. Copyright (2017), with permission from Elsevier.

	Non-specific	Specific
Morning hypertension (Exaggerated morning BP surge)	Long-acting drug	Bedtime dosing of Calcium channel blocker, RAS inhibitors, alpha-blocker
Nocturnal hypertension (Riser/non-dipper)	Long-acting drug	Diuretics (thiazides, aldosterone blocker) Bedtime dosing of RAS inhibitors, Calcium channel blocker, Alpha-blocker Sacubitril/valsartan (LCZ696) SGLT2 inhibitor

Figure 12.2 Antihypertensive treatment on morning and nocturnal hypertension. BP, blood pressure; RAS, renin-angiotensin system; SGLT2, sodium/glucose cotransporter 2.
Source: modified from Kario. 2015 [10]

Antihypertensive strategy

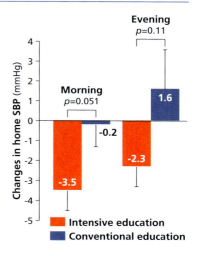

24-hour urine NaCl, g/24h	Intensive education n=51	Conventional education n=44	p-values
Baseline	8.6	8.1	0.47
After 12 weeks	6.8	8.6	0.006
Change after 12 weeks	-1.8	0.5	0.002

Figure 12.3 Effect of strict salt restriction by nutritionist on urinaly NaCl excretion and home systolic blood pressure (SBP) in medicated hypertensive patients (a prospective, randomised, open-label intervention study). *Source:* Nakano et al. 2016 [216]

Salt restriction

Salt restriction is the most effective non-pharmacological approach in hypertensive patients, regardless of antihypertensive medication. A recent intervention study demonstrated that strict salt restriction by a nutritionist lowered salt intake (estimated by 24-hour urine sodium excretion) by an additional 1.8 g/day in medicated hypertensive patients compared with conventional education by doctors. As a result, morning home SBP was marginally reduced (**Figure 12.3**) [216], and ambulatory BP was significantly reduced throughout the 24-hour period, including daytime, nighttime, and morning (**Figure 12.4**) [216]. The difference in the reduction of 24-hour systolic BP between the two groups was 7 mmHg or more.

Drug treatment

Selecting an antihypertensive drug also needs to take into account any concomitant conditions (**Figure 12.5**) [5]. Characteristics of antihypertensive drugs on the central pressure and pulse wave form (augmentation index) are shown (**Figure 12.6**) [217]. Vasodilators such as nitrates, RAS inhibitors and CCB preferentially reduce central pressure over brachial pressure.

A recent meta-analysis of data from 123 studies (n=613,815) showed that, regardless of baseline BP, a 10 mmHg reduction in SBP significantly reduced the rate of major cardiovascular events by 20%, coronary artery disease by 17%, stroke by 27%, heart failure by 28% and all-cause death by 13%. No effect of BP reduction on chronic kidney disease was identified (**Figure 12.7**) [218].

When looking at the event controlling effect of antihypertensive drug classes,

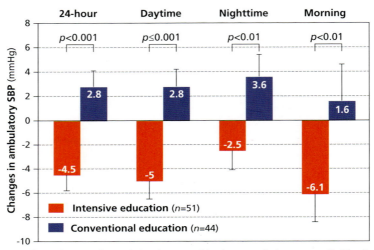

Figure 12.4 Effect of strict salt restriction by a nutritionist on ambulatory systolic blood pressure (SBP) in medicated hypertensive patients (a prospective, randomised, open-label intervention study). *Source:* Nakano et al. 2016 [216]

		CCB	ARB/ACE inhibitor	Diuretics	β-blocker
Left ventricular hypertrophy		●	●		
Congestive heart failure			●*1	●	●*1
Tachycardia		● (nonDHP)*4			●
Angina pectoris		●			●*2
Old myocardial infarction			●		●
Chronic kidney disease	Proteinuria −	●	●	●	
	Proteinuria +		●		
Chronic stroke		●	●	●	
Diabetes/MetS*3			●		
Osteoporosis				● (thiazide)	
Aspiration pneumonia			● (ACE inhibitor)		

*1: Administration should be started at a low dose, and the dose should be gradually increased carefully.
*2: Caution is needed in patients with coronary spastic angina pectoris.
*3: Metabolic syndrome. *4: Non-dihydropyridine.

Figure 12.5 JSH2014 guidelines recommendation. ACE, angiotensin-converting enzyme; ARB, angiotensin receptor blocker; CCB, calcium channel blocker. *Source:* Shimamoto, et al. 2014 [5]

	AI	Central-SBP
ACE inhibitors	↓↓	↓↓
ARBs	↓↓	↓↓
DRI	↓↓	↓↓
Calcium channel blockers	↓↓	↓↓
Beta-blockers (non-vasodilating)	↑	↔
Beta-blockers (vasodilating)	↔	↓
Thiazide diuretics	↓	↓
Nitrates	↓↓↓	↓↓↓

Figure 12.6 Comparative effect of antihypertensive drugs and nitrates on central systolic pressure and AI. ACE, angiotensin-converting enzyme; AI, augmentation index; ARB, angiotensin II receptor blocker; DRI, direct renin inhibitor; SBP, systolic blood pressure. Created based on data from Matsui et al. 2012 [217]

beta-blockers have less of a preventative effect in relation to major cardiovascular events and stroke compared with other antihypertensive drugs, while CCBs and ARBs are the most effective agents for reducing the risk of stroke (**Figure 12.8**) [218]. However, CCBs were not very effective at preventing the development of heart failure, while diuretics showed a superior preventative effect (**Figure 12.8**) [218]. The beta-blocker studies included in the meta-analysis used conventional beta-blockers from the 1980s through to the early 2000s, such as propranolol and atenolol. The effects of newer beta-blockers such as carvedilol and bisoprolol should be tested also.

	Studies	Intervention		Control		RR (95% CI) per 10 mmHg reduction in systolic blood pressure
		Events	Participants	Events	Participants	
Major cardiovascular events	55	13,209	137,319	14,068	128,259	0.80 (0.77–0.83)
Coronary heart disease	56	4,862	136,986	5,301	128,548	0.83 (0.78–0.88)
Stroke	54	4,635	136,682	5,378	128,641	0.73 (0.68–0.77)
Heart failure	43	3,284	115,411	3,760	107,440	0.72 (0.67–0.78)
Renal failure	16	890	39,888	834	39,043	0.95 (0.84–1.07)
All-cause mortality	57	9,775	138,298	9,998	129,700	0.87 (0.84–0.91)

RR per 10 mmHg reduction in systolic blood pressure
← Favours intervention   Favours control →

Figure 12.7 Event-controlling effect of a 10 mmHg reduction in systolic blood pressure. RR, relative risk.
Reprinted from the *Lancet*, Vol. 387, Ettehad D et al., Blood pressure lowering for prevention of cardiovascular disease and death: a systematic review and meta-analysis, pp.957-967., Copyright (2016), with permission from Elsevier. Ref. [218]

	Studies	Intervention		Control			RR (95% CI)
		Events	Participants	Events	Participants		
Major cardiovascular events							
ACE inhibitor	10	5,379	31,652	9,766	50,805		1.03 (1.00–1.06)
ARB	8	3,647	27,140	3,779	29,331		0.98 (0.93–1.02)
β blocker	9	2,863	25,989	2,520	27,231		1.17 (1.11–1.24)
CCB	21	7,857	63,693	12,808	82,904		0.97 (0.94–0.99)
Diuretic	11	5,830	38,353	6,782	42,410		0.97 (0.94–1.00)
Coronary heart disease							
ACE inhibitor	13	1,718	33,054	3,355	52,157		0.95 (0.90–1.01)
ARB	9	1,135	27,593	1,080	28,654		1.06 (0.98–1.15)
β blocker	11	1,579	39,864	1,544	39,966		1.03 (0.96–1.10)
CCB	25	2,955	76,465	4,576	95,725		0.98 (0.94–1.03)
Diuretic	11	2,041	40,531	2,246	43,508		1.02 (0.97–1.09)
Stroke							
ACE inhibitor	14	1,502	33,355	2,297	52,460		1.08 (1.01–1.16)
ARB	10	1,150	28,703	1,265	30,837		0.92 (0.85–0.99)
β blocker	12	1,199	40,953	989	42,170		1.24 (1.14–1.35)
CCB	26	2,245	76,768	3,470	96,026		0.90 (0.85–0.95)
Diuretic	12	1,215	41,625	1,409	45,707		0.97 (0.90–1.05)
Heart failure							
ACE inhibitor	13	1,494	32,304	2,706	50,277		0.98 (0.92–1.05)
ARB	8	1,141	26,418	1,187	26,311		0.96 (0.89–1.04)
β blocker	8	652	33,953	634	34,185		1.04 (0.93–1.16)
CCB	22	2,104	72,323	2,955	90,403		1.17 (1.11–1.24)
Diuretic	8	1,108	32,580	1,570	35,435		0.81 (0.75–0.88)
Renal failure							
ACE inhibitor	6	220	19,589	503	34,992		0.85 (0.72–0.99)
ARB	5	160	19,634	185	19,599		0.85 (0.69–1.05)
β blocker	3	526	10,417	468	10,692		1.19 (1.05–1.34)
CCB	12	787	45,024	1,022	61,117		1.02 (0.93–1.12)
Diuretic	3	220	20,992	277	23,827		0.93 (0.78–1.11)
All-cause mortality							
ACE inhibitor	14	3,321	33,104	5,865	52,263		1.01 (0.97–1.05)
ARB	11	2,546	29,282	2,638	31,404		0.99 (0.94–1.04)
β blocker	12	2,805	40,953	2,688	42,170		1.06 (1.01–1.12)
CCB	26	5,602	76,672	8,428	95,932		0.97 (0.94–1.00)
Diuretic	12	3,425	41,625	3,806	45,707		1.02 (0.97–1.06)

0.5　　　1　　　2
Class superior　　Class inferior
to pooled comparators　to pooled comparators

Figure 12.8 Event-controlling effect by antihypertensive drug class. ACE, angiotensin-converting enzyme; ARB, angiotensin receptor blockers; CCB, calcium channel blockers; RR, relative risk.
Reprinted from the *Lancet*, Vol. 387, Ettehad D et al., Blood pressure lowering for prevention of cardiovascular disease and death: a systematic review and meta-analysis, pp.957-967., Copyright (2016), with permission from Elsevier. Ref. [218]

CHAPTER 13
24-hour BP-lowering characteristics of drugs

Diuretics

Diuretics provide a sustained blood pressure (BP)-lowering effect and their effectiveness for the prevention of cardiovascular events, especially heart failure (**Figure 12.8**) [218], is well established, even in elderly hypertensive patients. Diuretics are specific drugs for reducing nighttime BP. When morning hypertension is treated using diuretics, non-dippers shift toward becoming dippers, while the dipping pattern of dippers remains unchanged or more extensively reduced [219]. This characteristic persists or is greater when diuretics are used in combination with renin-angiotensin system (RAS) inhibitors because the RAS inhibitors increase salt sensitivity (see "Evidence of RAS inhibitor-based combination" in Chapter 14).

Calcium channel blockers

Calcium channel blockers (CCBs) have potent BP-lowering effects on morning BP when their effect persists for 24 hours. The most important characteristic of the BP-lowering effects of CCBs is that the extent of BP reduction almost always depends on pre-treatment baseline BP. The higher the baseline BP, the greater the BP reduction achieved. The fact that CCBs do not lower BP extensively when baseline levels are lower means that these agents are ideally suited to reducing BP variability. In patients with a morning-surge-type of morning hypertension, higher morning BP is reduced to a greater extent while lower nighttime BP does not reduce, resulting in improved circadian rhythm. In patients with nocturnal hypertension (non-dipper/riser type), both higher nighttime BP and daytime BP could be comparably reduced by CCBs.

Amlodipine

Amlodipine, the CCB with the longest half-life, is the best drug for facilitating morning BP control when it is administered once daily in the morning. Amlodipine monotherapy was more effective than valsartan, a short-acting RAS inhibitor, in controlling 24-hour ambulatory BP and morning BP in hypertensive patients (**Figure 13.1**) [220]. In addition, the prevalence of nonreactor patients (showing no reduction in morning BP) was reduced to a greater extent in the amlodip-

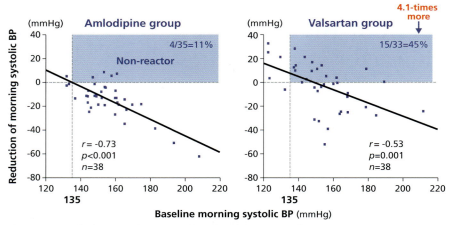

Figure 13.1 Ambulatory BP-lowering effect of amlodipine vs valsartan on morning BP. BP, blood pressure. *Source:* Eguchi et al. 2004 [220]

ine group than in the valsartan group. The higher the baseline morning BP, the greater the difference between the two agents in morning BP-lowering effect.

In a titration study of amlodipine 10 mg/day in an uncontrolled hypertensive patient treated with amlodipine 5 mg/day, similar characteristics of amlodipine were found even when the dose was increased [221]. The BP-lowering effect of amlodipine titration from 5 to 10 mg/day is highly dependent on baseline BP both for clinic BP and home BP (**Figure 13.2**) [221]. This clinic- and home-BP-lowering effect of amlodipine titration has been shown to be comparable in patients treated with amlodipine 5 mg monotherapy, amlodipine 5 mg + ARB combination, and amlodipine 5 mg + ARB + diuretics at baseline (**Figure 13.3**) [221] .

Amlodipine has been shown to significantly reduce higher daytime BP but not lower nighttime BP in extreme dippers, while in non-dippers amlodipine reduced higher nighttime BP as well as higher daytime BP (**Figure 13.4**) [222]. In a meta-analysis of Asian studies (two crossover and nine parallel controlled studies), where ten studies used amlodipine and one used nifedipine gastrointestinal therapeutic system (GITS), the ambulatory BP-lowering effect of CCBs was stronger than that of RAS inhibitors, and the slope of the regression lines was comparable for both nighttime and daytime BP measurements (**Figure 13.5**) [223].

The multicentre, multinational, randomised, double-blind, placebo-controlled X-CELLENT study of systolic BP (SBP) variability randomised hypertensive patients ($n=1,762$, aged 40–80 years) to placebo, indapamide (1.5 mg) sustained release, candesartan (8.0 mg) or amlodipine (5.0 mg) after a 4-week

24-hour BP-lowering characteristics of drugs

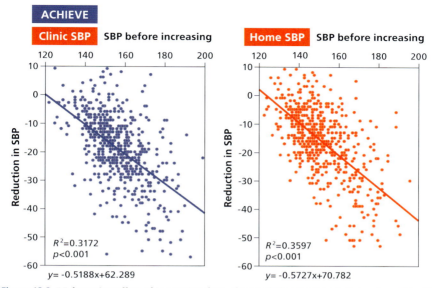

Figure 13.2 BP-lowering effect of increasing dose of once-daily use of amlodipine from 5 to 10 mg in 583 patients with uncontrolled hypertension. SBP, systolic blood pressure. Republished with permission of Bentham Science Publishers Ltd. Kario et al. 2011 [221]

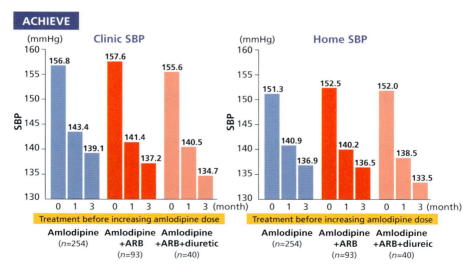

Figure 13.3 Effect of increasing dose of once daily use of amlodipine from 5 to 10 mg at the different baseline medication status in 583 patients with uncontrolled hypertension. ARB, angiotensin receptor blocker; SBP, systolic blood pressure. Republished with permission of Bentham Science Publishers Ltd. Kario et al. 2011 [221]

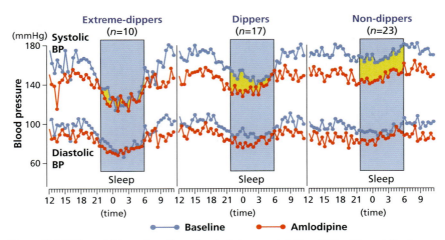

Figure 13.4 Differential lowering effect of amlodipine on nighttime BP in different dipping statuses. *Source:* Kario and Shimada. 1997 [222]

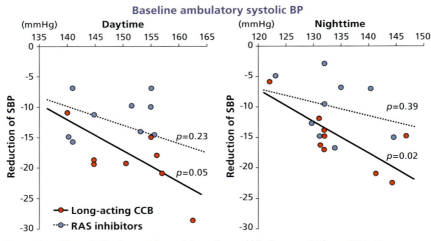

Figure 13.5 Effect of dihydropyridine calcium channel blockers on 24-hour BP in Eastern Asians. CCB, calcium channel blocker; RAS, renin-angiotensin system; SBP, systolic blood pressure. *Source:* Wang et al. 2011 [223]

selection and run-in placebo period. All treatments were given once daily in the morning for a treatment period of 12 weeks. Amlodipine was the most effective agent for reducing ambulatory BP variability (**Figure 13.6**) [224].

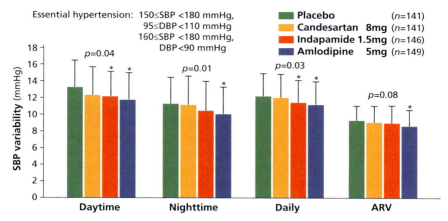

Figure 13.6 Comparisons of SBP variability after after three months of antihypertensive treatment in the X-CELLENT study, a multicentre, multinational, randomised, double-blind, placebo-controlled trial. SBP variability was assessed by the SD of 24-hour systolic blood pressure readings or read-to-read ARV mode. *p=0.05 for the subgroup comparison between subjects with treatment and those with placebo. ARV, read-to-read average real variability; BP, blood pressure; DBP, diastolic BP; SBP, systolic BP. *Source:* Zhang et al. 2011 [224]

Nifedipine

Nifedipine is a potent vasodilating drug that reduces nighttime BP and morning BP in hypertensive patients.

In the recent prospective, randomised, multicentre, open-label CARILLON study, the ambulatory BP-lowering of nifedipine controlled release (CR) (80 mg)/candesartan (8 mg) versus amlodipine (10 mg)/candesartan (8 mg) was investigated in uncontrolled hypertensive patients (n=51). Changes in 24-hour BP were comparable between the groups. The nifedipine group demonstrated a significant decrease in urinary albumin/creatinine ratio (UACR), whereas the amlodipine group demonstrated a significant decrease in N-terminal pro-brain natriuretic peptide (NT-proBNP) level. For patients with higher daytime and morning surge in SBP at the baseline, a greater reduction was found in the nifiedipine combination group than in the amlodipine group (**Figure 13.7**) [225].

In the Effects of Vasodilating vs. Sympatholytic Antihypertensives on Sleep Blood Pressure in Hypertensive Patients with Sleep Apnea Syndrome (VASSPS), a prospective, randomised, parallel-group crossover study [148], the effects of a nighttime dose of vasodilating (nifedipine CR 40 mg) versus sympatholytic (carvedilol 20 mg) antihypertensive agents on nighttime BP in 11 hypertensive obstructive sleep apnoea syndrome (OSAS) patients was evaluated using

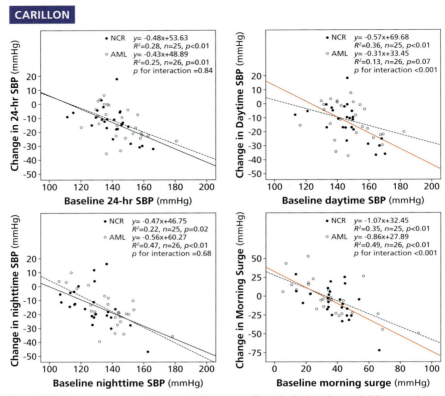

Figure 13.7 Comparison of ambulatory BP-lowering effects by higher doses of different calcium antagonists in uncontrolled hypertension: The Calcium Antagonist Controlled-Release High-Dose Therapy in Uncontrolled Refractory Hypertensive Patients (CARILLON) study. NCR = Nifedipine CR 80 mg + Candesartan 8 mg, AML = Amlodipine 10 mg + Candesartan 8 mg. SBP, systolic blood pressure. *Source:* Mizuno et al. 2017 [225]. Copyright © Skandinaviska Stiftelsen för Hjärt-och Kärlforskning, reprinted by permission of Taylor & Francis Ltd, www.tandfonline.com on behalf of Skandinaviska Stiftelsen för Hjärt-och Kärlforskning.

the recently developed trigger nighttime home BP monitor (TNP) with an oxygen-triggered function that initiates BP measurement when oxygen desaturation falls. The BP-lowering effects of nifedipine on the mean ($p<0.05$) and minimum nighttime SBP readings ($p<0.01$) as well as morning SBP ($p<0.001$) were greater than those of carvedilol (**Figure 7.30**) [148]. Nighttime systolic BP surge (difference between the hypoxia-peak SBP measured by oxygen-triggered function and SBP readings within 30 minutes before and after the peak SBP) was only significantly reduced by carvedilol ($p<0.05$). The nighttime dosing of both vasodilating and sympatholytic antihypertensive drugs is effective to reduce nighttime

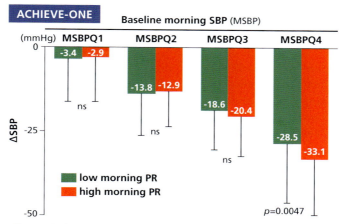

Figure 13.8 Changes in home morning BP in different status of morning BP and pulse rate at baseline by cilnidipine. Quartile of morning SBP (MSBP); MSBPQ1: MSBP <142.7 mmHg; MSBPQ2: MSBP ≥142.7 mmHg but <151.7 mmHg; MSBPQ3: MSBP ≥151.7 mmHg but <161.3 mmHg; MSBPQ4: MSBP ≥161.3 mmHg. Low morning PR: <70 bpm; high morning PR: ≥70 bpm. PR, pulse rate; SBP, systolic blood pressure. *Source:* Kario et al. 2013 [226]

BP, but with different BP-lowering profiles.

Cilnidipine

Cilnidipine, a unique *L/N-type CCB*, suppresses sympathetic activity by inhibiting N-type Ca^{2+} channel-associated norepinephrine release from peripheral sympathetic nerve endings.

The Ambulatory Blood Pressure Control and Home Blood Pressure (Morning and Evening) Lowering By N-Channel Blocker Cilnidipine (ACHIEVE-ONE) trial is a large-scale clinical study of 2,319 hypertensive patients treated with cilnidipine. After 12 weeks' therapy, both morning SBP and pulse rate (PR) self-measured at home reduced to a greater extent in patients with higher baseline morning SBP (-3.2 mmHg and -1.3 beats per minute [bpm] in the first quartile of morning SBP; -30.9 mmHg and -3.2 bpm in the fourth quartile), and also reduced both home morning PR and SBP more markedly in patients with higher baseline morning PR (0.6 bpm and -15.6 mmHg when PR was <70 bpm, and -9.7 bpm and -20.2 mmHg when PR was ≥85 bpm). When the study subjects were separated into two groups based on higher (≥70 bpm) and lower (<70 bpm) PR within each quartile of morning SBP, the highest quartile, higher PR groups had a greater morning SBP reduction (by 4.6 mmHg) than the lower PR group (**Figure 13.8**) [226]. These results suggest that cilnidipine significantly reduced

BP and PR in hypertensive patients with morning hypertension with increased sympathetic activity.

In another study, ambulatory blood pressure monitoring (ABPM) data were obtained from 615 patients and classified according to their nighttime dipping status as extreme dippers, dippers, non-dippers, or risers. Twelve weeks' treatment with cilnidipine significantly reduced 24-hour BP in all groups ($p<0.001$ vs baseline). Changes in nighttime SBP from baseline were -17.9 mmHg from 154.6 mmHg, -11.9 mmHg from 142.1 mmHg, -6.6 mmHg from 128.5 mmHg, and 0.1 mmHg from 115.8 mmHg in risers, non-dippers, dippers, and extreme dippers, respectively. Changes from baseline in nighttime SBP reduction rate were 8.2% in risers ($p<0.001$) but -7.0% in extreme dippers ($p<0.001$), while no change was observed in the nocturnal systolic BP reduction rate overall (**Figure 13.9**) [227]. Cilnidipine partially, but significantly, restored abnormal nighttime dipping status toward a normal dipping pattern in hypertensive patients.

Azelnidipine

Azelnidipine, another CCB, restored baroreflex sensitivity and significantly lowered the heart rate to reduce morning BP compared with amlodipine [215, 228].

Angiotensin-converting enzyme inhibitors

The RAS is activated in the morning and could contribute to the morning BP surge and the morning increase in cardiovascular risk. Long-acting angiotensin-converting enzyme (ACE) inhibitors have been reported to lower ambulatory BP without disruption of diurnal BP variation. Recently, it has been demonstrated that, in addition to circulating factors in the cardiovascular system, tissue RAS also exhibits diurnal variation, possibly in relation to a clock gene [100, 229]. In addition to the reduction of morning BP, morning activation of the tissue RAS could be effectively suppressed, resulting in increased protection against organ damage and cardiovascular events in hypertensive patients.

Trandolapril is an ACE inhibitor with one of the longest-acting activity profiles, and therefore BP-lowering effects, due to its lipophilic nature [230]. The effects of bedtime versus morning dosing of trandolapril on morning BP were studied. In the bedtime-administered group, pre-wakening and morning systolic BP levels were significantly decreased (**Figure 13.10**) [230]. On the other hand, the reduction of pre-wakening SBP and morning SBP did not reach statistical significance in the morning-administered group. There was no additional reduction in nighttime lowest BP in either group. Thus, bedtime administration of trandolapril appears to control morning BP without causing excessive nighttime falls in BP.

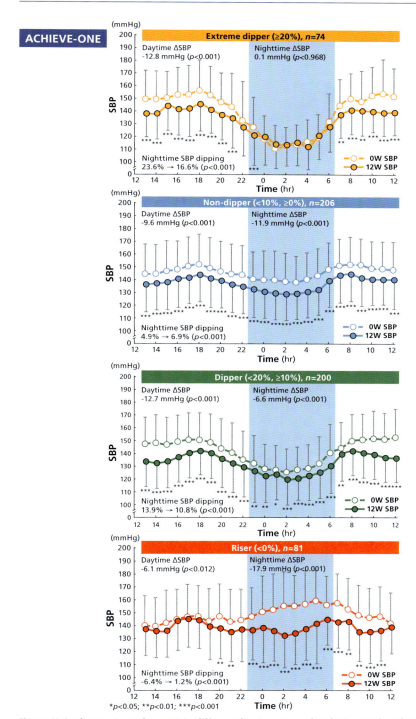

Figure 13.9 Changes in 24-hour BP in different dipping status of nighttime BP by cilnidipine. BP, blood pressure; SBP, systolic BP. *Source:* Kario et al. 2013 [227]

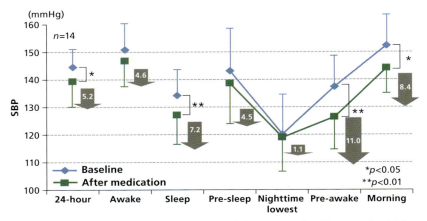

Figure 13.10 Bedtime dose of the long-acting ACE inhibitor, trandolapril on morning BP in hypertensive patients. SBP, systolic blood pressure. *Source:* Kuroda et al. 2004 [230]

Angiotensin-receptor blockers (ARBs)

As well as ACE inhibitors, previous large clinical trials have shown that ARB treatment is associated with significant suppression of organ damage and cardiovascular events. However, different ARBs have markedly different effects on morning BP levels and morning BP surge. This is due to differences in plasma half-life and the characteristics of binding to and dissociation from the vascular angiotensin-II receptor.

Valsaratan

Valsartan is a short-acting ARB, and ideally it should be used twice a day. The morning BP-lowering effect of once-daily valsartan is weaker than that of long-acting amlodipine [220].

Telmisartan

Telmisartan is a lipophilic ARB with the longest half-life (24 hours) and a meta-analysis of its clinical efficacy has demonstrated superior BP reductions to other short-acting non-lipophilic ARBs in the morning hours.

Candesartan

A prospective crossover study was performed in 73 patients with essential hypertension to compare the effects of candesartan and lisinopril on ambulatory BP and early-morning BP [231]. 24-hour ABPM was performed at baseline and for

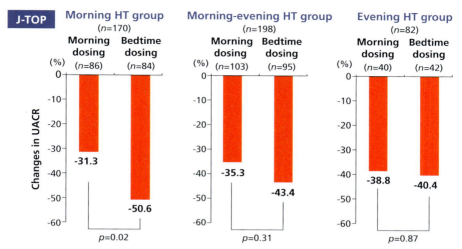

Figure 13.11 Effect of bedtime versus morning dose of candesartan on albuminuria hypertensive patients (*n*=450) (J-TOP study). HT, hypertension; UACR, urinary albumin/creatinine ratio. *Source:* Kario et al. 2010 [232]

each active treatment. Small doses of a thiazide diuretic were added as needed. The effects of both drugs on 24-hour BP were almost identical and satisfactory. Patients were classified into a morning surge group (the highest quartile of morning SBP surge; >36 mmHg) and a non-morning surge group (the remaining three quartiles of morning SBP surge); candesartan was superior to lisinopril for decreasing morning BP and morning SBP surge.

Another open-label multicentre trial, the Japan Target Organ Protection (J-TOP) study in 450 hypertensives with self-measured home SBP >135 mmHg, demonstrated that bedtime dosing of candesartan titrated by self-measured home BP was more effective for reducing albuminuria than morning dosing of an ARB in subjects with sufficiently well-controlled home BP levels both in the morning and in the evening [232]. This beneficial effect was stronger in subjects with morning-dominant hypertension with an morning and evening difference >15 mmHg for home SBP than in those with an morning and evening difference <15 mmHg (**Figure 13.11**) [232]. In the J-TOP study, even though the morning BP-lowering effect was similar between the bedtime-dosing and morning-dosing groups, bedtime dosing of an ARB may be more effective for reducing albuminuria because it may more potently suppress tissue RAS during the sleep-early morning period than morning dosing [232]. This possibility needs to be confirmed using a different class of antihypertensive drugs in the future.

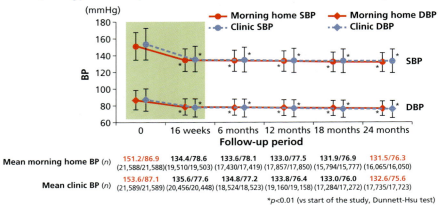

Figure 13.12 Change in clinic and morning home BP. At baseline, morning home BP was 151.2/86.9 mmHg, and clinic BP was 153.6/87.1 mmHg. Favourable BP control was maintained for 2 years. After 2 years, morning home BP was 131.5/76.3 mmHg, and clinic BP was 132.6/75.6 mmHg. *Source:* Kario et al. 2014 [21]

Olmesartan

Olmesartan is an ARB with not only potent but also persistent BP-lowering effects for 24 hours including the nocturnal and morning periods. Olmesartan can restore nighttime BP fall, as seen with diuretics and sodium restriction, possibly by enhancing daytime sodium excretion [233].

Once-daily use of olmesartan reduces morning home BP to a similar extent as clinic BP. The home BP-lowering effects of olmesartan were examined using data (n=21,341) from the Home BP measurement with Olmesartan Naive patients to Establish Standard Target blood pressure (HONEST) study, a prospective observational study of hypertensive patients. Olmesartan treatment reduced both the clinic and morning home BP levels to a similar extent, indicating that the BP-lowering effect of olmesartan persists for 24 hours (**Figure 13.12**) [21, 234]. The BP-lowering effect of olmesartan depends on the baseline BP level for both morning home and clinic BP readings (**Figure 13.13**) [235]. The slopes of BP reduction against the baseline BP were comparable between morning home and clinic SBP readings. The 16-week BP-lowering effects of olmesartan on clinic and morning home BP were comparable among hypertensive patients who were and were not on medication (**Figure 13.14**) [235].

When study subjects were stratified into the following four groups based on

HONEST

Morning home BP

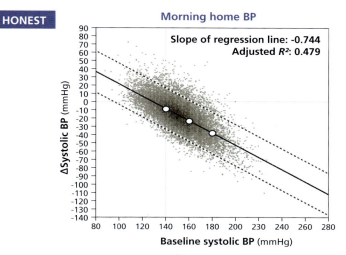

Slope of regression line: -0.744
Adjusted R^2: 0.479

Baseline BP (mmHg)	Predicted reduction (mmHg)	95% prediction interval (mmHg)	Predictive value after 16 weeks (mmHg)	Baseline dose of olmesartan (mg/day, mean ± SD)
140	-8.4	-33.5 to 16.8	131.6 (106.5 to 156.8)	18.1 ± 7.3
160	-23.2	-48.3 to 1.9	136.8 (111.7 to 161.9)	18.1 ± 6.7
180	-38.1	-63.2 to -13.0	141.9 (116.8 to 167.0)	18.9 ± 6.6

Clinic BP

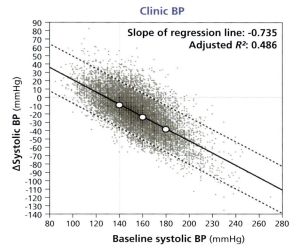

Slope of regression line: -0.735
Adjusted R^2: 0.486

Baseline BP (mmHg)	Predicted reduction (mmHg)	95% prediction interval (mmHg)	Predictive value after 16 weeks (mmHg)	Baseline dose of olmesartan (mg/day, mean ± SD)
140	-8.4	-36.6 to 20.0	131.6 (103.4 to 160.0)	18.2 ± 7.3
160	-23.1	-51.3 to 5.1	136.9 (108.7 to 165.1)	18.1 ± 6.9
180	-37.8	-66.0 to -9.6	142.2 (114.0 to 170.4)	18.3 ± 6.5

Figure 13.13 Changes in systolic blood pressure (BP) from baseline after 16 weeks of olmesartan-based treatment. *Source:* Kario et al. 2016 [235]

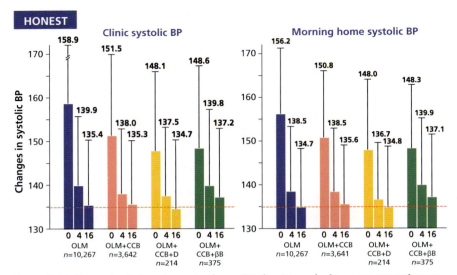

Figure 13.14 Change in clinic and morning home BP after 16-week olmesartan monotherapy or combination therapy (excluding patients who switched antihypertensive treatment). βB, beta-blocker; CCB, calcium channel blocker; D, diuretic; OLM, olmesartan. *Source:* Kario et al. 2016 [235]

baseline clinic and morning home BP readings at 16 weeks, the masked hypertension, white-coat hypertension, poorly controlled hypertension, and well-controlled hypertension groups showed changes in clinic SBP of -1.0, -15.2, -23.1, and 1.8 mmHg, respectively, and changes in morning home SBP of -12.5, 1.0, -20.3, and 2.0 mmHg, respectively (**Figure 13.15**) [234]. Thus, in real-world clinical practice, olmesartan-based treatment decreased high morning home BP or clinic BP without excessive decreases in normal morning home BP or clinic BP according to patients' BP status [236].

In addition, olmesartan may have enhanced BP-lowering effects by improving renal ischaemia in hypertensive chronic kidney disease (CKD) patients with potential increased sympathetic nerve activity. HONEST study data for hypertensive patients without antihypertensive medication at baseline were classified based on quartiles of baseline morning home SBP (MHSBP). In each group, patients were further classified based on baseline morning home pulse rate (MHPR). In the hypertensive CKD group, the patients in the fourth quartile of baseline MHSBP (≥165 mmHg) and with MHPR ≥70 bpm had a greater BP reduction (-36.9 mmHg) than those with MHPR<70 bpm (-30.4 mmHg) after 16 weeks of olmesartan treatment. An even greater BP reduction was observed in patients

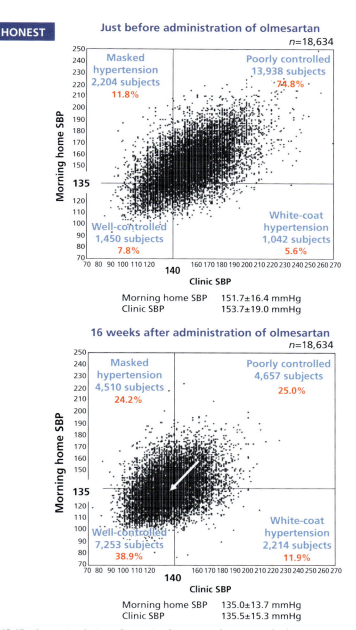

Figure 13.15 Change in clinic and morning home BP after 16-week olmesartan treatment in four groups. SBP, systolic blood pressure. *Source:* Kario et al. 2013 [234]

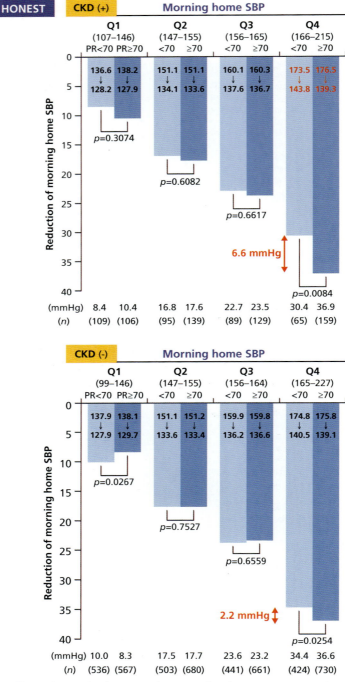

Figure 13.16 Change in morning home BP after 16 weeks' olmesartan treatment in quartiles of baseline morning BP and pulse rate. CKD, chronic kidney disease; PR, pulse rate; SBP, systolic blood pressure. *Source:* Kario et al. 2013 [237]

with versus without CKD in this group (-6.6 mmHg vs. -2.2 mmHg). (**Figure 13.16**) [237]. This shows that olmesartan was more effective in hypertensive patients with high MHSBP and MHPR ≥70 bpm, especially in those with CKD, suggesting that olmesartan may have enhanced BP-lowering effects by improving renal ischaemia in hypertensive CKD patients with potential increased sympathetic nerve activity.

Azilsartan

Azilsartan, a novel ARB, has been reported to be more effective for lowering BP than other ARBs, and to have a potent antihypertensive effect over 24 hours. A recent randomised, double-blind study of azilsartan (n=273, 20–40 mg once daily) and candesartan (n=275, 8–12 mg once daily) for 14 weeks in Japanese hypertensive patients demonstrated that azilsartan lowered nighttime BP in dippers (≥10% decrease from daytime SBP) more extensively than daytime BP in non-dippers. In addition, azilsartan reduced morning BP surge (MBPS) to a greater extent in those with exaggerated MBPS, produced a greater reduction from baseline in daytime than in nighttime SBP, and decreased daytime SBP to a significantly greater extent than candesartan (**Figure 13.17**) [238]. Thus, once daily azilsartan improved non-dipping nighttime SBP to a greater extent than candesartan in Japanese hypertensive patients.

We also compared the efficacy of azilsartan and candesartan for controlling morning SBP surges in patients with and without BP surges at baseline. In the

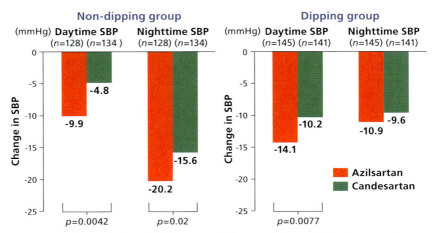

Figure 13.17 Differential effect of azilsartan on 24-hour ambulatory BP in dippers and non-dippers. *Source:* Rakugi et al. 2013 [238]. Copyright © Skandinaviska Stiftelsen för Hjärt-och Kärlforskning, reprinted by permission of Taylor & Francis Ltd, www.tandfonline.com on behalf of Skandinaviska Stiftelsen för Hjärt-och Kärlforskning.

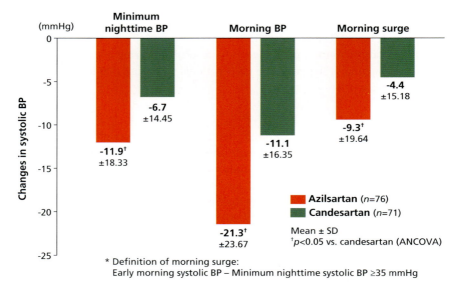

Figure 13.18 Azilsartan reduces morning BP preferentially in patients with morning surge. Of the hypertensive patients randomised into 16-week azilsartan treatment (20 mg for 8 weeks followed by an increased dose of 40 mg) and candesartan treatment groups (8 mg for 8 weeks followed by an increased dose of 12 mg), 147 patients whose morning surge was confirmed by ambulatory BP monitoring at weeks 0 and 14 were examined (double-blind controlled study). *Source:* Rakugi et al. 2014 [239]

morning surge group (n=147), defined as sleep-trough BP surge ≥35 mmHg, azilsartan significantly reduced both the sleep-trough surge and the pre-wakening surge at week 14 compared with candesartan (least squares means of the between-group differences -5.8 mmHg, p=0.0395; and -5.7 mmHg, p=0.0228, respectively) (**Figure 13.18**) [239]. Once-daily azilsartan improved the sleep-trough surge and pre-wakening surge to a greater extent than candesartan in Japanese hypertensive patients.

There are several characteristics of azilsartan that could account for its better 24-hour BP-lowering profiles compared with valsartan, including: (1) higher affinity for, and slower dissociation from, angiotensin II type-1 receptors; (2) more sustainable effect over 24 hours with a longer half-life of around 13 hours; and (3) increased lipophilicity.

In the multicentre, randomised, open-label, parallel ACS1 (Azilsartan Circadian and Sleep Pressure - the 1st) study, the nighttime BP-lowering effect of azilsartan 20 mmHg was weaker than that of amlodipine 5 mg, especially in older hypertensive patients [240]. In a post-hoc analysis, azilsartan significantly

24-hour BP-lowering characteristics of drugs

ACS1

Multivariate analysis in patients younger than 60 years

Variable	24-hour SBP ß	p-value
Azilsartan		
Intercept	12.31	0.2472
Baseline SBP	-0.18	0.0103
BMI ≥25 kg/m²	4.45	0.0208
Smoker	4.53	0.0451
Duration of hypertension <5 y	-4.86	0.0425
Drinking	ND	ND
Amlodipine		
Intercept	43.39	<0.0001
Baseline SBP	-0.42	<0.0001
Complication of type 2 diabetes mellitus	7.06	0.0028
Male	5.72	0.0010
Duration of hypertension <5 y	ND	ND
BMI ≥25 kg/m²	ND	ND

Multivariate analysis in patients older than 60 years

Variable	24-hour SBP ß	p-value
Azilsartan		
Intercept	35.60	0.0042
Baseline SBP	-0.31	0.0002
Smoker	7.25	0.0068
Duration of hypertension <5 y	-4.90	0.0189
BMI ≥25 kg/m²	ND	ND
Amlodipine		
Intercept	48.31	<0.0001
Baseline SBP	-0.47	<0.0001
Male	4.91	0.0004
BMI ≥25 kg/m²	3.68	0.0076

ND, not detectable

Figure 13.19 Variables that affect 24-hour SBP reduction by azilsartan. SBP, systolic blood pressure. BMI, body mass index. *Source:* modified from Kario et al. 2016 [241]

reduced diastolic BP compared with amlodipine in male patients aged <60 years, but amlodipine significantly reduced SBP in female patients aged ≥60 years versus azilsartan. In both younger and older hypertensive patients, shorter duration of hypertension history was significantly associated with greater 24-hour SBP reduction (**Figure 13.19**) [241].

Alpha-adrenergic blockers and beta-adrenergic blockers

Alpha-adrenergic and alpha/beta-adrenergic blockers are effective in reducing morning BP surge in hypertensive patients. In particular, nocturnal dosing of alpha-adrenergic blockers achieves peak effect in the mornings, providing greater BP reductions during these hours. In the Hypertension and Lipid Trial (HALT), bedtime administration of the alpha-1 blocker doxazosin predominantly reduced morning BP [111, 242]. In another study in hypertensive patients, morning BP and morning BP surge were shown to be reduced by bedtime dosing of doxazosin, when compared with ambulatory BP over other periods (**Figure**

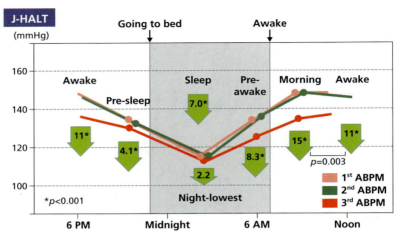

Figure 13.20 Effect of bedtime dose of doxazosin on 24-hour BP in J-HALT study (*n*=98). 1st and 2nd ABPMs were performed at the baseline, and the 3rd ABPM was performed after doxazosin therapy. *Source:* Kario et al. 2004 [71]

13.20) [71]. In addition, the alpha-adrenergic morning BP surge was defined as the reduction of morning BP surge by doxazosin. The alpha-adrenergic morning BP surge was closely associated with multiple silent cerebral infarcts (10 mmHg increase: odds ratio (OR) = 1.96, *p*=0.006), independent of age, MBPS, 24-hour SBP and other cofactors. **Figure 5.7** shows the scatter plots of morning BP surge and alpha-adrenergic morning BP surge, indicating that the slope of the regression lines was significantly different between those patients with versus without multiple silent cerebral infarcts [71]. This indicates that morning BP surge, particularly that which is dependent on alpha-adrenergic activity, is closely associated with advanced silent hypertensive cerebrovascular disease in elderly patients.

In addition, an open-label multicentre trial, the Japan Morning Surge-1 (JMS-1) study of 611 medicated patients with morning hypertension (self-measured morning SBP >135 mmHg) demonstrated that bedtime dosing of doxazosin on the top of baseline antihypertensive medication significantly reduced morning BP and albuminuria [243]. In this study, UACR decreased along with morning BP. However, decreases in UACR were independent of the reduction of morning BP. In addition, bedtime dosing of doxazosin improved the HOMA index, a measure of insulin resistance, independently of the reduction in morning BP [244]. In this study, doxazosin significantly restored orthostatic hypertension and the reduction in orthostatic BP increase was significantly associated with the reduction in UACR independently of sitting clinic and home BP read-

24-hour BP-lowering characteristics of drugs

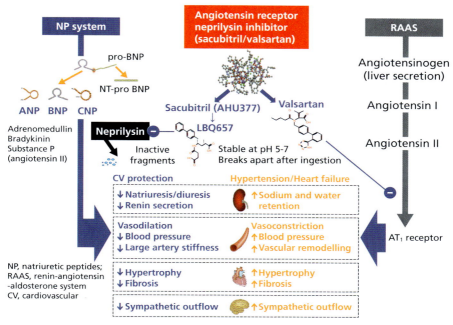

Figure 13.21 Mechanism of sacubitril/valsartan on cardiovascular system. *Source:* Kario. 2018 [245]. Reprinted by permission from Springer Nature.

ings (**Figure 9.27**) [191].

There is no evidence that beta-adrenergic blockers specifically reduce morning BP surge. Bedtime dosing of metoprolol, a pure beta-blocker, was inferior to carvedilol, a vasodilating beta-blocker with partial alpha-adrenergic blocking activity, for reducing morning BP [62]. In addition, bedtime dosing of carvedilol was effective for reducing both nighttime BP surge and nighttime heart rate in hypertensive patients with OSAS (**Figure 7.30**) [148]. Furthermore, the cardioprotective effects of beta-adrenergic blockers are well validated in hypertensive patients with coronary artery disease (CAD) and/or heart failure.

Sacubitril/valsartan

Sacubitril/valsartan (LCZ696) is a first-in-class, angiotensin receptor neprilysin inhibitor (ARNI) that inhibits neprilysin and the angiotensin (AT1) receptor, and has potential synergistic activity for cardiovascular protection (**Figure 13.21**) [245].

The recent PARADIGM-HF clinical trial demonstrated that this new agent

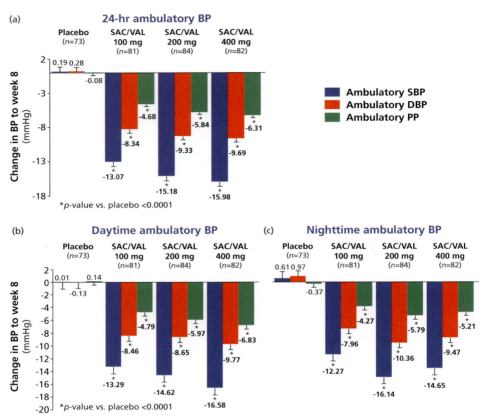

Figure 13.22 Effect of SAC/VAL on 24-hr BP in Asian hypertensive patients. (a) SAC/VAL showed a statistically significant reduction in 24-hour ambulatory BP and PP at endpoint compared with placebo. SAC/VAL showed a statistically significant reduction in (b) daytime and (c) nighttime ambulatory BP and PP at endpoint compared with placebo. BP, blood pressure; DBP, diastolic BP; PP, pulse pressure; SAC/VAL, sacubitril/valsartan; SBP, systolic BP. *Source:* Kario et al. 2014 [249].

was superior to ACE inhibitors for improving the prognosis of patients with heart failure. These results led to the drug being included in clinical practice guidelines for the management of heart failure with reduced ejection fraction (EF). [246]. In addition, sacubitril/valsartan is a drug not only for the treatment of heart failure but it is also likely to be a useful antihypertensive drug [247].

An ABPM study demonstrated that sacubitril/valsartan effectively reduced 24-hour BP, including nighttime BP, in both Western and Asian patients with hypertension [248, 249]. In the first randomised, double-blind, placebo-con-

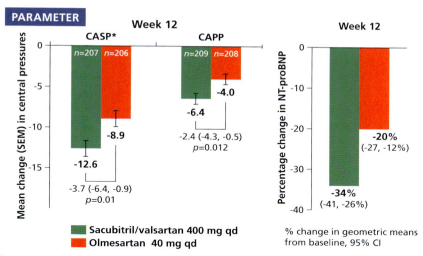

Figure 13.23 Change in central aortic systolic blood pressure (CASP) and central aortic pulse pressure (CAPP) and plasma NT-proBNP level after 12-week sacubitril/valsartan versus olmesartan therapy: The PARAMETER study - multicentre, randomised, double-blind, active-controlled study in elderly patients with isolated systolic hypertension (n=454, ≥60 years, systolic BP ≥150 mmHg, pulse pressure ≥60 mmHg). *CASP was the primary efficacy. BP, blood pressure; NT-proBNP, N-terminal pro-brain natriuretic peptide; SEM, standard error of mean. *Source:* Williams et al. 2017 [256]

trolled study of LCZ696 in Asia, hypertensive patients (n=389) were randomised to receive LCZ696 100 mg (n=100), 200 mg (n=101), or 400 mg (n=96), or placebo (n=92) for eight weeks [249]. Significant reductions in 24-hour daytime and nighttime ambulatory BP levels were seen with all doses of LCZ696 compared with placebo (p<0.0001) (**Figure 13.22**). LCZ696 was well tolerated and no cases of angioedema were reported. Data suggest that Asian patients with hypertension may respond particularly well to this agent. [250-255]

Sacubitril/valsartan significantly restores 24-hour central haemodynamics in the elderly with hypertension. A recent mechanistic study, PARAMETER, demonstrated that sacubitril/valsartan was superior to ARB monotherapy for reducing central aortic systolic pressure (primary endpoint) as well as for central aortic pulse pressure (secondary endpoint) (**Figure 13.23**) and nighttime BP (**Figure 13.24**) [256] preferentially. This may be due in part to the increases in atrial and brain natriuretic peptides with sacubitril/valsartan that would reduce circulating volume [256]. Therefore, sacubitril/valsartan could be effective in non-dippers with true resistant hypertension. Sacubitril/valsartan was also effective for reducing levels of NT-proBNP (**Figure 13.23**) [256], as found in heart

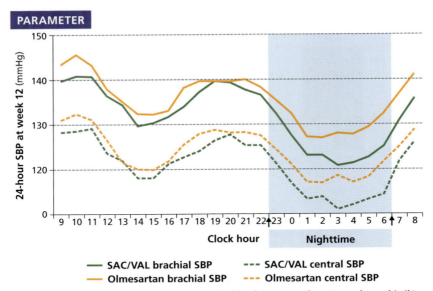

Figure 13.24 24-hour brachial and central systolic blood pressure after 12-week sacubitril/valsartan (400 mg) vs olmesartan (40 mg) therapy: The PARAMETER study – multicentre, randomised, double-blind, active-controlled study in elderly patients with isolated systolic hypertension (n=454, ≥60 years, systolic BP ≥150 mmHg, pulse pressure ≥60 mmHg). BP, blood pressure; SAC/VAL, sacubitril/valsartan; SBP, systolic BP. *Source:* Williams et al. 2017 [256]

failure patients with preserved left ventricular EF [257].

Aging increases arterial stiffness and salt sensitivity as well as decreasing glomerular filtration. Age-related increases in arterial stiffness cause systolic hypertension with higher pulse pressure and increased central pressure (structural hypertension), while age-related increases in salt sensitivity cause hypertension with diminished dipping in nighttime BP (non-dipper/riser pattern) (salt-sensitive hypertension). Structural and/or salt-sensitive hypertension phenotypes are likely to develop drug-uncontrolled (resistant) hypertension and heart failure with preserved EF. Sacubitril/valsartan restored this age-related cardiovascular change, resulting in effective prevention of heart failure (**Figure 13.25**) [245].

Considering these mechanisms, sacubitril/valsartan may be an attractive therapeutic agent to treat the elderly with age-related hypertension phenotypes such as drug-uncontrolled (resistant) hypertension characterised as systolic (central) hypertension (structural hypertension) and/or nocturnal hypertension (salt-sensitive hypertension) (**Figure 13.26**). These are high-risk hypertension phenotypes that are prone to develop heart failure with preserved EF and CKD.

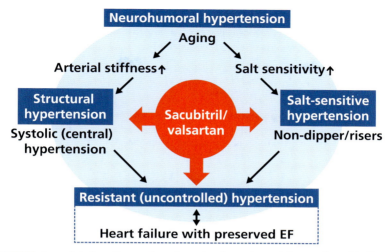

Figure 13.25 Age-related continuum from hypertension to heart failure and sacubitril/valsartan. Aging increases arterial stiffness and salt sensitivity as well as decreasing glomerular filtration. Age-related increase in arterial stiffness develop systolic hypertension with higher pulse pressure and increased central pressure (structural hypertension), while age-related increases in salt sensitivity develop hypertension with diminished dipping in nighttime blood pressure (non-dipper/riser pattern) (salt-sensitive hypertension). Structural and/or salt-sensitive hypertension phenotypes are likely to develop drug-uncontrolled (resistant) hypertension and heart failure with preserved ejection fraction (EF). The sacubitril/valsartan restored this age-related cardiovascular change, resulting in effective prevention of heart failure. *Source:* Kario. 2018 [245]. Reprinted by permission from Springer Nature.

SGLT2 inhibitor

Recent large randomised clinical trials have shown that inhibitors of sodium/glucose cotransporter 2 (SGLT2i) significantly reduce the rate of adverse cardiovascular outcomes (especially heart failure (HF)) and preserve renal function in patients with type 2 diabetes at high cardiovascular risk [258-260]. Several potential novel pathways associated with the cardiovascular effects of SGLT2i have been suggested by clinical and mechanistic studies. In addition to body weight reduction, risk factors such as glycaemia, BP, insulinaemia, and oxidative stress are reported to be improved by SGLT2 inhibition. However, the improvement of these factors does not completely explain the beneficial effects of SGLT2i. A recent Phase III study and a meta-analysis have shown that SGLT2i significantly reduces 24-hour ambulatory BP, with significant reductions in both daytime and nighttime BP [261]. It is now proposed that control of nocturnal hypertension is a particularly efficient haemodynamic mechanism underlying the beneficial effect of SGLT2i in reducing heart failure in diabetic patients [262].

1. Elderly hypertension (structural hypertension with increased pulse pressure ≥60 mmHg)

2. Central hypertension (central systolic BP ≥130 mmHg)

3. Nocturnal hypertension (salt-sensitive, non-dipper/riser)

4. Drug-resistant (uncontrolled) hypertension

5. Asian hypertension (higher salt sensitivity and higher salt intake)

Figure 13.26 Five target hypertension phenotypes of sacubitril/valsartan. *Source:* Kario. 2018 [245]. Reprinted by permission from Springer Nature.

The time-course of the haemodynamic consequences of SGLT2 inhibition in a 41-year old diabetic man with resistant hypertension, obstructive sleep apnoea, and shortness of breath who was newly initiated on the SGLT2i, canagliflozin are detailed. He had been previously treated with an ARB, a CCB, thiazides, and a dipeptidyl peptidase-4 inhibitor (candesartan 8 mg, hydrochlorothiazide 6.25 mg, and sitagliptin 25 mg). ABPM showed markedly elevated 24-hour BP, daytime, and nighttime BP levels at baseline (**Figure 13.27**) [262], and simultaneous nighttime pulse oximetry revealed mild/moderate sleep apnoea, with an oxygen desaturation index (ODI) of 12.7/h (**Figure 13.27**) [262]. After two months of daily 100 mg canagliflozin treatment, the patient's 24-hour BP, particularly nighttime BP, were significantly reduced, the ODI decreased markedly from to 2.6/h (**Figure 13.27**) [262], HbA_{1c} fell from 7.3% to 6.5%, and body weight decreased by 3.1 kg. Of note, daytime BP decreased by 3% whereas nighttime mean BP decreased to a greater extent (14%). Six months after canagliflozin initiation, daytime BP was 5% lower than at baseline and nighttime BP was still reduced by 12% compared with baseline. Serial cardiac MRIs demonstrated that the patient's left ventricular (LV) end-diastolic volume and stroke volume were decreased two months after initiation of canagliflozin, but had returned to baseline values at six months (**Figure 13.28**) [262]. Despite the transient nature of these haemodynamic changes, LV mass was consistently and progressively reduced (by 5% and 15% at 2 and 6 months, respectively), along with increased arterial dispensability of the ascending aorta (indexed as the percent increase of the cross-sectional area, as well as the percent increase in area per 1 mmHg of central pulse pressure as estimated by a SphygmoCor BP measurement device) (**Figure 13.29**) [262].

Figure 13.30 conceptualises the impact of nocturnal hypertension on HF, and suggests the decrease in nocturnal LV strain as a possible synergistic mechanism of SGLT2i-associated improvement [262]. The initial effect of an SGLT2i is a reduction in LV preload due to a reduction in the circulating volume (which

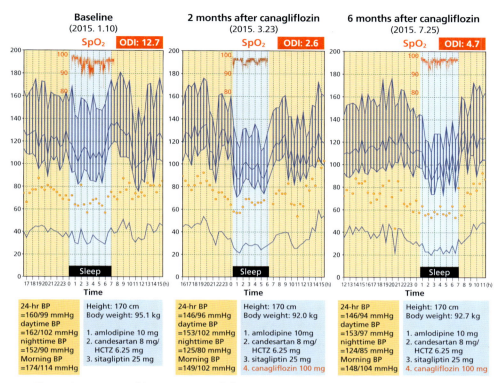

Figure 13.27 Nocturnal hypertension in diabetes: Potential target of sodium/glucose cotransporter 2 (SGLT2) inhibition. Change in the 24-hour ambulatory BP profile during daily treatment with 100 mg canagliflozin in the patient, a 41-year old diabetic man with resistant hypertension and obstructive sleep apnoea. After the baseline evaluation (left), canagliflozin was given for six months. ABPM was carried out at 2 months (middle) and 6 months (right) after the initiation of canagliflozin. ABPM, ambulatory blood pressure monitoring.
Source: Kario et al. 2018 [262]

resulted in a mean 3% increment in haematocrit sustained throughout the 3 years of treatment with empagliflozin in the EMPA-REG OUTCOME trial)[258]. In addition, a decrease in LV mass with an amelioration of aortic stiffness reduces LV afterload. The impact of higher BP on wall stress is stronger during sleep, because the supine position increases venous return from the lower body, LV wall stress being determined by both LV pressure and LV diameter (i.e., Laplace law). Thus, the nighttime BP-lowering effect of SGLT2 inhibition would be synergistic with the reduction in circulating volume. In addition, the fluid shift from the lower body to the upper body during sleep worsens obstructive sleep apnoea by increasing intrathoracic pressure. The effect of SGLT2 inhibition to contract

	Baseline (2015. 1.10)		2 months after canagliflozin (2015. 3.23)		6 months after canagliflozin (2015. 7.25)	

LV			LV		LV	
LV Ejection Fraction	72%		LV Ejection Fraction	69%	LV Ejection Fraction	69%
Stroke Volume	93.0 mL		Stroke Volume	69.9 mL	Stroke Volume	85.7 mL
End-Diastolic Vol Index	64.1 mL/m²		End-Diastolic Vol Index	50.3 mL/m²	End-Diastolic Vol Index	60.9 mL/m²
End-Systolic Vol Index	17.9 mL/m²		End-Systolic Vol Index	15.6 mL/m²	End-Systolic Vol Index	18.7 mL/m²
End-Diastolic Volume	129 mL		End-Diastolic Volume	101 mL	End-Diastolic Volume	124 mL
End-Systolic Volume	36.1 mL		End-Systolic Volume	31.3 mL	End-Systolic Volume	38.0 mL
Heart Rate	79 bpm		Heart Rate	92 bpm	Heart Rate	63 bpm
Mass ED	190 g		Mass ED	180 g	Mass ED	161 g
Peak Filling Rate	384 mL/s		Peak Filling Rate	513 mL/s	Peak Filling Rate	285 mL/s
Peak Ejection Rate	616 mL/s		Peak Ejection Rate	586 mL/s	Peak Ejection Rate	502 mL/s
Cardiac Output	7.3 L/min		Cardiac Output	6.4 L/min	Cardiac Output	5.4 L/min
Cardiac Index	3.65 L/min/m²		Cardiac Index	3.19 L/min/m²	Cardiac Index	2.66 L/min/m²
Stroke Volume Index	46.2 mL/m²		Stroke Volume Index	34.7 mL/m²	Stroke Volume Index	42.2 mL/m²
Mass	190 g		Mass	180 g	Mass	161 g
Mass ES	174 g		Mass ES	169 g	Mass ES	180 g
End Diastolic Epicardial Volume	310 mL		End Diastolic Epicardial Volume	273 mL	End Diastolic Epicardial Volume	277 mL
End-Systolic Epicardial Volume	202 mL		End-Systolic Epicardial Volume	192 mL	End-Systolic Epicardial Volume	210 mL
Standard Deviation Heart Rate	0 bpm		Standard Deviation Heart Rate	0 bpm	Standard Deviation Heart Rate	0 bpm

Figure 13.28 Cardiac MRI showing a significant reduction in stroke volume and end-diastolic volume after 2 months of daily 100 mg canagliflozin treatment. At 6 months after the initiation of treatment, these values had returned to the baseline levels. The LV mass was progressively reduced at 2 and 6 months. *Source:* Kario et al. 2018 [262]

extracellular fluid volume reduces intrathoracic pressure. Better control of nocturnal hypertension acts synergistically with fluid offload to decrease nighttime LV strain. In the longer term, this may lead to protection against both HF and renal failure, especially in diabetic patients with obstructive sleep apnoea and/or individuals with salt-sensitivity augmented by RAS inhibitors.

As a result of improved aortic stiffness, SGLT2i may be effective agents for treating systemic haemodynamic atherothrombotic syndrome (SHATS) . Clinical trials investigating the effects of SGLT2i therapy on BP variability and arterial stiffness in diabetic hypertensive patients would be of great interest.

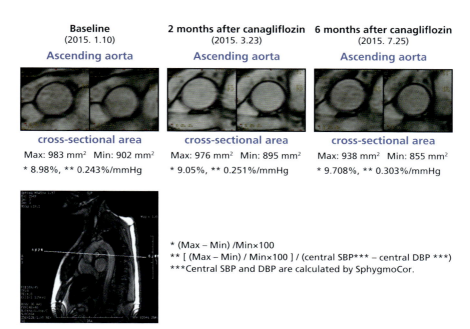

Figure 13.29 Aortic MRI demonstrating that the percent change in the ascending aortic cross-sectional area of 8.98% (0.243%/mmHg, when divided by the central pulse pressure) at baseline was significantly increased to 9.05% at 2 months and 9.78% at 6 months after the initiation of treatment with 100 mg canagliflozin. Source: Kario et al. 2018 [262]

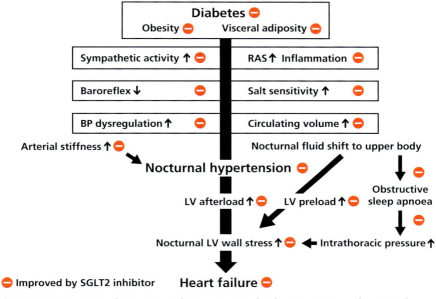

Figure 13.30 Synergistic decrease in nighttime LV strain by the management of nocturnal hypertension with reduced fluid retention as a possible mechanism of SGLT2i-associated cardiovascular protection in diabetes. BP, blood pressure; LV, left ventricle; RAS, renin-angiotensin system; SGLT2, sodium/glucose cotransporter 2. Source: Kario et al. 2018 [262]

CHAPTER 14

Combination therapy: Home and ambulatory BP-profile-based combination strategy

First-line therapy

An age-related approach for the management of hypertension would be reasonable. In younger hypertensive patients is characterised by obesity, multiple metabolic risk factors, and an increase in the activity of sympathetic nervous system and renin-angiotensin system (RAS) (metabolic neurohumoral hypertension), while in older patients systolic hypertension is characterised by the arterial stiffness of large and small arteries (structural hypertension), and salt-sensitivity. Thus, it is reasonable to use an RAS inhibitor at first for younger hypertensive patients, particularly those with metabolic risk factors, while a calcium channel blocker (CCB) is reasonable for older hypertensive patients, especially those with the characteristics of structural hypertension (**Figure 14.1**). Age-related first-line therapy recommendations are also included in the British Hypertension Society (**Figure 14.2**) [263] and the NICE guidelines.

Second-line therapy

To choose a second-line agent, it may be practical to consider the blood pressure (BP) variability profile separately for the arterial stiffness type characterised by increased BP variability, such as excess morning BP surge (MBPS), day-by-day home BP variability, visit-to-visit BP variability, and for the volume retention type characterised by non-dipper or riser nighttime BP patterns (**Figure 14.3**) [264].

Arterial stiffness type

For elderly patients with arterial stiffness type, exhibiting exaggerated BP variability, long-acting CCB in combination with an RAS inhibitor is the most effective drug for reducing BP and BP variability. The higher the baseline BP, the greater the BP-lowering effect to be expected from the CCB as described in Chapter 13. This property of CCB remains significant even when used in combination therapy with an RAS inhibitor. This ability of CCB to reduce BP variability is stronger at higher doses. The maximum dose of a long-acting CCB minimises the exaggerated morning BP surge because CCBs can decrease the highest morning BP more extensively than other drugs without causing any reduction in the lowest

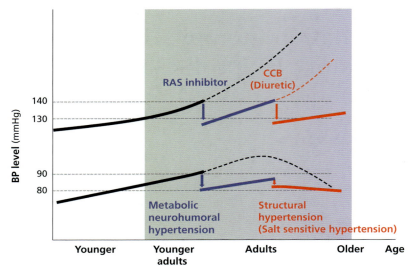

Figure 14.1 Age-related antihypertensive medication strategy. RAS inhibitor for younger metabolic (neurohumoral) hypertension, and CCB for older structural hypertension. BP, blood pressure; CCB, calcium channel blocker; RAS, renin-angiotensin system. *Source:* Kario K. *Essential Manual on Perfect 24-hour Blood Pressure Management from Morning to Nocturnal Hypertension: Up-to-date for Anticipation Medicine*. Wiley, 2018.

nighttime BP. To reduce BP variability, a combination of a long-acting CCB and a long-acting angiotensin-receptor blocker (ARB) is effective (**Figure 14.4**) [265].

Volume retention type

The non-dipping of nighttime BP is closely associated with increased circulating volume retention. Diuretics are the most effective class of antihypertensives for changing non-dipping nighttime BP to a dipping pattern, as described in Chapter 13. This property of diuretics is augmented when used in combination with RAS inhibitors. As salt sensitivity is already increased in hypertensive patients treated with RAS inhibitors, small doses of diuretics may be sufficient to reduce nighttime BP when combined with RAS inhibitors. Particularly in Asians, who are characterised by both increased salt sensitivity and salt intake, a small dose of diuretics in combination with RAS inhibitors is effective for reducing 24-hour BP levels, especially for nighttime BP [140]. As described in Chapter 13, sacubitril/valsartan and inhibitors of sodium/glucose cotransporter 2 (SGLT2i) are effective for this type (**Figure 14.4**) [265].

For patients with heart disease (coronary artery disease [CAD], heart failure), a beta-blocker is recommended in combination with RAS inhibitors at this stage.

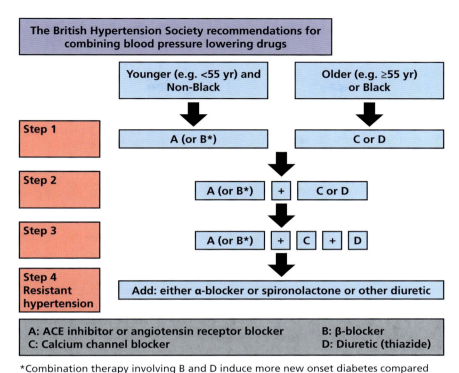

Figure 14.2 Strategy of antihypertensive medication. *Source:* Williams et al. 2004 [263]

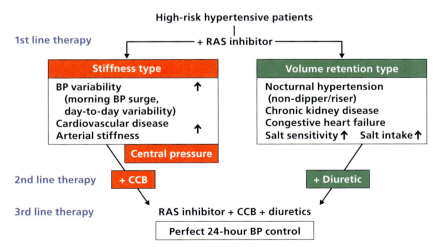

Figure 14.3 Home and ambulatory BP-based combination strategies for high-risk hypertension. CCB, calcium channel blocker; RAS, renin-angiotensin system. *Source:* Kario. 2010 [264]

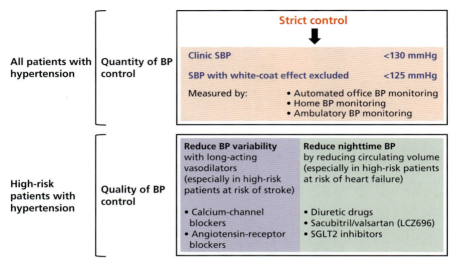

Figure 14.4 Precision medicine for the management of hypertension. The strict BP control (quantity of BP control) guided by white-coat effect excluded BP <125 mmHg, as well as clinic BP <130 mmHg for all the hypertensive patients. The perfect 24-hour BP control considering BP variability and nocturnal hypertension (quality of BP control) is recommended for high-risk patients with hypertension. Calcium-channel blockers and angiotensin receptor blockers may be protective against stroke via BP variability, while the drugs reducing circulating volume such as diuretics, sacubitril/valsartan, or SGLT2 inhibitors may be protective against heart failure via reducing nighttime blood pressure. BP, blood pressure; SBP, systolic BP; SGLT2, sodium-glucose cotransporter 2. *Source:* Kario. 2016 [265]

Third-line therapy

For uncontrolled hypertension, if therapy with an RAS inhibitor + CCB or RAS inhibitor + diuretics is not effective, triple combination therapy consisting of a CCB, RAS inhibitor and diuretics should be started (**Figure 14.3**) [264].

Evidence of RAS inhibitor-based combination

There are a lot of combination therapies and clinically available combination pills. RAS inhibitor-based combination is the most popular.

In the Japan-Combined Treatment with Olmesartan and a Calcium Channel Blocker versus Olmesartan and Diuretics Randomised Efficacy (J-CORE) study that investigated the effect of an ARB–CCB combination versus an ARB–diuretics combination on central pressure and ambulatory BP profile, the olmesartan (OLM)–azelnidipine (AZL) combination more extensively reduced central aor-

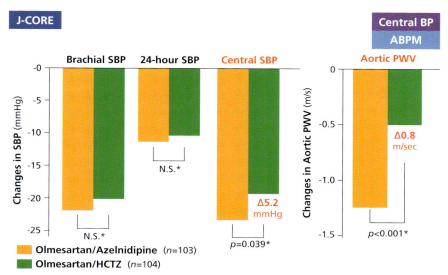

Figure 14.5 Changes in brachial, ambulatory and central SBP. BP, blood pressure; HCTZ, hydrochlorothiazide; PWV, pulse wave velocity; SBP, systolic BP. Created based on data from Matsui et al. 2009 [266]

tic pressure and aortic pulse wave velocity (PWV) (measured by SpygmoCore) than OLM–hydrochlorothiazide (HCTZ), even when brachial BP was comparably reduced in the two groups [155, 266] (**Figure 14.5**). In addition, the OLM–AZL combination more effectively reduced morning home SBP variability (SD) than the OLM–HCTZ combination, although mean home SBP was reduced to a similar extent in both groups (**Figure 14.6**) [169]. This reduction in home BP variability was correlated with the reduction in PWV.

On the other hand, even when the brachial clinic and 24-hour BP were reduced to the same extent in the two arms, nighttime BP was preferentially reduced in the OLM–HCTZ arm and daytime BP was preferentially reduced in the OLM–AZL arm, resulting in more significant reduction of nighttime BP dipping and urinary albumin/creatinine ratio (UACR) with OLM-HCTZ than with OLM-AZL (**Figure 14.7**) [267]. Even when a low dose of HCTZ (6.25 mg/day) was added to candesartan therapy, nighttime BP was significantly and more extensively reduced than daytime BP (**Figure 14.8**) [268]. Add-on therapy with eplerenone, an aldosterone antagonist, also reduced nighttime BP more extensively than daytime BP in uncontrolled hypertensive patients who are treated with ARB (**Figure 14.9**) [269].

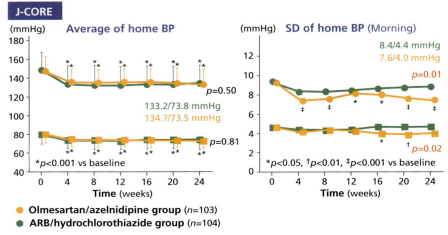

Figure 14.6 Differential effect of ARB (angiotensin receptor blocker) combinations with CCB (calcium channel blocker) or diuretics on average and standard deviation (SD) of morning home BP in hypertensive patients. BP, blood pressure. *Source:* Matsui et al. 2012 [169]

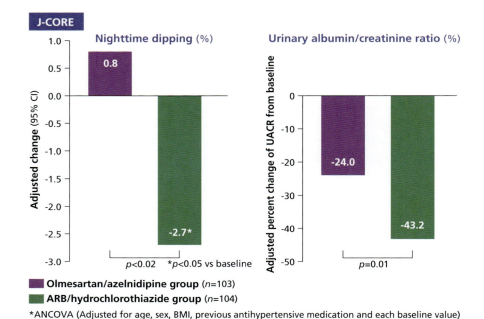

*ANCOVA (Adjusted for age, sex, BMI, previous antihypertensive medication and each baseline value)

Figure 14.7 Changes in nighttime dipping and urinary albumin/creatinine ratio (UACR). ARB, angiotensin II receptor blocker. Created based on data from Matsui et al. 2011 [267]

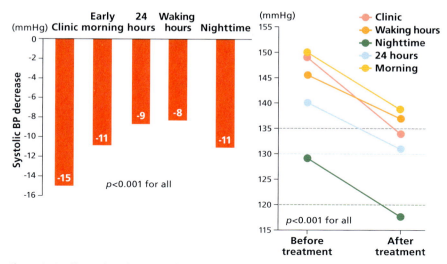

Figure 14.8 Effects of candesartan + hydrochlorothiazide (HCTZ) 6.25 mg on 24-hour BP (*n*=40). *Source:* Eguchi et al. 2010 [268]

In the ALPHABET study, an open-label multicentre trial, the effects of losartan/HCTZ fixed combination therapy and high-dose amlodipine monotherapy were investigated. After 8 weeks, losartan/HCTZ and high-dose amlodipine had similar effects on clinic, home, and ambulatory (24-hour, daytime, and nighttime) BP control and brain natriuretic peptide (BNP) reduction, whereas losartan/HCTZ was associated with greater reductions in UACR (**Figure 14.10**) [270].

In a prospective, randomised, multicentre, open-label ambulatory blood pressure monitoring (ABPM) study, 105 elderly patients with uncontrolled hypertension medicated with amlodipine 5 mg were randomly allocated to aliskiren (150–300 mg)/amlodipine (5 mg) (ALI/AML, *n*=53) or high-dose amlodipine (10 mg) (h-dAML, *n*=52). After 16 weeks' treatment, both groups showed a similar reduction in mean 24-hour, daytime, and nighttime BPs and brachial-ankle PWV (baPWV) [271]. The UACR reduction was significantly greater in the ALI/AML group. In addition, improvement of brachial flow-mediated dilation (FMD) was found in the ALI/AML group (from 2.6% to 3.7%, *p*=0.001) but not in the h-dAML group, while nitroglycerin-mediated vasodilation (NMD) did not change in either group [272]. However, ALI/AML was significantly less effective in reducing early-morning BP (*p*=0.002) and morning BP surge (*p*=0.001) compared with h-dAML (**Figure 14.11**) [271].

The ACROBAT study, a multicentre, prospective, randomised, open-label clinical trial, investigated differences in the 3-month effect of morning versus

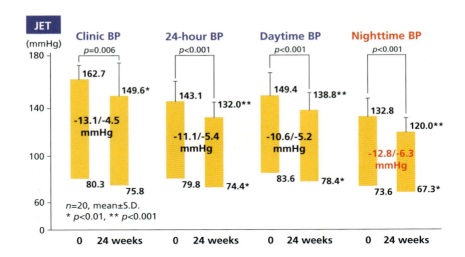

Figure 14.9 Changes in clinic and 24-hour BP levels in ARB (angiotensin receptor blocker)-treated uncontrolled hypertensive patients after eplerenone add-on treatment ($n=20$) Jichi-Eplerenone Treatment (JET) study. *Source:* Yano et al. 2011 [269]

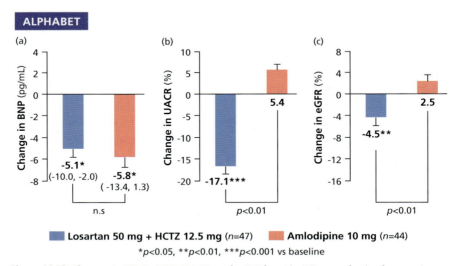

Figure 14.10 Changes in NT-ProBNP, UACR, and eGFR by strict BP control using losartan/HCTZ combination and high-dose amlodipine (ALPHABET study). BP, blood pressure; eGFR, estimate glomerular filtration rate; HCTZ, hydrochlorothiazide; NT-proBNP, N-terminal pro-brain natriuretic peptide; UACR, urinary albumin/creatinine ratio. Created based on data from Fukutomi et al. 2012 [270]

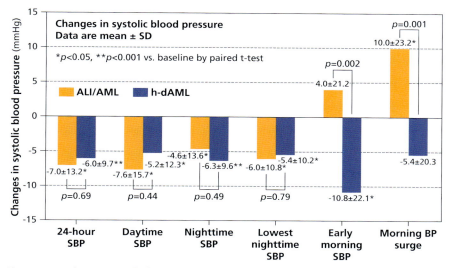

Figure 14.11 Changes in ambulatory blood pressure. ALI/AML, aliskiren/amlodipine; h-dAML, high-dose amlodipine; BP, blood pressure; SBP, systolic blood pressure. Created based on data from Mizuno et al. 2016 [271]

bedtime administration of telmisartan 40 mg/amlodipine 5 mg combination tablets on ambulatory and home BP in hypertensive patients with paroxysmal atrial fibrillation. During treatment, clinic, home, 24-hour, nighttime, pre-wakening, and morning BP were significantly reduced, and antihypertensive effects were similar regardless of the timing of the drug administration. The SD of day-by-day home systolic BP (SBP) and the maximum home SBP were also significantly reduced, and these effects were similar regardless of the treatment timing (**Figure 14.12**) [273]. This indicated that the BP-lowering effect of the combination of both long-acting drugs persisted for 24-hours [273].

In the CPET study (ChronotheraPy for ambulatory cEnTral pressure), a 16-week prospective, multicentre, randomised, open-label, crossover, noninferiority clinical trial, the effects of morning and bedtime administration of valsartan/amlodipine combination therapy (80/5 mg) on nighttime brachial and central BP measured by ABPM capable of measuring ambulatory central pressure in patients with hypertension were compared. Twenty-three patients (mean 68.0 years) were studied. The difference in nighttime brachial SBP between morning and bedtime administrations of valsartan/amlodipine was -3.2 mmHg (**Figure 14.13**), and the two-sided 95% confidence interval [CI] ranged from -6.8 to 0.4 mmHg. The difference in nighttime central SBP was -4.0 mmHg (95% CI, -7.6 to -0.4 mmHg). The upper limit of the 95% CI was below the margin of 3.0 mmHg

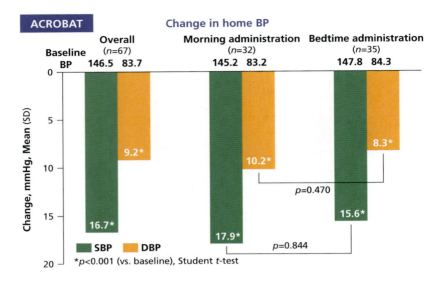

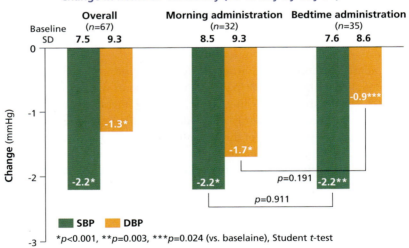

Figure 14.12 Three-month home BP-lowering effect of different time of telmisartan 40 mg/amlodipine 5 mg dosing in hypertensive patients with paroxysmal atrial fibrillation. The ARB and CCB longest combination treatment on ambulatory and home BP in hypertension with atrial fibrillation multicenter study on time of dosing (ACROBAT) study. ARB, angiotensin-receptor blocker; BP, blood pressure; CCB, calcium channel blocker; DBP, diastolic BP; SBP, systolic BP; SD, standard deviation. Created based on data from Kario et al. 2016 [273]

CPET

- Hypertensive patients (*n*=23, mean 68.0 years)
- A 16-week prospective, randomised, open-label, **crossover**, **non-inferiority** clinical trial
- Valsartan/amlodipine combination (80/5 mg): morning vs. bedtime administration
  → the effect on **nighttime brachial and central SBP** measured by **24-hr ABPM (Mobil-O-Graph)**

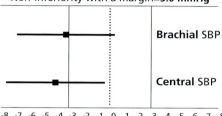

Difference in the changes of nighttime brachial and central SBP from baseline
Non-inferiority with a margin=3.0 mmHg

Brachial SBP
Central SBP

Brachial SBP
mean: -3.2±1.7 mmHg
95% CI: -6.8 to 0.4 mmHg

Central SBP
mean: -4.0±1.7 mmHg
95% CI: -7.6 to -0.4 mmHg

-8 -7 -6 -5 -4 -3 -2 -1 0 1 2 3 4 5 6 7 8 (mmHg) Data is presented as mean change (SEM).

← Morning administration better   Bedtime administration better →

The upper limit of the 95% CI: below the margin in **both nighttime brachial and central SBP** → **non-inferiority** of morning administration to the bedtime administration

Figure 14.13 CPET (ChronotheraPy for ambulatory cEnTral pressure) study. ABPM, ambulatory blood pressure monitoring; SBP, systolic blood pressure. *Source:* Fujiwara et al. 2017 [274]

in both nighttime brachial and central systolic BP, confirming the non-inferiority of morning administration to bedtime administration of valsartan/amlodipine combination therapy [274].

Taken together, the results of the ACROBAT and CPET studies show that combination therapies including at least one long-acting drug have BP-lowering effects that persist throughout a 24-hour period.

The NOCTURNE study, a multicentre randomised controlled trial (RCT) using the recently developed ICT-based nocturnal home BP monitoring (HBPM) device, was performed to compare the nighttime home BP-lowering effects of differential ARB-based combination therapies in 411 Japanese patients with nocturnal hypertension. Patients with nighttime BP ≥120/70 mmHg at baseline even under ARB therapy (100 mg irbesartan daily) were enrolled (**Figure 14.14**) [275]. The ARB/CCB combination therapy (irbesartan 100 mg + amlodipine 5 mg) was associated with a significantly greater reduction in nighttime home SBP (primary endpoint) than the ARB/diuretic combination (daily irbesartan 100 mg + trichlormethiazide 1 mg) (-14.4 vs. -10.5 mmHg, $p<0.0001$) (**Figure 14.15**) [275], independent of urinary sodium excretion and/or nighttime BP dipping

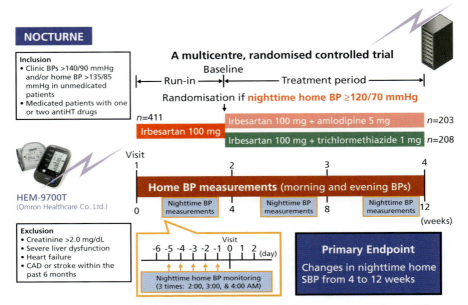

Figure 14.14 Nocturne study design. BP, blood pressure; CAD, coronary artery disease; HT, hypertensive; SBP, systolic blood pressure. *Source:* Kario et al. 2017 [275]

status. The change in nighttime home SBP was comparable among the post-hoc subgroups with higher salt sensitivity (diabetes, chronic kidney disease, and elderly patients) (**Figure 14.16**) [275]. Both combinations significantly reduced UACR and N-terminal pro-BNP (NT-proBNP) levels, while the reduction in NT-proBNP was greater in the ARB/CCB arm (**Figure 14.17**) [275]. This is the first RCT demonstrating the feasibility of clinical assessment of nighttime BP by ICT-nighttime HBPM. The ARB/CCB combination was shown to be superior to ARB/diuretic in patients with uncontrolled nocturnal hypertension independently of sodium intake, despite the similar impact of the two combinations in patients with higher salt sensitivity.

The SUNLIGHT (Study on Uncontrolled Morning Surge for N-type CCB and Low Dose of HCTZ, Using the Internet Through Blood Pressure Data Transmission System) study was an 8-week prospective, multicentre, randomised, open-label clinical trial conducted in 129 patients with morning hypertension (≥135/85 mmHg measured using the self-measuring information and communications technology (ICT)-based HBPM device). The hypothesis that a valsartan/cilnidipine combination would suppress the morning home BP surge more effectively than a valsartan/hydrochlorothiazide (HCTZ) combination was tested. Nighttime

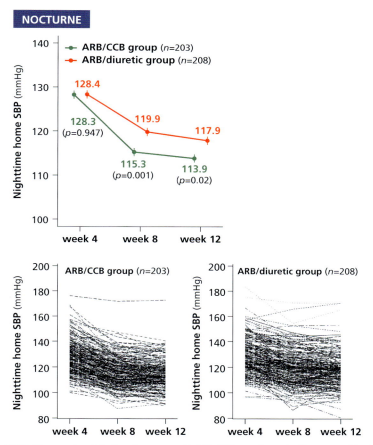

Figure 14.15 Changes in nighttime home systolic BP. ARB, angiotensin II receptor blocker; CCB, calcium-channel blocker; SBP, systolic blood pressure. *Source:* Kario et al. 2017 [275]

and morning SBP were significantly reduced from baseline in both the valsartan/cilnidipine and valsartan/HCTZ groups ($p<0.001$). Morning home BP surge, which is a new index defined as the mean morning SBP minus the mean nighttime SBP was significantly decreased from baseline in both groups ($p<0.001$), but there was no significant difference between the two groups: 14.4 vs. 14.0 mmHg ($p=0.892$) (**Figure 14.18**) [276]. The achieved morning and home SBP levels were around 132 mmHg and 119 mmHg, respectively, in the valsartan/cilnidipine combination group (**Figure 14.19**) [276].

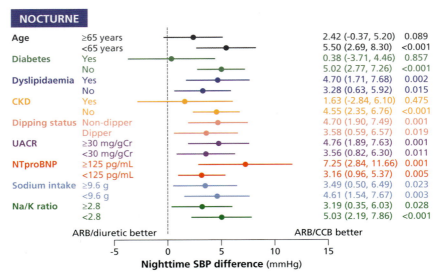

Figure 14.16 Forest plot of nighttime BP-lowering effects of combination therapy with ARB/diuretic vs. ARB/CCB in the NOCTURNE study. Sodium intake (g/day) was estimated by urinary sodium and creatinine concentrations. ARB, angiotensin-receptor blocker; CCB, calcium channel blocker; CKD, chronic kidney disease (eGFR < 60 mL/min/1.73 m^2); Na/K ratio, urinary sodium/potassium ratio; NT-proBNP, N-terminal pro-B-type natriuretic peptide; UACR, urinary albumin/creatinine ratio. *Source:* Kario et al. 2017 [275]

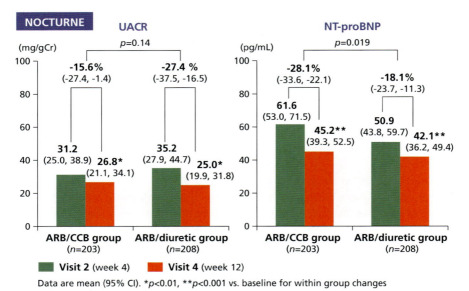

Figure 14.17 Changes in UACR and NT-proBNP. ARB, angiotensin II receptor blocker; CCB, calcium-channel blocker; NT-proBNP, N-terminal pro-brain natriuretic peptide; SBP, systolic blood pressure; UACR, urinary albumin/creatinine ratio. Created based on data from Kario et al. 2017 [275]

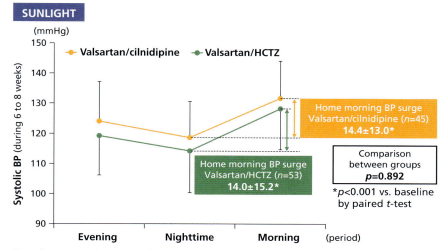

Figure 14.18 The comparison of morning systolic BP surge at the end of treatment period between valsartan/cilnidipine combination and valsartan/HCTZ combination. BP, blood pressure; HCTZ, hydrochlorothiazide; SD, standard deviation. *Source:* Fujiwara et al. 2018 [276]

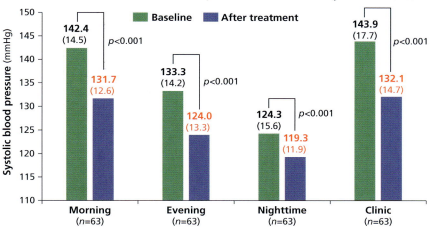

Figure 14.19 SUNLIGHT (Study on Uncontrolled Morning Surge for N-type CCB and Low Dose of HCTZ, Using the Internet through Blood Pressure Data Transmission System) study. The comparison of morning SBP surge at the end of treatment period between valsartan/cilnidipine combination and valsartan/HCTZ combination. CCB, calcium channel blocker; DBP, diastolic blood pressure; HCTZ, hydrochlorothiazide; SBP, systolic BP. Created base on data from Fujiwara et al. 2018 [276]

CHAPTER 15

Resistant hypertension and renal denervation

Uncontrolled hypertension despite treatment with three or more drugs including diuretics is diagnosed as resistant hypertension. Recent increases in the aging population, the prevalence of chronic kidney disease (CKD), and epidemic obesity in hypertension patients have been contributing to the prevalence of drug-resistant hypertension [277]. The prevalence of resistant hypertension is around 10–15% in all hypertensive patients.

The strategies for the management of resistant hypertension

An effective approach for the management of blood pressure (BP) control is required for high-risk patients with resistant hypertension (**Figure 15.1**) [140]. In cases of suspected resistant hypertension, causes of secondary hypertension (**Figure 15.2**) [1] should first be excluded. Obstructive sleep apnoea, primary aldosteronism, renal artery stenosis, drugs, and renal parenchymal disease are the most common (**Figure 15.3**) [278]. Ambulatory blood pressure monitoring (ABPM) is recommended to exclude white-coat hypertension and diagnose true resistant hypertension.

For patients with true resistant hypertension, lifestyle and medication changes should be considered. Strict salt restriction would be very effective for Asian patients with resistant hypertension [279], because even mild obesity and high salt intake are important risk factors for resistant hypertension in Asians with high salt sensitivity. In one study, salt restriction changed patients' night-time BP dipping status from non-dipper to dipper [280].

Fourth-line therapy

There are several options for controlling resistant hypertension based on the BP variability profile. An increase in the dose of renin-angiotensin system (RAS) inhibitor is usually ineffective for reducing BP, while an increase in the dose of diuretics worsens the glucometabolic profile and increases uric acid. Thus, among the three classes of antihypertensives (calcium channel blocker [CCB], RAS inhibitors), an increase in the CCB dose is recommended, especially for hypertensive patients with arterial stiffness type, while diuretics are the most

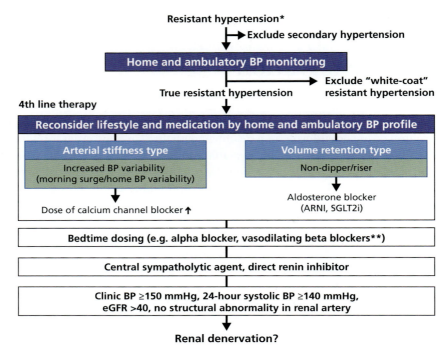

Figure 15.1 Management of resistant hypertension based on home and ambulatory BP. *Already treated by calcium channel blocker, RAS inhibitors (angiotensin receptor blocker, ACE inhibitor), diuretics (thiazide, thiazide-like). **Carvedilol, nebivolol (unavailable in Japan). ARNI, angiotensin receptor neprilysin inhibitor; BP, blood pressure; SGLT2i, inhibitors of sodium/glucose cotransporter 2. *Source:* modified from Kario. 2013 [140]

effective option for reducing BP without adverse effects, especially for patients with volume reduction type hypertension (**Figure 15.1**) [140].

Aldosterone blockers are preferable as fourth-line therapy, especially for the volume-retention type, because these agents reduce circulating volume without impairing glucose metabolism (**Figure 15.1**). Low-dose spironolactone clearly reduced BP in subjects with resistant hypertension [281]. Eplerenone has been shown to predominantly reduce nighttime BP compared with daytime BP in uncontrolled hypertensive patients already being treated with RAS inhibitors [269]. Angiotensin receptor neprilysin inhibitor (ARNI) may also be effective in non-dippers with true resistant hypertension [248, 249].

In a recent double-blind, placebo-controlled, crossover trial in patients with resistant hypertension (**Figure 15.4**) [282], patients rotated, in a preassigned, randomised order, through 12 weeks of once-daily treatment with each of

Resistant hypertension and renal denervation

Common causes
Renal parenchymal disease
Renovascular disease
Primary aldosteronism
Obstructive sleep apnoea
Drug or alcohol induced
Uncommon causes
Pheochromocytoma/paraganglioma
Cushing's syndrome
Hypothyroidism
Hyperthyroidism
Aortic coarctation (undiagnosed or repaired)
Primary hyperparathyroidism
Congenital adrenal hyperplasia
Mineralocorticoid excess syndromes other than primary aldosteronism
Acromegaly

Figure 15.2 Causes of secondary hypertension with clinical indications. Reprinted from Whelton et al. 2017 [1]. Copyright (2017), with permission from Elsevier.

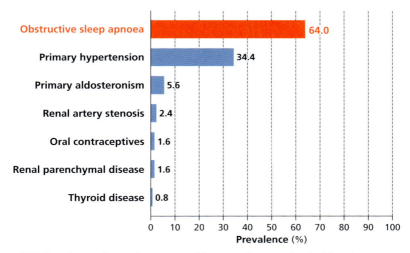

Figure 15.3 Prevalence of secondary causes of hypertension associated with resistant hypertension (n=125). *Source:* Pedrosa et al. 2011 [278]

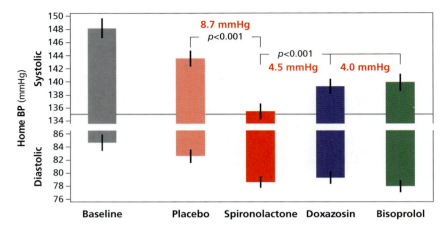

Aldosterone blocker was the most effective in patients with resistant hypertension medicated with A + C + D drugs

Figure 15.4 Home systolic BP in PATHWAY–2. A + C + D, angiotensin-converting-enzyme inhibitor or an angiotensin II receptor blocker (A), a calcium channel blocker (C), and diuretic (D). *Source:* Williams et al. 2015 [282]

spironolactone (25–50 mg), bisoprolol (5–10 mg), doxazosin modified release (4–8 mg), or placebo, in addition to their baseline BP medication. Drug dosages were doubled after 6 weeks of each cycle. The average reduction in home systolic BP (SBP) by spironolactone was superior to placebo (-8.70 mm Hg, $p<0.0001$), superior to the mean of the other two active treatments (doxazosin and bisoprolol; -4.26; $p<0.0001$), and superior to the individual treatments; versus doxazosin (-4.03; $p<0.0001$) and versus bisoprolol (-4.48; $p<0.0001$). Spironolactone was the most effective BP-lowering treatment.

Era of renal denervation

For patients with resistant hypertension being treated with the aforementioned ambulatory BP-based medication strategy, two new device approaches have recently been introduced into clinical practice. One is catheter-based renal sympathetic denervation and the other is electrical stimulation of the carotid baroreceptor (baroreceptor activation therapy). The renal sympathetic nerves, both efferent and afferent, are located in the adventitia of the renal arteries. The first Symplicity™ catheter-based renal sympathetic denervation system is designed to deliver low-level radiofrequency energy through the wall of the renal artery to achieve renal denervation (**Figure 15.5**).

Resistant hypertension and renal denervation

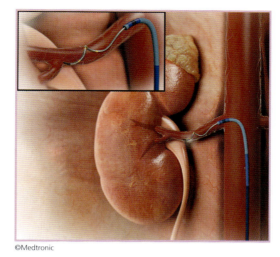

Figure 15.5 Catheter-based renal denervation (Symplicity Spyral™). CVD, cardiovascular disease; eGFR, estimated glomerular filtration rate. *Source:* Medtronic plc. ©Medtronic. Reproduced with permission.

Hypothesis of perfect 24-hour BP control by renal denervation

As the mechanism of renal denervation, efferent denervation reduces renal catecholamine production and beta-1 adrenergic renin production. These changes increase renal blood flow and reduce circulating volume, thus explaining the shift from non-dipping to dipping of nighttime BP in patients with resistant hypertension. In addition, afferent denervation decreases central sympathetic activity in response to increased baroreceptor sensitivity, thus potentially explaining the reduced variability in BP, including the morning BP surge (MBPS) and the 24-hour BP reduction, resulting from decreases in peripheral resistance and cardiac workload. It is hypothesised that renal denervation could achieve perfect 24-hour ambulatory BP control consisting of a strict reduction in the 24-hour BP level, a dipper pattern of nighttime BP, and an adequate morning BP surge (**Figure 15.6**). Thus, renal denervation should be effective for nocturnal hypertension and morning hypertension [140].

Evidence for renal denervation

Symplicity HTN-1 (the first in-man clinical trial without control) and Symplicity HTN-2 (observational study with control) demonstrated that renal dener-

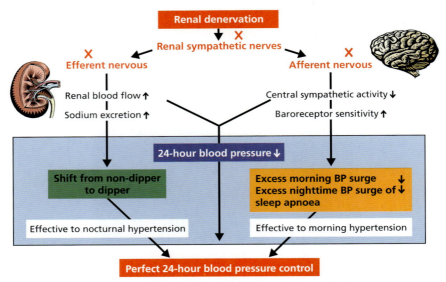

Figure 15.6 Hypothesis of perfect 24-hour BP control by renal denervation in resistant hypertension. *Source:* Kario. 2013 [140]

vation reduces clinic SBP by 30 mmHg, self-measured home BP by 20 mmHg, and 24-hour ambulatory BP by 10 mmHg [283, 284]. However, the Symplicity HTN-3 trial with a sham operation arm demonstrated that there were no significant differences between the renal denervation arm and sham operation arm [285].

A randomised clinical trial of renal denervation with a control arm, HTN-Japan (HTN-J), was initiated to evaluate the efficacy and safety of catheter-based renal denervation in Japanese patients with resistant hypertension in August 2012 until March 2014. The target of renal denervation of previous studies, including HTN-J, is resistant hypertension regardless of pathogenesis of hypertension, and the inclusion and exclusion criteria are almost the same: (1) high clinic SBP ≥160 mmHg and high 24-hour SBP ≥135 mmHg, even when treated with three or more different classes of antihypertensive drugs, including diuretics; (2) a maintained estimated glomerular filtration rate ≥45 mL/min/1.73m^2; and (3) no structural abnormality in the renal artery (**Figure 15.5**). 41 cases were enrolled in HTN-J, and Jichi Medical University conducted nine cases including the first two cases in Japan with no complications. The first patient with Symplicity™-based renal denervation in Japan in this institution exhibited marked reduction of 24-hour ambulatory BP one month after the procedure (**Figure 15.7**). The HTN-J was stopped because of the negative result of Symplicity HTN-

Resistant hypertension and renal denervation

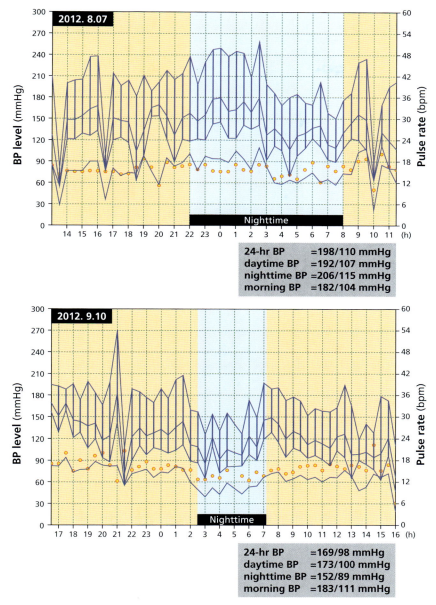

Figure 15.7 First case of renal denervation in Japan, a 38-year-old hypertensive man with diabetes (calcium channel blocker, angiotensin II receptor blocker, diuretics, β-blocker). BP, blood pressure. *Source:* Kario K. *Essential Manual on Perfect 24-hour Blood Pressure Management from Morning to Nocturnal Hypertension: Up-to-date for Anticipation Medicine.* Wiley, 2018.

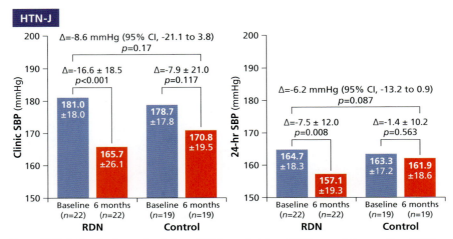

Figure 15.8 6 Month-change in clinic and 24-hr ambulatory SBP by renal denervation (HTN-J). The percentage of patients with medication changes are 9.1% for the RDN group and 5.3% for the control group in HTN-J. RDN, renal denervation; SBP, systolic blood pressure. *Source:* Kario et al. 2015 [286]

3. Available data showed that the reduction in 24-hour SBP tended to be greater in the renal denervation arm than in the control arm (**Figure 15.8**) [286].

Morning BP

In a recent analysis of combined data from HTN-J and Symplicity HTN-3, morning and nighttime BP levels were reduced to a greater extent in the renal denervation group than in the control group (combined sham operation group in the HTN-3, and observational control group in the HTN-J) (**Figure 15.9**) [287]. In addition to the 2-hour average of morning BP, the maximum (the highest in the morning) and moving peak (the highest moving average of three consecutive BP readings in the morning) BP levels were more significantly reduced in the renal denervation versus control group.

Nighttime BP

In addition, all nighttime BP measures were more significantly reduced in the renal denervation group than in the control group (**Figure 15.9**) [287]. These results indicate the important clinical implication of renal denervation in the strategy of obtaining perfect 24-hour BP control, because the nighttime and morning BP readings are the blind spot of antihypertensive drugs, which may not have BP-lowering effects that persist throughout the nighttime and until the next morning.

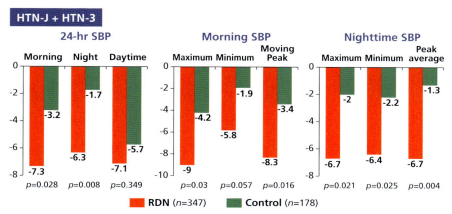

Figure 15.9 Six-month change in ambulatory BP index assessed by ABPM after renal denervation. HTN-J + HTN-3 pooled data. RDN, renal denervation. *Source:* Kario et al. 2015 [287]

Sleep apnoea

Obstructive sleep apnoea (OSA) is associated with activation of the sympathetic nervous system, and patients with this condition often experience elevated BP, increased BP variability, and nighttime BP surges [147]. In a post-hoc analysis of Symplicity HTN-3 data, the reduction in nighttime BP levels, especially peak (the average to the highest three nighttime BP readings) and maximum (highest BP) nighttime BP readings, by renal denervation were greater in patients with versus without OSA (**Figure 15.10**) [288]. Renal denervation seems effective to reduce the peak and maximum nighttime BP levels which depend on the sympathetic drive induced by sleep apnoea episodes in OSA patients. In fact, hypoxia-induced peak nighttime BP detected by nighttime HBPM was significantly reduced after renal denervation in a patient with OSA (**Figure 15.11**) [289].

Isolated systolic hypertension

The effect of renal denervation may be limited in the patients with isolated systolic hypertension (**Figure 15.12**) [290]. Isolated systolic hypertension is the phenotype of structural hypertension. Diastolic BP ≥90 mmHg seems to be a good indicator by which to detect responders to renal denervation. The improvement of vascular stiffness and subsequent reduction of pulse pressure may take longer after renal denervation.

Potential beyond-BP effect

Previous studies have also demonstrated that renal denervation improves insu-

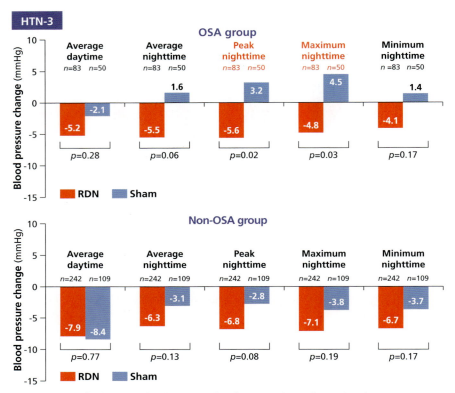

Figure 15.10 Nighttime BP reduction 6 months after RDN. OSA, obstructive sleep apnoea; RDN, renal denervation. *Source:* Kario et al. 2016 [288].

lin resistance (HOMA index) [291], renal resistive index and microalbuminuria values without reducing the glomerular filtration rate [292], and it improves hypertensive heart disease (left ventricular hypertrophy [LVH] and diastolic dysfunction) [293]. These target organ protection effects are predominantly caused by the extensive BP-lowering effect but may partly result from a direct sympatholytic effect on the target organ.

The Symplicity Spyral™ and evidence

The Symplicity Spyral™ renal denervation catheter is depicted in illustration (**Figure 15.13** upper panel) [294]. The Symplicity Spyral™ catheter includes a 4-electrode array mounted on a 4F catheter that self-expands into a helical configuration with electrodes located at 90 degrees from each other circumferentially. Radiofrequency energy treatment is delivered simultaneously to all four renal artery quadrants for 60 seconds.

	-1–0 month	0–1 month	1–2 month
n	19 nights	22 nights	20 nights
Nighttime BP			
Fixed-interval function			
Mean SBP (mmHg)	134.2±12.2	127.7±7.2*	123.1±6.3***†
Mean DBP (mmHg)	76.5±4.6	75.1±3.5	72.5±2.6**†
Mean PR (bpm)	52.9±3.3	55.4±2.9**	56.5±3.1***
Basal nighttime SBP (mmHg)	113.3±8.8	108.5±6.6*	106.5±5.7**
Oxygen-triggered function			
Hypoxia-peak SBP (mmHg)	164.2±19.4	152.9±17.6*	153.5±16.1*
Mean SBP (mmHg)	144.1±16.8	132.3±10.4**	132.2±8.6**
Mean DBP (mmHg)	78.5±6.1	76.5±4.8	76.5±5.1
Mean PR (bpm)	52.4±3.5	54.7±2.8*	56.0±2.6***
Nighttime SBP surge (mmHg)	29.7±10.4	24.5±14.0	26.9±12.5
Morning BP			
SBP (mmHg)	169.2±15.4	160.1±8.4*	145.6±10.1***††
DBP (mmHg)	90.1±5.9	89.7±3.6	83.0±3.5***††
PR (bpm)	55.1±4.5	59.6±4.6**	59.4±3.4**
Oxygen Desaturation Index (per hour)	9.2±3.3	11.1±4.5	13.0±5.6**

*$p<0.05$, **$p<0.01$, ***$p<0.001$ vs. before 1 month, by t-test;
†$p<0.05$, ††$p<0.001$, vs. after 1 month, by t-test

Figure 15.11 Changes in nighttime BP parameters repeatedly measured by trigger nighttime BP monitoring after renal denervation: Patient 1. DBP, diastolic blood pressure; SBP, systolic blood pressure; PR, pulse rate. *Source:* Kario et al. 2016 [289]

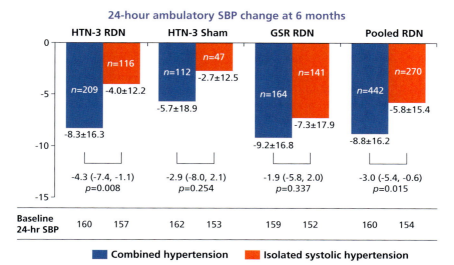

Figure 15.12 Differential 24-hour ambulatory blood pressure lowering effect of renal denervation between isolated systolic hypertension and combined systolic-diastolic hypertension. GSR, Global SYMPLICITY Registry; HTN-3, SYMPLICITY HTN-3 trial; RDN, catheter-based renal denervation; SBP, systolic blood pressure. *Source:* Mahfoud et al. 2017 [290]

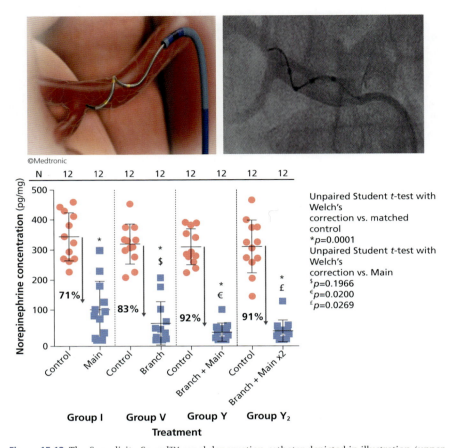

Figure 15.13 The Symplicity Spyral™ renal denervation catheter depicted in illustration (upper left panel) and under fluoroscopy (upper right panel). Upper left: The Symplicity Spyral™ catheter includes a 4-electrode array mounted on a 4F catheter that self-expands into a helical configuration with electrodes located at 90° from each other circumferentially. Radiofrequency energy treatment is delivered simultaneously to all four renal artery quadrants for 60 seconds. Upper right: After guide wire withdrawal, the catheter adopts a spiral conformation in the renal artery. Lower panel: Renal norepinephrine(NE) concentration after renal denervation in the main renal artery (I), in the renal artery branches (V), and in both the main renal artery and branches (Y). The variation in response of renal NE on renal norepinephrine is larger when the renal artery branches are untreated (I) or undertreated (V). Combination treatment of renal artery branches and main artery provided the best and most consistent reduction of NE (Y). *Source:* Upper figures: Kandzari et al. 2016 [294]. Reprinted with permission from Elsevier. Lower figure: Mahfoud et al [295]

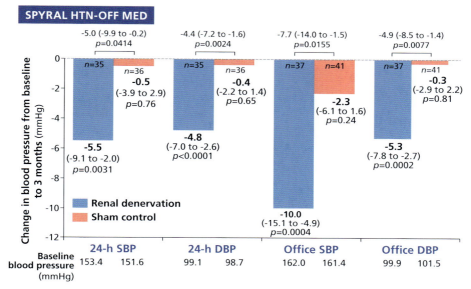

Figure 15.14 Changes at 3 months in office and ambulatory SBP and DBP for renal denervation and sham control groups. 95% CIs and unadjusted p values shown. DBP, diastolic blood pressure; SBP, systolic blood pressure. Reprinted from the *Lancet*, Vol.390 (10108), Townsend RR et al., Catheter-based renal denervation in patients with uncontrolled hypertension in the absence of antihypertensive medications (SPYRAL HTN-OFF MED): a randomised, sham-controlled, proof-of-concept trial, pp.2160-2170. Copyright (2017), with permission from Elsevier. [296]

In an experimental study to compare the reduction of renal norepinephrine concentration after renal denervation, combination treatment of renal artery branches and the main artery provided the best and most consistent reduction in norepinephrine levels [295]. In a recent study using the Symplicity Spyral™, renal denervation significantly reduced 24-hour ambulatory SBP by 5.5 mmHg and clinic SBP by 7.7 mmHg compared with the sham operation in hypertensive patients not receiving medication (**Figure 15.14**) [296]. The estimated clinical impact of this BP reduction corresponds to a 20–25% decrease in stroke and heart failure events [294].

Current potential candidates

The number of individuals with drug-resistant hypertension – possible candidates for renal denervation – was estimated when this treatment was introduced into Japan. Data from the nationwide Ambulatory Blood Pressure Prospective

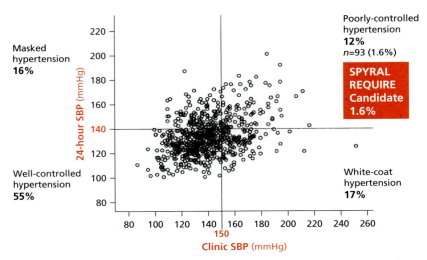

Figure 15.15 JAMP (Japan Ambulatory Blood Pressure Monitoring) study ($n=6,114$). The possible candidates for renal denervation in Japan. Hypertensive patietns medicated with ≥3 drugs including diuretics ($n=749$). SBP, systolic blood pressure. *Source:* Kario et al. 2016 [297]. Republished with permission of Bentham Science Publishers Ltd.

(JAMP) registry, which enrolled outpatients with cardiovascular risks from every region of the country, was analysed. 6,450 patients were registered from 37 prefectures and 120 medical institutions between January 2009 and September 2015. The prevalence of resistant hypertension (clinic SBP ≥150 mmHg and 24-hour SBP ≥140 mmHg despite treatment with three antihypertensive drugs including diuretics) was 1.6% (**Figure 15.15**) [297]. In Japan, three clinical trials of catheter-based renal denervation are now ongoing: SPYRAL (using the Symplicity Spyral™ multielectrode renal denervation catheter, Medtronic, Santa Rosa, CA) [294]; REQUIRE (using an ultrasound based renal denervation system, PARADISE™, ReCor Medical, Palo Alto, CA, USA) (**Figure 15.16**) [298] and IBERIS® (using TCD-16164 multielectrode renal denervation system, Terumo Corporation, Tokyo, Japan) (**Figure 15.17**).

Asians may respond to renal denervation. Ethnicity-related differences in the effectiveness of renal denervation for reducing both BP and cardiovascular events needs to be confirmed in future studies. Considering ethnic differences in the demographics of hypertension and related cardiovascular disease, it will be important to achieve consensus on the positioning of renal denervation in the hypertension management strategy in Asian countries.

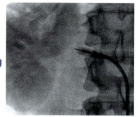
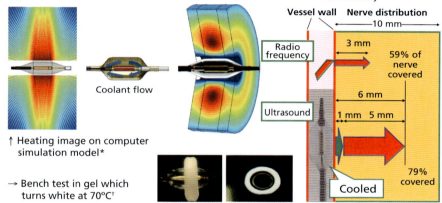

Figure 15.16 Catheter-based ultrasound renal denervation: major differences from radiofrequency. *Mauri et al. 2018 [298]. Reprinted from *American Heart Journal*, Vol. 195, Mauri L et al., A multinational clinical approach to assessing the effectiveness of catheter-based ultrasound renal denervation: The RADIANCE-HTN and REQUIRE clinical study designs, pp.115-129., Copyright (2018), with permission from Elsevier. †Reprinted from Sakakura K et al. Controlled circumferential renal sympathetic denervation with preservation of the renal arterial wall using intraluminal ultrasound: a next-generation approach for treating sympathetic overactivity. *EuroIntervention*. 2015; 10: 1230-1238. Copyright (2015), with permission from Europa Digital & Publishing. ‡Reprinted from *EuroIntervention*, Vol. 8(1), Mabin T et al., First experience with endovascular ultrasound renal denervation for the treatment of resistant hypertension. pp.57-61., Copyright (2012), with permission from Europa Digital & Publishing.

Iberis® Renal Denervation System
Radiofrequency ablation catheter & Generator

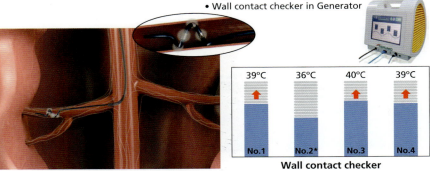

Safe deliverability
- Good trackability for branch ablation
- One size fits for 3–8 mm diameter
- TRI type catheter (developing now)

Good wall contact
- Optimised catheter design to ablate nerves more efficiency and ease
- Four radiofrequency electrodes for circumferential ablation
- High radial force for good wall contact
- Wall contact checker in Generator

Ablation in branch artery through trans radial (TRI)

Wall contact checker
*No.2 is not good contact.

Figure 15.17 Iberis® Renal Deneravation System using RF energy (TERUMO CORPORATION, Tokyo, Japan) has CE marked approval. Clinical studies are ongoing in Japan and China. Reproduced with permission from TERUMO CORPORATION Copyright ©Shanghai AngioCare Medical Technology Ltd, All Rights Reserved.

Responders and future indication of renal denervation

The indication for renal denervation in previous trials has been BP control status regardless of pathogenesis of hypertension. In near future, there are two possible clinical indications for renal denervation in the hypertension management strategy (**Figure 15.18**): the first is based on BP control status [299]. The SPYRAL HTN Global Clinical Trial Program for studies of renal denervation in the absence (SPYRAL HTN-OFF MED) and presence (SPYRAL HTN-ON MED) of antihypertensive medications is now ongoing [294]. The target of all these clinical studies of renal denervation, except the OFF MED trial, is to focus on drug-resistant hypertension, which may be expanded to drug-uncontrolled hypertension because the cardiovascular prognosis of uncontrolled hypertension medicated by two drugs was comparable to that of hypertension uncontrolled by three or more drugs (J-HOP study). The OFF MED trial demonstrated the effectiveness of renal denervation in unmedicated hypertensive patients [296]. Therefore,

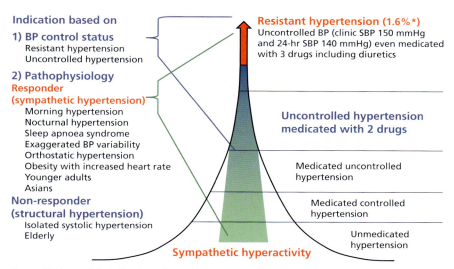

Figure 15.18 Possible indication of renal denervation. *Prevalence in all hypertensives (Kario, et al. *Curr Hypertens Rev*. 2016; 12: 156-163). BP, blood pressure; SBP, systolic BP. *Source:* Kario. 2017 [299]. Republished with permission of Bentham Science Publishers Ltd.

renal denervation may be an alternative to antihypertensive medication for some responders. Ideally, the clinical indication for this therapy would be based on the underlying pathogenesis of hypertension. **Figure 15.18** shows possible responders with sympathetic hyperactivity and non-responders with structural hypertension plus vascular disease [299]. Additionally, patients with structural hypertension (such as isolated systolic hypertension, already with advanced large artery disease) appear to be non-responders to renal denervation [290], while patients with OSA appear to be the most likely to respond.

CHAPTER 16

HOPE Asia Network

There are significant ethnic differences in the cardiovascular-renal demographics around the world, and hypertension is one of the most powerful risk factors associated with these demographic differences.

HOPE Asia Network formation

The Hypertension, brain, cardiovascular and renal Outcome Prevention and Evidence in Asia (HOPE Asia) Network has recently been established [300]. Its mission is to improve the management of hypertension and organ protection with the ultimate goal of achieving zero cardiovascular events in Asia. Activity is based on three initiatives: (1) the examination and analysis of all of the existing evidence related to hypertension, (2) formation of a consensus regarding hot clinical topics in hypertension, and (3) conducting Asia-wide clinical studies of hypertension (**Figure 16.1**). The HOPE Asia Network is proud to now be a member organisation of The World Hypertension League (WHL) and looks forward to contributing actively to the WHL's mission of confronting the global epidemic of hypertension and the high burden of premature death and disability that results from this condition [301-303].

As the first activity, we studied the current prevalence and awareness of hypertension, and the percentage of treated and controlled hypertension in each Asian country (**Figure 16.2**) [304]. It was again recognised that the situation and requirements in each country were very different. There is continuing focus

To improve the management of hypertension and organ protection for zero cardiovascular events in Asia

1. To know the current evidence

2. To achieve consensus

3. To conduct clinical studies based on current local practice

Figure 16.1 Mission of HOPE Asia Network (Hypertension, brain, cardiovascular and renal Outcome Prevention and Evidence in Asia). *Source:* Kario. 2018 [300]

	Prevalence (%)	Awareness (%)	Treated (%)	Controlled (%)
China[1]	25.2	46.5	41.1	13.8
Hong Kong[2]	31.6	46.2	69.7	25.8
India[3]	29.8	25.1 (rural) 41.9 (urban)	24.9 (rural) 37.6 (urban)	10.7 (rural) 20.2 (urban)
Indonesia[4]	26.5	35.8	NR	NR
Japan[5]	60.0 (men) 45.0 (women)	NR	52.8 (men) 52.8 (women)	31.7 (men) 42.0 (women)
Korea[6]	32.9 (men) 23.7 (women)	58.5 (men) 76.1 (women)	51.7 (men) 71.3 (women)	36.9 (men) 49.4 (women)
Malaysia[7]	30.3	43.2	81.2	26.3
Pakistan[8]	50.3	29.6	18.0	5.5
Philippines[9]	28.0	67.8	75.0	27.0
Singapore[10]	23.5	73.7	NR	69.1
Taiwan[11]	20.8	72.1	89.4	70.2
Thailand[12]	24.7	55.3	49.2	60.4

1. National Health and Family Planning Commission. 2015 Report on Chinese Nutrition and Chronic Disease. 2015.
2. Leung GM, Ni MY, Wong PT, et al. Cohort Profile: FAMILY Cohort. *Int J Epidemiol*. 2017; 46: e1.
3. Anchala R, Kannuri NK, Pant H, et al. Hypertension in India: a systematic review and meta-analysis of prevalence, awareness, and control of hypertension. *J Hypertens*. 2014; 32:1170-1177. https://journals.lww.com/jhypertension/
4. RISKESDAS. 2013. http://www.depkes.go.id/resources/download/general/Hasil%20Riskesdas%202013.pdf Accessed November 2, 2016.
5. *Hypertens Res*. 2014; 37: 253-390 [5]
6. Shin J, Park JB, Kim K, et al., Guideline Committee of the Korean Society of Hypertension. 2013 Korean Society of Hypertension guidelines for the management of hypertension: part I—epidemiology and diagnosis of hypertension. *Clin Hypertens*. 2015; 21: 1.
7. Ministry of Health Malaysia. National Health and Morbidity Survey, 2015: Non-communicable diseases, risk factors and other health problems. http://www.iku.gov.my/images/IKU/Document/REPORT/nhmsreport2015vol2.pdf. Accessed November 2, 2016; Ministry of Health Malaysia. National Health and Morbidity Survey, 2006: Non-communicable diseases, risk factors and other health problems. http://www.iku.gov.my/images/IKU/Document/REPORT/2006/ExecutiveSummary.pdf. Accessed November 2, 2016.
8. Non-communicable Diseases Risk Factors Survey—Pakistan. Pakistan Health Research Council. 2016. Islamabad, Pakistan: World Health Organization. ISBN 978-969-499-008-8.
9. Sison JA. Philippine Heart Association—Council on Hypertension Report on Survey of Hypertension (PRESYON 3). A report on prevalence of hypertension, awareness and treatment profile. 2013. http://philheart.org/44/images/sison.pdf. Accessed December 15, 2016.
10. Singapore Ministry of Health. National Health Survey, 2010. https://www.moh.gov.sg/content/moh_web/home/Publications/Reports/2011/national_health_survey2010.html. Accessed November 2, 2016.
11. NHANES, 2013–2016, unpublished data.
12. NHES, 2014–2015, unpublished data.

Figure 16.2 Prevalence, awareness, treatment and control of hypertension in Asia.
Source: Chia et al. 2017 [304]

HOPE Asia Network

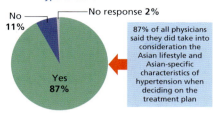

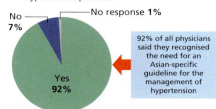

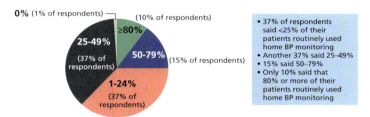

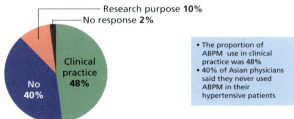

Figure 16.3 Asian physicians' knowledge of hypertension management ($n=133$). A total of 133 physicians responded to the questionnaire. The respondents were attendees of an Asian Stroke Conference in Tokyo ($n=11$); a conference titled Protection Along the Cardiovascular Continuum in China ($n=5$); and meetings of the Taiwan Society of Cardiology in Taiwan ($n=24$), the OCC 2014 in China ($n=20$), the Hypertension Forum in Singapore ($n=47$), and the International Society of Hypertension in Greece ($n=26$), which were separately held in the period of March to May 2014. The nationality of them were as follows: China ($n=33$), Taiwan ($n=29$), Indonesia ($n=8$), Thailand ($n=7$), Vietnam ($n=7$), Myanmar ($n=7$), Pakistan ($n=4$), Korea ($n=3$), Philippines ($n=3$), Malaysia ($n=1$), Egypt ($n=1$), Hong Kong ($n=1$), Saudi Arabia ($n=1$), and unknown ($n=28$). BP, blood pressure; ABPM, ambulatory BP monitoring. *Source:* Hoshide et al. 2016 [305]. Republished with permission of Bentham Science Publishers Ltd.

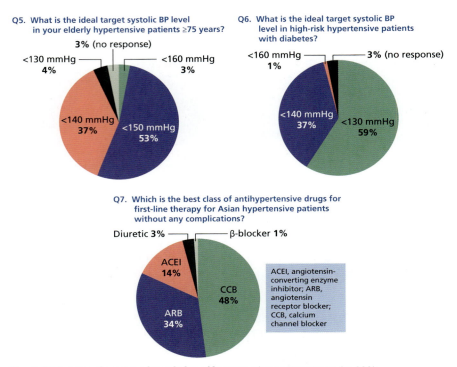

Figure 16.4 Asian physicians' knowledge of hypertension management (*n*=133).
Source: Hoshide et al. 2016 [305]. Republished with permission of Bentham Science Publishers Ltd.

on the clinically important Asian 'hot topics' concerning the management of hypertension and the prevention of cardiovascular-renal disease, focussing on evidence, pathogenesis, and treatment.

In a previous survey of awareness of hypertension management in Asia (**Figures 16.3** and **16.4**), 87% of all physicians who responded said that they did take the Asian lifestyle and Asian-specific characteristics of hypertension into consideration, and 92% recognised the need for an Asian-specific guideline for the management of hypertension [305]. As groups of Asian hypertension researchers (e.g. the Asia BP@Home investigators and the COME Asia-MHDG [Characteristics On the ManagEment of hypertension in the Asia-Morning Hypertension Discussion Group]), the characteristics of hypertension and cardiovascular-renal disease in Asian populations have been studied [223, 249, 306-309]. Collaboration between these groups was instrumental in forming the HOPE Asia Network.

1. Stroke, especially haemorrhagic stroke, more common than myocardial infarction

2. Steeper association between blood pressure and cardiovascular disease

3. Higher salt intake with higher salt sensitivity

4. Obesity and metabolic syndrome epidemic

5. Morning and nocturnal hypertension more common

Figure 16.5 Characteristics of hypertension in Asia. *Source:* Modified from Kario et al. 2013 [140]

Characteristics of cardiovascular disease in Asia

It is well established that the characteristics of hypertension and its related diseases are markedly different in Asians compared with Caucasians and Blacks (**Figure 16.5**) [4, 140, 157]. For example, the phenotypes of cardiovascular disease, stroke and heart failure that are closely associated with blood pressure (BP) are more common in Asia (**Figure 16.6**) [310]. Even in the recent prospective HONEST study in an Asian population, the incidence of stroke in on-treatment hypertensive patients was around 2.8-times higher than that of myocardial infarction (2.92 vs 1.03 per 1,000 person-years) (**Figure 16.7**) [21]. The incidence of coronary artery disease (composite of myocardial infarction and angina pectoris with intervention) (2.80 per 1,000 person-years) was almost comparable to that of stroke. The slope of the association between higher BP levels and cardiovascular events is also steeper in Asians compared with Western populations (**Figures 16.8** and **16.9**) [311, 312]. Thus, the impact of 24-hour hypertension control would be greater in Asians [4, 11, 157].

Obesity and salt intake in Asia

The impact of obesity on high BP may be different between Asian and Caucasian individuals. Asians are likely to develop high BP even with mild obesity. Looking at the risk of elevated BP/stage 1 hypertension (2017 AHA/ACC; previously known as prehypertension), the impact of BMI 25 kg/m^2 in a Japanese population was almost comparable to that of a BMI of 30 kg/m^2 in a U.S. population (**Figure 16.10**) [313, 314].

Obesity is known to increase salt sensitivity. Asians are genetically more likely to have salt sensitivity [315]. In addition, Asian individuals tend to have a higher dietary salt intake (**Figure 16.11**) [316]. Thus, the increase in salt sensi-

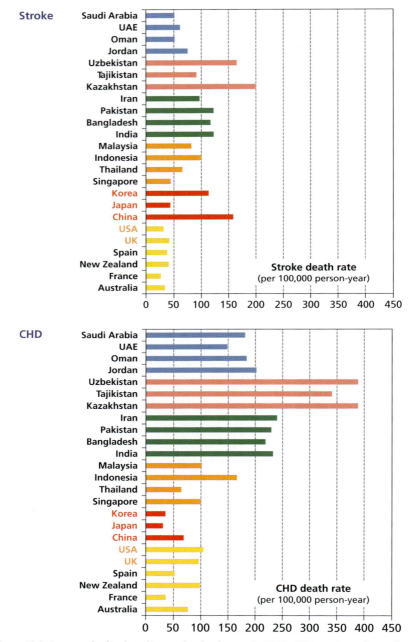

Figure 16.6 Age-standardised cardiovascular death rates in 2002. CHD, coronary heart disease. *Source:* Ueshima et al. 2008 [310]

HONEST

Cardiovascular events	No. of events	Incidence, events/1,000 patient-years (95% CI)
Primary end point	280	6.46 (5.75–7.27)
Secondary end point	336	7.76 (6.98–8.64)
Stroke events*	127	2.92 (2.46–3.48)
Atherothrombotic cerebral infarction	43	0.99 (0.73–1.33)
Lacunar infarction	40	0.92 (0.67–1.25)
Cerebral haemorrhage	17	0.39 (0.24–0.63)
Unclassified cerebral infarction	13	0.30 (0.17–0.51)
Subarachnoid haemorrhage	8	0.18 (0.09–0.37)
Cardiogenic cerebral infarction	4	0.09 (0.03–0.24)
Unclassified stroke	3	0.07 (0.02–0.21)
Cardiac events	167	3.85 (3.30–4.48)
Coronary revascularisation procedure for angina pectoris*	77	1.77 (1.42–2.21)
Myocardial infarction*	45	1.03 (0.77–1.38)
Hospitalisation for heart failure	36	0.83 (0.60–1.15)
Hospitalisation for angina pectoris	13	0.30 (0.17–0.51)
All death	190	4.36 (3.78–5.02)
Cardiovascular death	46	1.05 (0.79–1.41)
Sudden death*	35	0.80 (0.58–1.12)
Aortic dissection	5	0.11 (0.05–0.28)
Arteriosclerosis obliterans	12	0.28 (0.16–0.48)

Figure 16.7 Cardiovascular disease in medicated hypertensives. HONEST study (21,591 hypertensive patients were followed for >2 years). *Events comprising the primary end point. Cardiovascular death comprised fatal stroke, fatal myocardial infarction, and sudden death. *Source:* Kario et al. 2014 [21]

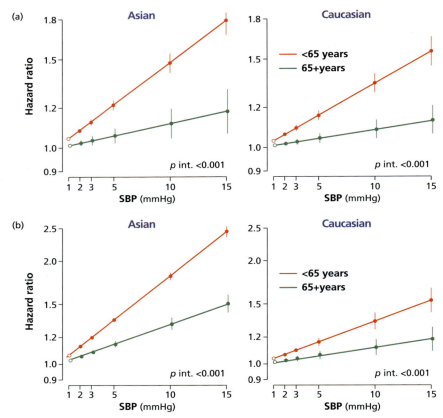

Figure 16.8 Asian populations are at greater cardiovascular risk related to hypertension. Risk of (a) fatal and nonfatal coronary heart disease, or (b) stroke. SBP, systolic blood pressure. *Source:* Perkovic et al. 2007 [311]

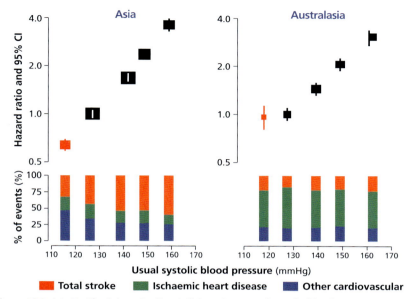

Figure 16.9 Asia Pacific Cohort Studies Collaboration. Usual systolic blood pressure and risks of cardiovascular death in Asia and Australasia. The study analysed a total of 425,325 study participants who were followed up for 3 million person-years. *Source:* Lawes et al. 2003 [312]

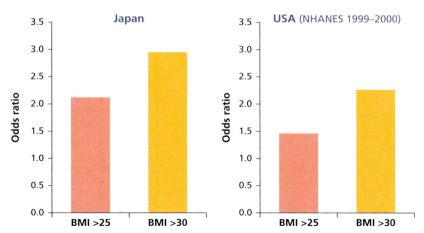

Figure 16.10 Racial difference in impact of obesity on prehypertension (JMS Cohort, n=12,000). Odds ratio (prehypertensives vs normotensives) adjusted for age and sex. Left: Created based on data from Ishikawa et al. 2008 [313]. Right: Created based on data from Greenlund et al. 2004 [314]

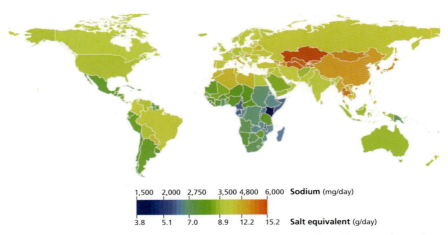

Figure 16.11 Salt intake in 2010 (age >20 years, men/women). Reprinted from Powles et al. 2013 [316]. with permission from BMJ Publishing Group Ltd.

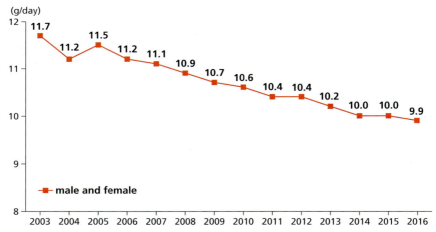

Figure 16.12 Salt intake in Japan. Created based on data from 2016 National Health and Nutrition Survey. (Ministry of Health, Labour and Welfare; http://www.mhlw.go.jp/bunya/kenkou/kenkou_eiyou_chousa.html) accessed on December 20, 2017.

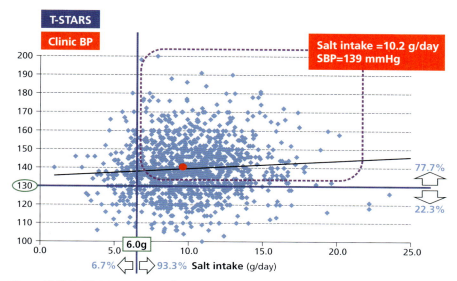

Figure 16.13 T-STARS on Japanese hypertensive patients. Tochigi Salt Cardiovascular Risk Study (T-STARS; *n*=4,511). *Source:* Kario K. *Essential Manual on Perfect 24-hour Blood Pressure Management from Morning to Nocturnal Hypertension: Up-to-date for Anticipation Medicine.* Wiley, 2018.

tivity caused by mild obesity is enough to cause high BP in Asians who already have high salt sensitivity and high salt intake.

Salt intake is gradually decreasing in Japan. However, it still remains high, above 10 g/day (**Figure 16.12**). In a survey of hypertensive patients recruited from general practitioner-based clinics in Tochigi prefecture, the average salt intake (estimated by concentrations of sodium and creatinine in the spot urine) was 10.2 g/day. The prevalence of well-controlled patients with an intake of <6 g/day was only 6.7% (**Figure 16.13**).

Salt restriction and maintaining a BMI <25 kg/m² are the two key prophylactic strategies against high BP, especially in Asian populations.

24-hour ambulatory BP profile in Asia

A 24-hour BP profile is determined partly by an individual's genetic factors, but it is also strongly affected by a variety of cultural factors (e.g. food, lifestyle, and traditions) and environmental factors (e.g. temperature, atmospheric pressure, humidity, and seasonal changes) [4, 9, 10]. BP variability may be greater in Asian populations than Western populations. Recent analysis of the International ambulatory blood pressure monitoring (ABPM) registry, ARTEMIS,

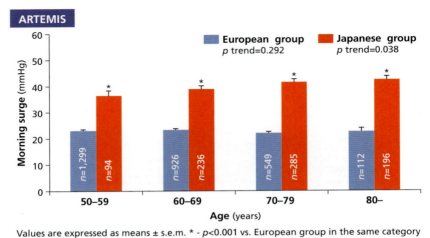

Figure 16.14 Ethnic differences in the degree of morning BP surge in the ARTEMIS study (811 Japanese vs 2,887 Caucasians). *Source:* Hoshide et al. 2015 [318].

demonstrated that the prevalence of masked hypertension was higher in Asians than in Westerners [317].

In the same database, when clinic BP was comparable, Japanese hypertensive patients had a more exaggerated morning BP surge than similar Western patients (**Figure 16.14**) [318]. In patients with drug-resistant hypertension, who were recruited using the same global entry criteria of Simplicity HTN-3 and HTN-J for catheter-based renal denervation, Japanese patients had higher morning BP levels and greater morning BP surges than the patients from other ethnic backgrounds, even when clinic BP was comparable (**Figure 16.15**) [319]. In a population cohort, the nighttime BP fall may be less in Asians than in Westerners (**Figure 16.16**) [320].

Facilitation of a home BP-guided approach in Asia

The HOPE Asia Network has initially focused on home BP values, because we consider the home BP-guided approach to be the most effective practical approach in clinical practice. In particular, the morning home BP-guided approach is the most effective strategy to achieve zero cardiovascular events in Asia [11, 321].

Asian data from two prospective observational studies (Ohasama study [25], J-HOP [29]) and two intervention studies (HOMED-BP [30], HONEST [21]) clearly demonstrated that morning home BP is the most important predictor of cardiovascular events, especially stroke, independent of clinic BP.

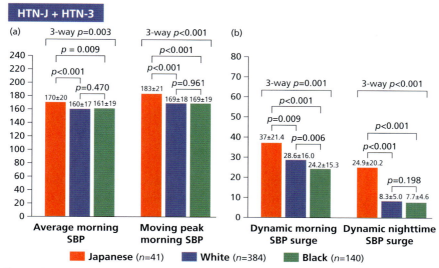

Figure 16.15 ABPM parameters stratified by ethnicity. ABPM, ambulatory blood pressure monitoring; SBP, systolic blood pressure *Source:* Kario et al. 2017 [319]

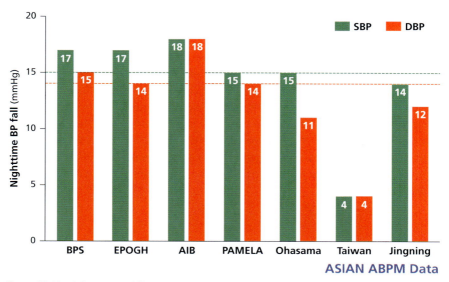

Figure 16.16 Nighttime BP fall across populations. BPS, Belgian population study; EPOGH, European Project on Genes of Hypertension; AIB, Allied Irish Bank study; PAMELA, Pressioni Arteriose Monitorate E Loro Associazioni, Monza, Italy; Ohasama, survey conducted in Ohasama, Iwate Prefecture, 100 km north of Sendai, Japan; Taiwan, study conducted on the Taiwan and Kinmen (Quemoy) islands; Jingning, six villages of the Jingning County, China. Created based on data from Li et al. 2005 [320]

In Asia in particular, because of the local lifestyle, individuals are unlikely to measure their evening home BP before dinner, and measuring the evening home BP just before going to bed is therefore recommended [5]. The importance of morning home BP as standard clinical practice was stressed, because morning home BP has shown better reproducibility than evening home BP or clinic BP [322]. However, the measurement of evening home BP just before going to bed is strongly influenced by the individual's dinner (including alcohol consumption) and evening behaviour (e.g. bathing in the evening is common in Asia) [26].

Asia BP@Home study

Across Asia there are significant country-specific, regional, and ethnic differences in BP control status. To achieve effective protection against cardiovascular-renal events in Asia, it is important that Asian characteristics of hypertension-related cardiovascular-renal disease are identified at the regional, national and ethnic levels.

As the initial project conducted by the HOPE Asia Network, the current status and evidence regarding home BP in the medical literature published in 12 Asian countries was evaluated [304]. Subsequently, several meetings were held with the purpose of achieving a consensus on home BP-guided clinical management of hypertension in Asia [321, 323]. In addition, the Asia BP@Home study is underway, which will determine the prevalence of masked uncontrolled morning home BP and the characteristics of home BP variability in medicated hypertensive patients living in 12 Asian counties [324]. As noted above, among the countries that comprise Asia, there are expected to be significant regional, country-based, and ethnic differences in BP characteristics. The Asia BP@Home study is the first study of home BP in Asia that uses the same protocol and the same home BP monitoring device across all participating countries. It is hoped that through this HOPE Asia Network activity, continuing advances in the management of hypertension and the prevention of cardiovascular-renal disease will be made, and contribute towards reaching the goal of zero cardiovascular events in Asia.

CHAPTER 17

Disaster hypertension and ICT-based home BP monitoring

Damage as a result of natural disasters is growing worldwide. A major disaster triggers serial cardiovascular events (**Figure 17.1**) [325]. An increase in thrombophilic tendency and blood pressure (BP) is the leading cause of disaster-induced cardiovascular events such as stroke, cardiac events, and heart failure. (**Figure 17.2**) [325]. Based on previous experience, a disaster cardiovascular risk score was developed to identify patients who are at high risk of developing disaster-induced cardiovascular events, along with a prevention score (**Figure 17.3**) [325].

Disaster hypertension

Disaster hypertension was defined as hypertension found in the disaster area, including newly-developed hypertension, and hypertension with deteriorated BP control in the disaster area [325].

At the time of the Great Hanshin-Awaji earthquake in 1995, the author was working for the Awaji-Hokudan Public Clinic in the area near the epicentre of the earthquake, and found a disaster-associated increase in BP. Borderline hypertensive patients developed uncontrolled hypertension, but their BP levels returned to previous levels after one month. However, some patients, especially those with microalbuminuria, developed persistent uncontrolled disaster hypertension (**Figure 17.4**) [326, 327]. At the time of the Great East Japan earthquake in 2011, marked, uncontrolled disaster hypertension was again found in people who were residing in temporary shelters (**Figure 17.5**).

High salt intake and increased salt sensitivity caused by disrupted circadian rhythms are suggested as the two leading causes of this disaster hypertension through neurohumoral activation under stressful conditions [325, 328, 329] (**Figure 17.6**).

Disaster cardiovascular prevention (DCAP) network

To better assess and reduce the risks for disaster-associated cardiovascular events, the web-based disaster cardiovascular prevention (DCAP) network (which consists of DCAP risk and prevention score assessment and self-measured BP monitoring at both a shelter and the home) was established to help survivors of the

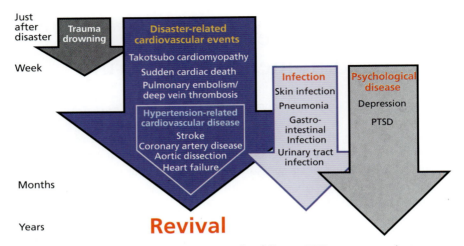

Figure 17.1 Time course of the onset of disaster-related disease. PTSD, post-traumatic stress disorder. *Source:* Kario. 2012 [325]

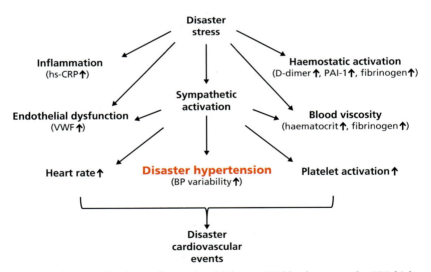

Figure 17.2 Disaster-activating cardiovascular risk factors. BP, blood pressure; hs-CRP, high-sensitivity C-reactive protein; VWF, von Willebrand factor; PAI-1, plasminogen activator inhibitor-1. *Source:* Kario. 2012 [325]

DCAP - AFHCHDC7 Risk Score and DCAP - SEDWITMP8 Prevention Score		✓
1 Age (A)	>75 years	☐
2 Family (F)	death or hospitalisation (partner, parents, or children)	☐
3 Housing (H)	completely destroyed	☐
4 Community (C)	completely destroyed	☐
5 Hypertension (H)	Positive (under medication, or systolic blood pressure >160mmHg)	☐
6 Diabetes (D)	Positive	☐
7 Cardiovascular disease (C)	Positive (coronary artery disease, stroke, heart failure)	☐
	Average total score*	_____
DCAP - SEDWITMP8 Prevention Score#		
1 Sleep (S)	Sleep duration >6 hr, arousal <3 times during sleep	☐
2 Physical activity (E)	Walking >20 min/day	☐
3 Diet (D)	Reduce salt intake with high potassium intake (3 serves of green vegetable, fruit, or seaweed/day)	☐
4 Body weight (W)	change < ±2 kg	☐
5 Infection prevention (I)	regular face mask use and washing hands	☐
6 Thrombosis (T)	sufficient water intake >1,000 mL per day	☐
7 Medication (M)	continuous use of antihypertensive medication and antiplatelet agents and/or anticoagulation	☐
8 Blood pressure control (P)	<140 mmHg systolic (clinic, shelter, or self-measured)	☐
	Average total score#	_____

Figure 17.3 Disaster cardiovascular prevention (DCAP) risk score (AFHCHDC7) and prevention score (SEDWITMP8). *Total number of each risk factor as the individual risk score (0–7 points). The individual with 4 points or more is in the high-risk group. #Total number of each prevention factor as the individual prevention score (0–8 points). Recommended prevention score is six or more, particularly in high-risk patients. *Source:* Kario. 2012 [325]

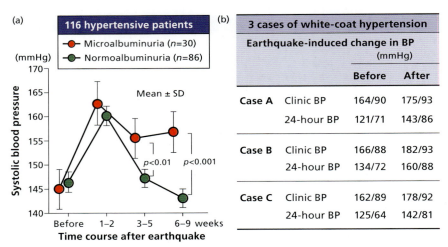

Figure 17.4 Earthquake-induced BP increase (Hanshin-Awaji earthquake 1995). *Source:* (a) Kario et al. 2001 [326], (b) Kario et al. 1995 [327].

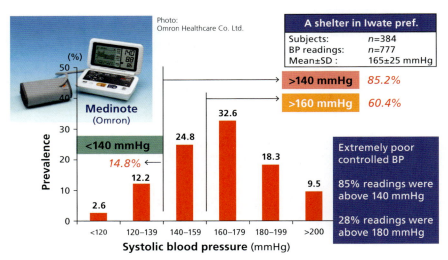

Figure 17.5 BP values recorded in indivduals housed in shelter (First Jichi Medical University Supporting Team) March 25–April 1, 2011. *Source:* Kario. 2015 [10]

Disaster hypertension and ICT-based home BP monitoring

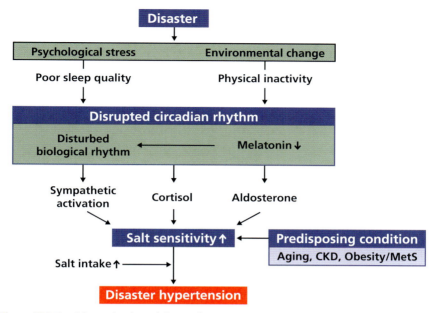

Figure 17.6 Possible mechanism of disaster hypertension. CKD, chronic kidney disease; MetS, metabolic syndrome. *Source:* Kario. 2012 [325]

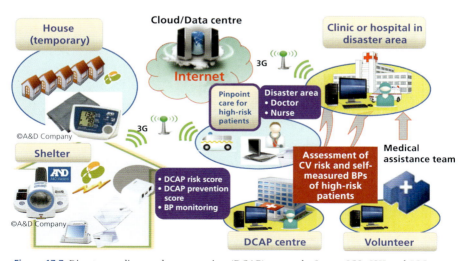

Figure 17.7 Disaster cardiovascular prevention (DCAP) network. *Source:* JCS, JSH and JCC Joint Working Group. Guidelines for disaster medicine for patients with cardiovascular diseases (JCS 2014/JSH 2014/JCC 2014) - digest version. *Circ J.* 2016; 80: 261-284.

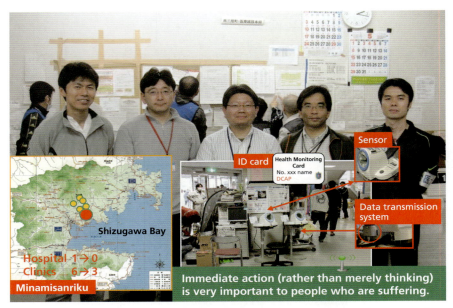

Figure 17.8 Introduction of disaster cardiovascular prevention (DCAP) network system to the shelter in Minamisanriku area (April 29, 2011). From left, Satoshi Hoshide, Masahisa Shimpo, Masafumi Nishizawa (center), Kazuomi Kario, and Yuichiro Yano. Lower left: Shizugawa bay; Reduction in the number of hospital and clinics after the earthquake. Source: *Kario*. 2015 [10]

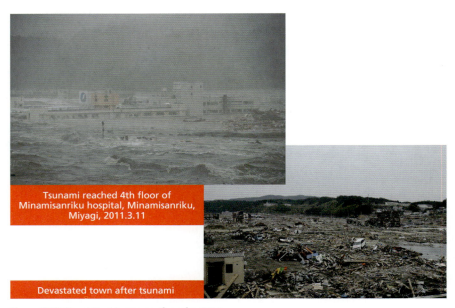

Figure 17.9 Great East Japan earthquake 2011.

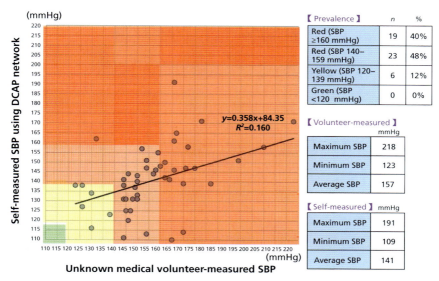

Figure 17.10 Unknown medical volunteers-measured versus self-measured BP using DCAP network (Minami-Sanriku, April 29–May 6, 2011). DBP, diastolic blood pressure; SBP, systolic blood pressure. *Source:* Kario. 2012 [325]

2011 disaster (**Figure 17.7**) [330, 331]. The DCAP network system was developed using cloud-based computing on the internet to monitor individual BP data self-measured at home or at a shelter.

This DCAP network system was introduced into the major shelter in Minamisanriku town where Dr Masafumi Nishizawa had been working hard for victims since just after the Great East Japan earthquake (**Figure 17.8**). The town of Minanisanriku was severely damaged by the direct hit of the earthquake and the subsequently triggered tsunami (**Figure 17.9**).

Disaster-induced increases in BP have been shown to be influenced by the white-coat effect (clinic BP minus home BP) [326]. Thus, BP measurement by the disaster medical assistance team (DMAT) or unknown medical volunteers under stressful conditions in a shelter may overestimate BP, and thus self-measured BP could be considered better for guiding adequate antihypertensive medication under such conditions [325, 332]. In fact, the results showed that there are marked differences between volunteer-measured BP and BP self-measured in conjunction with the DCAP system (**Figure 17.10**) [325].

In most patients, the increases in clinic BP and self-measured BP were transient and BP levels returned to the pre-earthquake baseline levels within four weeks [325-329]. This characteristic of disaster-induced BP increase is important, because persistent intensive antihypertensive treatment for subjects with

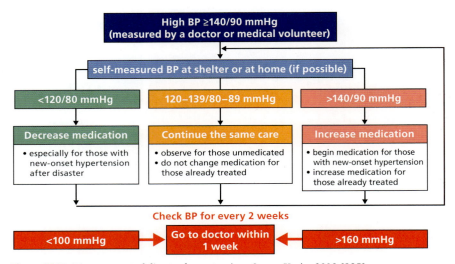

Figure 17.11 Management of disaster hypertension. *Source:* Kario. 2012 [325]

high BP at the time of a disaster could result in excessive BP reduction, as was observed in a patient who had started treatment with antihypertensive agents just after the Great Hanshin-Awaji earthquake [332]. She was referred to the clinic because she developed dizziness 3 months later. Her antihypertensive medication was discontinued and ambulatory BP was taken. This was found to be normal, and her symptoms disappeared. Thus, it is recommended that BP should be monitored and the dose of antihypertensive medication reconsidered every two weeks during a disaster situation (**Figure 17.11**) [325, 332].

In disaster victims, the memory of the major earthquake and its damage may have augmented the pressor effect of the aftershock even though it occurred 19 months after the major earthquake. Ambulatory blood pressure monitoring (ABPM) was used in eight hypertensive patients who lived in the Minamisanriku town, the disaster area at the time of the first major aftershock. A pressor effect of ambulatory BP was found just after the aftershock. A persistent pressor effect generated a non-dipper pattern of nighttime BP and exaggerated morning BP surge in the patients living in temporary housing (**Figure 17.12**) [333].

ICT-based BP control: successful model of telemedicine

Successful home BP control was achieved in the DCAP participants following the 2011 Great East Japan earthquake (**Figure 17.13**) [334]. After four years, home SBP had decreased from 151 mmHg to 125 mmHg in the winter and 120

Disaster hypertension and ICT-based home BP monitoring

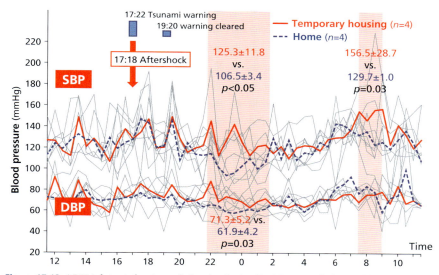

Figure 17.12 ABPM data at the time of aftershocks ($n=8$). ABPM, ambulatory blood pressure monitoring; DBP, diastolic BP; SBP, systolic BP. *Source:* Nishizawa et al. 2015 [333]

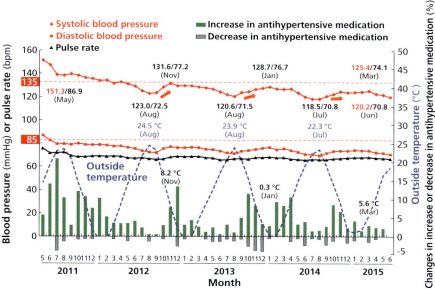

Figure 17.13 Changes in home blood pressure in DCAP participants ($n=351$) after 2011 Great East Japan earthquake. *Source:* Nishizawa et al. 2017 [334]

mmHg in the summer. This BP control status is almost identical to the ideal levels of the SPRINT study [2] and less than the universal BP goal of 2017 AHA/ACC guidelines [1]. Importantly, the seasonal variation had decreased to within 5 mmHg even in patients living in the severely damaged area. In addition, the duration from the summer bottom to the winter peak of home BP had decreased year-on-year. This may have been due to timely and appropriate titration of antihypertensive medication. As shown in the lower panel of **Figure 17.3**, the dose of antihypertensive medication was increased from October 2012, then the winter BP peak was suppressed even during December to February (the coldest temperature). In the following year (2013), drug titration was initiated in September, and the winter BP peak was suppressed. This proactive adjustment of drug dosages can only be achieved when the doctor and patient both recognise the seasonal variation in BP over the previous year. Thus, this is one of the most successful models of anticipation medicine using telemedicine and telecare.

CHAPTER 18
Anticipation telemedicine

Haemodynamic biomarker-initiated anticipation medicine is the future of cardiovascular disease management. The key haemodynamic biomarker is blood pressure (BP) surge, a pressor component of BP variability [4, 9].

Anticipation medicine

The concept of anticipation medicine presents a unique and exciting challenge in the era of Information Communication Technology (ICT) and Internet of Things (IoT)-based big data. In the context of cardiovascular disease, anticipation medicine is defined as medicine that predicts the time and place of the onset of cardiovascular events, based on a time-series of data, and provides a patient or doctor with advanced warning of potential risk factors, resulting in proactive, real-time risk reduction.

The field of individualised medicine is currently split into two distinct approaches (**Figure 18.1**) [4]. One is precision medicine, utilising population-based big data such as genomic information, and the other is anticipation medicine, using individual-based big data such as time-series data. While there is a huge body of evidence on the relation between hypertension and cardiovascular disease risk based on population-based big data, there is less available information on the use of anticipation medicine to predict the time and place of cardiovascular events in individual subjects using time-series data for BP and its effectors.

Concept of event management

The management of hypertension should move from BP control to event management. It is a shift away from focussing on BP level to that of focusing on BP surge. BP surge management will lead to the effective prevention of cardiovascular event onset, especially in high-risk subjects with vascular disease.

The BP surge management strategy based on the resonance hypothesis consists of the following three goals: (1) minimising triggers of BP surge, (2) reducing the amplitude of each peak, (3) avoiding the synchronisation of peaks of different time phases (**Figure 18.2**) [9]. The aim of this strategy is to avoid the generation of a large dynamic BP surge that could trigger cardiovascular events.

In practical terms, to reduce the amplitude of morning BP surge, it is rec-

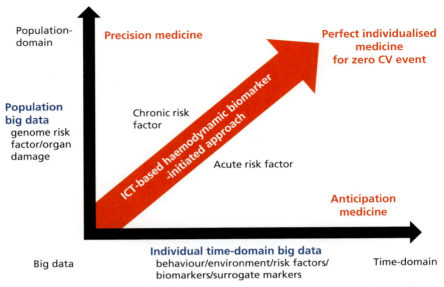

Figure 18.1 Anticipation medicine of cardiovascular disease. CV, cardiovascular. Reprinted from Kario. 2016 [4] with permission from Elsevier.

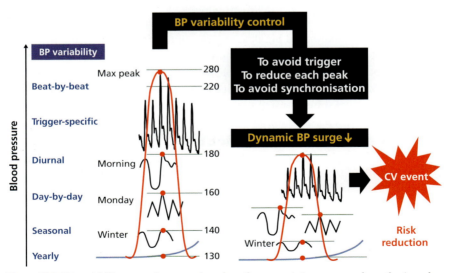

Figure 18.2 BP variability control strategy based on the synergistic resonance hypothesis and aiming at the prevention of cardiovascular-event onset. BP, blood pressure; CV, cardiovascular. Reprinted from Kario et al. 2017 [9] with permission from Elsevier.

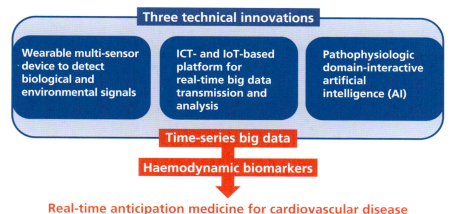

Figure 18.3 Three technical innovations to establish real-time anticipation medicine for cardiovascular disease. The key biomarker of real-time anticipation medicine for cardiovascular disease is BP variability. BP, blood pressure. Reprinted from Kario et al. 2017 [9] with permission from Elsevier.

ommended that patients reduce their alcohol and salt intake at dinner. In winter, abrupt high intensity running just after rising without adequate protection against the cold weather should be avoided to protect against winter morning BP surge. Regular physical exercise is recommended, especially low intensity running, to improve cardiorespiratory fitness, which is associated with a reduction in BP variability due to a decrease in arterial stiffness and BP level [335-337].

Monotherapy or combination therapy using long-acting antihypertensive drugs, or bedtime dosing of drugs is recommended to reduce the peak of BP surge [308]. In addition, renal denervation reduces sympathetic tonus resulting in the suppression of morning and nighttime BP peaks [140, 287, 296, 338], especially in patients with obstructive sleep apnoea [288, 289].

Innovation technology

To establish real-time anticipation medicine, several technical innovations are needed as follows: (1) a wearable multi-sensor device to detect biological and environmental signals; (2) an ICT- and IoT-based platform for real-time big data transmission and analysis; and (3) pathophysiologic domain-interactive artificial intelligence (AI). With these technologies in hand, time-series big data collection with short-term intervals could be performed in the context of a prospective study (**Figure 18.3**) [9].

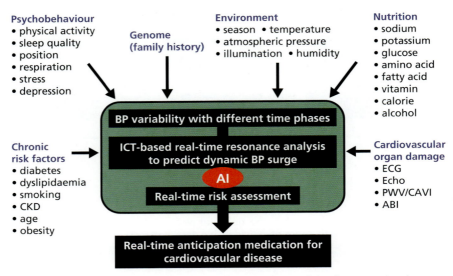

Figure 18.4 Haemodynamic biomarker-initiated anticipation medicine for preventing the onset and aggravation of cardiovascular events. BP, blood pressure CKD, chronic kidney disease; ECG, electrocardiography; Echo, cardiac and carotid echography; PWV, pulse wave velocity; CAVI, cardio ankle vascular index; ABI, ankle-brachial index; AI, artificial intelligence. Reprinted from Kario. 2016 [4] with permission from Elsevier.

The BP surge-initiated anticipation medicine, when combined with the data on organ damage and psychobehavioural, genomic, environmental, and nutritional risk factors, has the potential to achieve a perfect individualised medicine regimen for zero cardiovascular events (**Figure 18.4**) [4].

Telemedicine and telecare

Haemodynamic biomarker-initiated anticipation medicine that can predict BP surge based on individual haemodynamic profiles, and provide early intervention by an ICT-based real-time feedback system, could prevent or combat the onset, recurrence, and aggravation of cardiovascular events.

In the near future, telemedicine and telecare using an ICT- and IoT-based anticipation approach could dramatically reduce the incidence of cardiovascular events, and improve the healthy longevity of patients worldwide (**Figure 18.5**) [9].

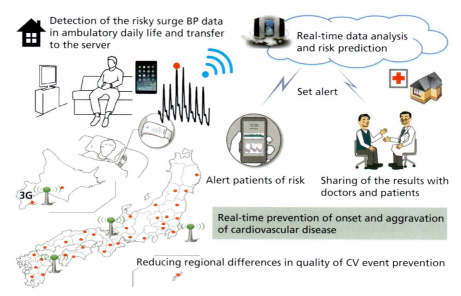

Figure 18.5 The model of ICT-based real-time anticipation medicine of cardiovascular disease. Reprinted from Kario et al. 2017 [9] with permission from Elsevier.

References

1 Whelton PK, Carey RM, Aronow WS, Casey DE, Jr., Collins KJ, Dennison Himmelfarb C, DePalma SM, Gidding S, Jamerson KA, Jones DW, MacLaughlin EJ, Muntner P, Ovbiagele B, Smith SC, Jr., Spencer CC, Stafford RS, Taler SJ, Thomas RJ, Williams KA, Sr., Williamson JD, Wright JT, Jr. 2017 ACC/AHA/AAPA/ABC/ACPM/AGS/APhA/ASH/ASPC/NMA/PCNA Guideline for the prevention, detection, evaluation, and management of high blood pressure in adults: a report of the American College of Cardiology/American Heart Association task force on clinical practice guidelines. *J Am Coll Cardiol*. 2017. [in press].
2 SPRINT research group, Wright JT, Jr., Williamson JD, Whelton PK, Snyder JK, Sink KM, Rocco MV, Reboussin DM, Rahman M, Oparil S, Lewis CE, Kimmel PL, Johnson KC, Goff DC, Jr., Fine LJ, Cutler JA, Cushman WC, Cheung AK, Ambrosius WT. A randomized trial of intensive versus standard blood-pressure control. *N Engl J Med*. 2015; 373: 2103-2116.
3 Kario K. PREFACE: "The Lower the better" Association between white-coat effect-excluded blood pressure and cardiovascular events in high-risk hypertension: insights from SPRINT. *Curr Hypertens Rev*. 2016; 12: 2-10.
4 Kario K. Evidence and perspectives on the 24-hour management of hypertension: hemodynamic biomarker-initiated 'anticipation medicine' for zero cardiovascular event. *Prog Cardiovasc Dis*. 2016; 59: 262-281.
5 Shimamoto K, Ando K, Fujita T, Hasebe N, Higaki J, Horiuchi M, Imai Y, Imaizumi T, Ishimitsu T, Ito M, Ito S, Itoh H, Iwao H, Kai H, Kario K, Kashihara N, Kawano Y, Kim-Mitsuyama S, Kimura G, Kohara K, Komuro I, Kumagai H, Matsuura H, Miura K, Morishita R, Naruse M, Node K, Ohya Y, Rakugi H, Saito I, Saitoh S, Shimada K, Shimosawa T, Suzuki H, Tamura K, Tanahashi N, Tsuchihashi T, Uchiyama M, Ueda S, Umemura S; Japanese Society of Hypertension Committee for Guidelines for the Management of Hypertension. The Japanese Society of Hypertension guidelines for the management of hypertension (JSH 2014). *Hypertens Res*. 2014; 37: 253-390.
6 Mancia G, Fagard R, Narkiewicz K, Redon J, Zanchetti A, Bohm M, Christiaens T, Cifkova R, De Backer G, Dominiczak A, Galderisi M, Grobbee DE, Jaarsma T, Kirchhof P, Kjeldsen SE, Laurent S, Manolis AJ, Nilsson PM, Ruilope LM, Schmieder RE, Sirnes PA, Sleight P, Viigimaa M, Waeber B, Zannad F; Task Force Members. 2013 ESH/ESC guidelines for the management of arterial hypertension: the task force for the management of arterial hypertension of the European Society of Hypertension (ESH) and of the European Society of Cardiology (ESC). *J Hypertens*. 2013; 31: 1281-1357. https://journals.lww.com/jhypertension/
7 Krause T, Lovibond K, Caulfield M, McCormack T, Williams B; Guideline Development Group. Management of hypertension: summary of NICE guidance. *BMJ*. 2011; 343: d4891.
8 Kario K. Perfect 24-h management of hypertension: clinical relevance and per-

spectives. *J Hum Hypertens.* 2017; 31: 231-243.
9. Kario K, Tomitani N, Kanegae H, Yasui N, Nishizawa M, Fujiwara T, Shigezumi T, Nagai R, Harada H. Development of a new ICT-based multisensor blood pressure monitoring system for use in hemodynamic biomarker-initiated anticipation medicine for cardiovascular disease: the national IMPACT program project. *Prog Cardiovasc Dis.* 2017; 60: 435-449.
10. Kario K. *Essential Manual of 24-hour Blood Pressure Management from Morning to Nocturnal Hypertension.* UK: Wiley Blackwell; 2015: 1-138.
11. Kario K. Global impact of 2017 AHA/ACC hypertension guidelines: a perspective from Japan. *Circulation.* 2018; 137: 543-545. http://circ.ahajournals.org/
12. Kario K. *Clinician's Manual on Early Morning Risk Management in Hypertension.* London, UK: Science Press; 2004: 1-68.
13. Muller JE, Tofler GH, Stone PH. Circadian variation and triggers of onset of acute cardiovascular disease. *Circulation.* 1989; 79: 733-43. http://circ.ahajournals.org/
14. Kario K, Pickering TG, Umeda Y, Hoshide S, Hoshide Y, Morinari M, Murata M, Kuroda T, Schwartz JE, Shimada K. Morning surge in blood pressure as a predictor of silent and clinical cerebrovascular disease in elderly hypertensives: a prospective study. *Circulation.* 2003; 107: 1401-1406. http://circ.ahajournals.org/
15. Kario K. Time for focus on morning hypertension: pitfall of current antihypertensive medication. *Am J Hypertens.* 2005; 18: 149-151.
16. Kario K, Ishikawa J, Pickering TG, Hoshide S, Eguchi K, Morinari M, Hoshide Y, Kuroda T, Shimada K. Morning hypertension: the strongest independent risk factor for stroke in elderly hypertensive patients. *Hypertens Res.* 2006; 29: 581-587.
17. Li Y, Thijs L, Hansen TW, Kikuya M, Boggia J, Richart T, Metoki H, Ohkubo T, Torp-Pedersen C, Kuznetsova T, Stolarz-Skrzypek K, Tikhonoff V, Malyutina S, Casiglia E, Nikitin Y, Sandoya E, Kawecka-Jaszcz K, Ibsen H, Imai Y, Wang J, Staessen JA; International Database on Ambulatory Blood Pressure Monitoring in Relation to Cardiovascular Outcomes Investigators. Prognostic value of the morning blood pressure surge in 5645 subjects from 8 populations. *Hypertension.* 2010; 55: 1040-1048. http://hyper.ahajournals.org
18. Kario K. Morning surge in blood pressure and cardiovascular risk: evidence and perspectives. *Hypertension.* 2010; 56: 765-773. http://hyper.ahajournals.org
19. Nishinaga M, Takata J, Okumiya K, Matsubayashi K, Ozawa T, Doi Y. High morning home blood pressure is associated with a loss of functional independence in the community-dwelling elderly aged 75 years or older. *Hypertens Res.* 2005; 28: 657-663.
20. Asayama K, Ohkubo T, Kikuya M, Obara T, Metoki H, Inoue R, Hara A, Hirose T, Hoshi H, Hashimoto J, Totsune K, Satoh H, Imai Y. Prediction of stroke by home "morning" versus "evening" blood pressure values: the Ohasama study. *Hypertension.* 2006; 48: 737-743. http://hyper.ahajournals.org
21. Kario K, Saito I, Kushiro T, Teramukai S, Ishikawa Y, Mori Y, Kobayashi F, Shimada K. Home blood pressure and cardiovascular outcomes in patients during antihypertensive therapy: primary results of HONEST, a large-scale prospective, real-world observational study. *Hypertension.* 2014; 64: 989-996. http://hyper.ahajournals.org
22. Chobanian AV, Bakris GL, Black HR, Cushman WC, Green LA, Izzo JL, Jr., Jones DW, Materson BJ, Oparil S, Wright JT, Jr., Roccella EJ; National Heart, Lung, and

Blood Institute Joint National Committee on Prevention, Detection, Evaluation, and Treatment of High Blood Pressure; National High Blood Pressure Education Program Coordinating Committee. The Seventh report of the Joint National Committee on prevention, detection, evaluation, and treatment of high blood pressure: the JNC 7 report. *JAMA*. 2003; 289: 2560-2572.

23 Julius S, Nesbitt SD, Egan BM, Weber MA; Michelson EL, Kaciroti N, Black HR, Grimm RH, Jr., Messerli FH, Oparil S, Schork MA, Trial of Preventing Hypertension (TROPHY) Study Investigators. Feasibility of treating prehypertension with an angiotensin-receptor blocker. *N Engl J Med*. 2006; 354: 1685-1697.

24 Kanegae H, Oikawa T, Kario K. Should pre-hypertension be treated? *Curr Hypertens Rep*. 2017; 19: 91.

25 Imai Y, Ohkubo T, Sakuma M, Tsuji II, Satoh H, Nagai K, Hisamichi S, Abe K. Predictive power of screening blood pressure, ambulatory blood pressure and blood pressure measured at home for overall and cardiovascular mortality: a prospective observation in a cohort from Ohasama, northern Japan. *Blood Press Monit*. 1996; 1: 251-254.

26 Fujiwara T, Hoshide S, Nishizawa M, Matsuo T, Kario K. Difference in evening home blood pressure between before dinner and at bedtime in Japanese elderly hypertensive patients. *J Clin Hypertens (Greenwich)*. 2017; 19: 731-739.

27 Pickering TG, Miller NH, Ogedegbe G, Krakoff LR, Artinian NT, Goff D; American Heart Association; American Society of Hypertension; Preventive Cardiovascular Nurses Association. Call to action on use and reimbursement for home blood pressure monitoring: executive summary: a joint scientific statement from the American Heart Association, American Society of Hypertension, and Preventive Cardiovascular Nurses Association. *Hypertension*. 2008; 52: 1-9. http://hyper.ahajournals.org

28 Fujiwara T, Kario K. Comparison of waiting room and examination room blood pressure with home blood pressure level in a rural clinical practice. *J Clin Hypertens (Greenwich)*. 2017; 19: 1051-1053.

29 Hoshide S, Yano Y, Haimoto H, Yamagiwa K, Uchiba K, Nagasaka S, Matsui Y, Nakamura A, Fukutomi M, Eguchi K, Ishikawa J, Kario K; J-HOP Study Group. Morning and evening home blood pressure and risks of incident stroke and coronary artery disease in the Japanese general practice population: the Japan Morning Surge-Home Blood Pressure study. *Hypertension*. 2016; 68: 54-61. http://hyper.ahajournals.org/

30 Asayama K, Ohkubo T, Metoki H, Obara T, Inoue R, Kikuya M, Thijs L, Staessen JA, Imai Y; Hypertension Objective Treatment Based on Measurement by Electrical Devices of Blood Pressure (HOMED-BP). Cardiovascular outcomes in the first trial of antihypertensive therapy guided by self-measured home blood pressure. *Hypertens Res*. 2012; 35: 1102-1110.

31 Kario K, Saito I, Kushiro T, Teramukai S, Tomono Y, Okuda Y, Shimada K. Morning home blood pressure is a strong predictor of coronary artery disease: the HONEST study. *J Am Coll Cardiol*. 2016; 67: 1519-1527.

32 Kushiro T, Kario K, Saito I, Teramukai S, Sato Y, Okuda Y, Shimada K. Increased cardiovascular risk of treated white coat and masked hypertension in patients with diabetes and chronic kidney disease: the HONEST study. *Hypertens Res*. 2017; 40: 87-95.

33 Saito I, Kario K, Kushiro T, Teramukai S, Yaginuma M, Mori Y, Okuda Y, Shimada K. Home blood pressure and cardiovascular risk in treated hypertensive patients: the prognostic value of the first and second measurements and the difference between them in the HONEST study. *Hypertens Res.* 2016; 39: 857-862.
34 Kario K, Shimada K, Schwartz JE, Matsuo T, Hoshide S, Pickering TG. Silent and clinically overt stroke in older Japanese subjects with white-coat and sustained hypertension. *J Am Coll Cardiol.* 2001; 38: 238-245.
35 Kario K, Matsuo T, Kobayashi H, Imiya M, Matsuo M, Shimada K. Nocturnal fall of blood pressure and silent cerebrovascular damage in elderly hypertensive patients. Advanced silent cerebrovascular damage in extreme dippers. *Hypertension.* 1996; 27: 130-135. http://hyper.ahajournals.org/
36 Kario K, Pickering TG, Matsuo T, Hoshide S, Schwartz JE, Shimada K. Stroke prognosis and abnormal nocturnal blood pressure falls in older hypertensives. *Hypertension.* 2001; 38: 852-857. http://hyper.ahajournals.org/
37 Kario K, Schwartz JE, Pickering TG. Ambulatory physical activity as a determinant of diurnal blood pressure variation. *Hypertension.* 1999; 34: 685-691. http://hyper.ahajournals.org/
38 Kabutoya T, Imai Y, Hoshide S, Kario K. Diagnostic accuracy of a new algorithm to detect atrial fibrillation in a home blood pressure monitor. *J Clin Hypertens (Greenwich).* 2017; 19: 1143-1147.
39 Kario K. Hemodynamic biomarker-initiated anticipation medicine in the future management of hypertension. *Am J Hypertens.* 2017; 30: 226-8.
40 Kario K. Morning surge in blood pressure in hypertension: clinical relevance, prognostic significance and therapeutic approach. In: *Special Issues in Hypertension* (AE Berbari, G Manccia, eds). Springer Inc., pp. 71-89, 2012.
41 Kario K. Morning surge in blood pressure: a phenotype of systemic hemodynamic atherothrombotic syndrome. *Am J Hypertens.* 2015; 28: 7-9.
42 Kario K. Orthostatic hypertension-a new haemodynamic cardiovascular risk factor. *Nat Rev Nephrol.* 2013; 9: 726-738.
43 Bombelli M, Fodri D, Toso E, Macchiarulo M, Cairo M, Facchetti R, Dell'Oro R, Grassi G, Mancia G. Relationship among morning blood pressure surge, 24-hour blood pressure variability, and cardiovascular outcomes in a white population. *Hypertension.* 2014; 64: 943-950. http://hyper.ahajournals.org/
44 Parati G, Vrijens B, Vincze G. Analysis and interpretation of 24-h blood pressure profiles: appropriate mathematical models may yield deeper understanding. *Am J Hypertens.* 2008; 21: 123-125; discussion 7-9.
45 Head GA, Chatzivlastou K, Lukoshkova EV, Jennings GL, Reid CM. A novel measure of the power of the morning blood pressure surge from ambulatory blood pressure recordings. *Am J Hypertens.* 2010; 23: 1074-1081.
46 Gosse P, Lasserre R, Minifie C, Lemetayer P, Clementy J. Blood pressure surge on rising. *J Hypertens.* 2004; 22: 1113-1118. https://journals.lww.com/jhypertension/
47 Metoki H, Ohkubo T, Kikuya M, Asayama K, Obara T, Hashimoto J, Totsune K, Hoshi H, Satoh H, Imai Y. Prognostic significance for stroke of a morning pressor surge and a nocturnal blood pressure decline: the Ohasama study. *Hypertension.* 2006; 47: 149-154. http://hyper.ahajournals.org/
48 Sheppard JP, Hodgkinson J, Riley R, Martin U, Bayliss S, McManus RJ. Prognostic significance of the morning blood pressure surge in clinical practice: a systematic

review. *Am J Hypertens*. 2015; 28: 30-41.

49 Verdecchia P, Angeli F, Mazzotta G, Garofoli M, Ramundo E, Gentile G, Ambrosio G, Reboldi G. Day-night dip and early-morning surge in blood pressure in hypertension: prognostic implications. *Hypertension*. 2012; 60: 34-42. http://hyper.ahajournals.org/

50 Israel S, Israel A, Ben-Dov IZ, Bursztyn M. The morning blood pressure surge and all-cause mortality in patients referred for ambulatory blood pressure monitoring. *Am J Hypertens*. 2011; 24: 796-801.

51 Pierdomenico SD, Pierdomenico AM, Di Tommaso R, Coccina F, Di Carlo S, Porreca E, Cuccurullo F. Morning blood pressure surge, dipping, and risk of coronary events in elderly treated hypertensive patients. *Am J Hypertens*. 2016; 29: 39-45.

52 Pierdomenico SD, Pierdomenico AM, Coccina F, Lapenna D, Porreca E. Prognostic value of nondipping and morning surge in elderly treated hypertensive patients with controlled ambulatory blood pressure. *Am J Hypertens*. 2017; 30: 159-165.

53 Xie JC, Yan H, Zhao YX, Liu XY. Prognostic value of morning blood pressure surge in clinical events: a meta-analysis of longitudinal studies. *J Stroke Cerebrovasc Dis*. 2015; 24: 362-369.

54 Cheng HM, Wu CL, Sung SH, Lee JC, Kario K, Chiang CE, Huang CJ, Hsu PF, Chuang SY, Lakatta EG, Yin FCP, Chou P, Chen CH. Prognostic utility of morning blood pressure surge for 20-year all-cause and cardiovascular mortalities: results of a community-based study. *J Am Heart Assoc*. 2017; 6.

55 Kuwajima I, Mitani K, Miyao M, Suzuki Y, Kuramoto K, Ozawa T. Cardiac implications of the morning surge in blood pressure in elderly hypertensive patients: relation to arising time. *Am J Hypertens*. 1995; 8: 29-33.

56 Marfella R, Gualdiero P, Siniscalchi M, Carusone C, Verza M, Marzano S, Esposito K, Giugliano D. Morning blood pressure peak, QT intervals, and sympathetic activity in hypertensive patients. *Hypertension*. 2003; 41: 237-243. http://hyper.ahajournals.org/

57 Kaneda R, Kario K, Hoshide S, Umeda Y, Hoshide Y, Shimada K. Morning blood pressure hyper-reactivity is an independent predictor for hypertensive cardiac hypertrophy in a community-dwelling population. *Am J Hypertens*. 2005; 18: 1528-1533.

58 Yano Y, Hoshide S, Inokuchi T, Kanemaru Y, Shimada K, Kario K. Association between morning blood pressure surge and cardiovascular remodeling in treated elderly hypertensive subjects. *Am J Hypertens*. 2009; 22: 1177-1182.

59 Soylu A, Yazici M, Duzenli MA, Tokac M, Ozdemir K, Gok H. Relation between abnormalities in circadian blood pressure rhythm and target organ damage in normotensives. *Circ J*. 2009; 73: 899-904.

60 Caliskan M, Caliskan Z, Gullu H, Keles N, Bulur S, Turan Y, Kostek O, Ciftci O, Guven A, Aung SM, Muderrisoglu H. Increased morning blood pressure surge and coronary microvascular dysfunction in patient with early stage hypertension. *J Am Soc Hypertens*. 2014; 8: 652-659.

61 Zakopoulos NA, Tsivgoulis G, Barlas G, Papamichael C, Spengos K, Manios E, Ikonomidis I, Kotsis V, Spiliopoulou I, Vemmos K, Mavrikakis M, Moulopoulos SD. Time rate of blood pressure variation is associated with increased common carotid artery intima-media thickness. *Hypertension*. 2005; 45: 505-512. http://hyper.ahajournals.org/

62. Marfella R, Siniscalchi M, Nappo F, Gualdiero P, Esposito K, Sasso FC, Cacciapuoti F, Di Filippo C, Rossi F, D'Amico M, Giugliano D. Regression of carotid atherosclerosis by control of morning blood pressure peak in newly diagnosed hypertensive patients. *Am J Hypertens*. 2005; 18: 308-318.
63. Marfella R, Siniscalchi M, Portoghese M, Di Filippo C, Ferraraccio F, Schiattarella C, Crescenzi B, Sangiuolo P, Ferraro G, Siciliano S, Cinone F, Mazzarella G, Martis S, Verza M, Coppola L, Rossi F, D'Amico M, Paolisso G. Morning blood pressure surge as a destabilizing factor of atherosclerotic plaque: role of ubiquitin-proteasome activity. *Hypertension*. 2007; 49: 784-791. http://hyper.ahajournals.org/
64. Shimizu M, Ishikawa J, Yano Y, Hoshide S, Shimada K, Kario K. The relationship between the morning blood pressure surge and low-grade inflammation on silent cerebral infarct and clinical stroke events. *Atherosclerosis*. 2011; 219: 316-321.
65. Kario K. Treatment of early morning surges in blood pressure. In: *Clinical Challenges in Hypertension Management* (D Sicca D, P Toth, eds). Atlas Medical Publishing, Oxford, UK, pp. 27-38, 2010.
66. Chen CT, Li Y, Zhang J, Wang Y, Ling HW, Chen KM, Gao PJ, Zhu DL. Association between ambulatory systolic blood pressure during the day and asymptomatic intracranial arterial stenosis. *Hypertension*. 2014; 63: 61-67. http://hyper.ahajournals.org/
67. Polonia J, Amado P, Barbosa L, Nazare J, Silva JA, Bertoquini S, Martins L, Carmona J. Morning rise, morning surge and daytime variability of blood pressure and cardiovascular target organ damage. A cross-sectional study in 743 subjects. *Rev Port Cardiol*. 2005; 24: 65-78.
68. Pucci G, Battista F, Anastasio F, Schillaci G. Morning pressor surge, blood pressure variability, and arterial stiffness in essential hypertension. *J Hypertens*. 2017; 35: 272-278. https://journals.lww.com/jhypertension/
69. Pregowska-Chwala B, Prejbisz A, Kabat M, Pucilowska B, Paschalis-Purtak K, Florczak E, Klisiewicz A, Kusmierczyk-Droszcz B, Hanus K, Bursztyn M, Januszewicz A. Morning blood pressure surge and markers of cardiovascular alterations in untreated middle-aged hypertensive subjects. *J Am Soc Hypertens*. 2016; 10: 790-798 e2.
70. Alpaydin S, Turan Y, Caliskan M, Caliskan Z, Aksu F, Ozyildirim S, Buyukterzi Z, Kostek O, Muderrisoglu H. Morning blood pressure surge is associated with carotid intima-media thickness in prehypertensive patients. *Blood Press Monit*. 2017; 22: 131-136.
71. Kario K, Pickering TG, Hoshide S, Eguchi K, Ishikawa J, Morinari M, Hoshide Y, Shimada K. Morning blood pressure surge and hypertensive cerebrovascular disease: role of the alpha adrenergic sympathetic nervous system. *Am J Hypertens*. 2004; 17: 668-675.
72. Kimura G. Kidney and circadian blood pressure rhythm. *Hypertension*. 2008; 51: 827-828. http://hyper.ahajournals.org/
73. Fukuda M, Mizuno M, Yamanaka T, Motokawa M, Shirasawa Y, Nishio T, Miyagi S, Yoshida A, Kimura G. Patients with renal dysfunction require a longer duration until blood pressure dips during the night. *Hypertension*. 2008; 52: 1155-1160. http://hyper.ahajournals.org/
74. Lurbe E, Redon J, Kesani A, Pascual JM, Tacons J, Alvarez V, Batlle D. Increase in nocturnal blood pressure and progression to microalbuminuria in type 1 diabetes.

N Engl J Med. 2002; 347: 797-805.
75 Caramori ML, Pecis M, Azevedo MJ. Increase in nocturnal blood pressure and progression to microalbuminuria in diabetes. *N Engl J Med*. 2003; 348: 260-264; author reply -4.
76 Kawai T, Kamide K, Onishi M, Yamamoto-Hanasaki H, Baba Y, Hongyo K, Shimaoka I, Tatara Y, Takeya Y, Ohishi M, Rakugi H. Usefulness of the resistive index in renal Doppler ultrasonography as an indicator of vascular damage in patients with risks of atherosclerosis. *Nephrol Dial Transplant*. 2011; 26: 3256-3262.
77 Turak O, Afsar B, Siriopol D, Ozcan F, Cagli K, Yayla C, Oksuz F, Mendi MA, Kario K, Covic A, Kanbay M. Morning blood pressure surge as a predictor of development of chronic kidney disease. *J Clin Hypertens (Greenwich)*. 2016; 18: 444-448.
78 Shimizu M, Ishikawa J, Eguchi K, Hoshide S, Shimada K, Kario K. Association of an abnormal blood glucose level and morning blood pressure surge in elderly subjects with hypertension. *Am J Hypertens*. 2009; 22: 611-616.
79 Ishikawa J, Kario K, Eguchi K, Morinari M, Hoshide S, Ishikawa S, Shimada K; J-MORE Group. Regular alcohol drinking is a determinant of masked morning hypertension detected by home blood pressure monitoring in medicated hypertensive patients with well-controlled clinic blood pressure: the Jichi Morning hypertension Research (J-MORE) study. *Hypertens Res*. 2006; 29: 679-686.
80 Ohira T, Tanigawa T, Tabata M, Imano H, Kitamura A, Kiyama M, Sato S, Okamura T, Cui R, Koike KA, Shimamoto T, Iso H. Effects of habitual alcohol intake on ambulatory blood pressure, heart rate, and its variability among Japanese men. *Hypertension*. 2009; 53: 13-19. http://hyper.ahajournals.org/
81 Murakami S, Otsuka K, Kubo Y, Shinagawa M, Yamanaka T, Ohkawa S, Kitaura Y. Repeated ambulatory monitoring reveals a Monday morning surge in blood pressure in a community-dwelling population. *Am J Hypertens*. 2004; 17: 1179-1183.
82 Modesti PA, Morabito M, Bertolozzi I, Massetti L, Panci G, Lumachi C, Giglio A, Bilo G, Caldara G, Lonati L, Orlandini S, Maracchi G, Mancia G, Gensini GF, Parati G. Weather-related changes in 24-hour blood pressure profile: effects of age and implications for hypertension management. *Hypertension*. 2006; 47: 155-161. http://hyper.ahajournals.org/
83 Murakami S, Otsuka K, Kono T, Soyama A, Umeda T, Yamamoto N, Morita H, Yamanaka G, Kitaura Y. Impact of outdoor temperature on prewaking morning surge and nocturnal decline in blood pressure in a Japanese population. *Hypertens Res*. 2011; 34: 70-73.
84 Kario K. Caution for winter morning surge in blood pressure: a possible link with cardiovascular risk in the elderly. *Hypertension*. 2006; 47: 139-140. http://hyper.ahajournals.org/
85 Amin R, Somers VK, McConnell K, Willging P, Myer C, Sherman M, McPhail G, Morgenthal A, Fenchel M, Bean J, Kimball T, Daniels S. Activity-adjusted 24-hour ambulatory blood pressure and cardiac remodeling in children with sleep disordered breathing. *Hypertension*. 2008; 51: 84-91. http://hyper.ahajournals.org/
86 Sheng CS, Cheng YB, Wei FF, Yang WY, Guo QH, Li FK, Huang QF, Thijs L, Staessen JA, Wang JG, Li Y. Diurnal blood pressure rhythmicity in relation to environmental and genetic cues in untreated referred patients. *Hypertension*. 2017; 69: 128-135. http://hyper.ahajournals.org/
87 Kario K. Vascular damage in exaggerated morning surge in blood pressure. *Hyper-*

tension. 2007; 49: 771-772. http://hyper.ahajournals.org/

88 Otto ME, Svatikova A, Barretto RB, Santos S, Hoffmann M, Khandheria B, Somers V. Early morning attenuation of endothelial function in healthy humans. *Circulation*. 2004; 109: 2507-2510. http://circ.ahajournals.org/

89 Linsell CR, Lightman SL, Mullen PE, Brown MJ, Causon RC. Circadian rhythms of epinephrine and norepinephrine in man. *J Clin Endocrinol Metab*. 1985; 60: 1210-1215.

90 Johnson AW, Hissen SL, Macefield VG, Brown R, Taylor CE. Magnitude of morning surge in blood pressure is associated with sympathetic but not cardiac baroreflex sensitivity. *Front Neurosci*. 2016; 10: 412.

91 Kawasaki T, Cugini P, Uezono K, Sasaki H, Itoh K, Nishiura M, Shinkawa K. Circadian variations of total renin, active renin, plasma renin activity and plasma aldosterone in clinically healthy young subjects. *Horm Metab Res*. 1990; 22: 636-639.

92 Kario K, Yano Y, Matsuo T, Hoshide S, Eguchi K, Shimada K. Additional impact of morning haemostatic risk factors and morning blood pressure surge on stroke risk in older Japanese hypertensive patients. *Eur Heart J*. 2011; 32: 574-580.

93 Kario K, Yano Y, Matsuo T, Hoshide S, Asada Y, Shimada K. Morning blood pressure surge, morning platelet aggregation, and silent cerebral infarction in older Japanese hypertensive patients. *J Hypertens*. 2011; 29: 2433-2439. https://journals.lww.com/jhypertension/

94 Kario K. Preceding linkage between a morning surge in blood pressure and small artery remodeling: an indicator of prehypertension? *J Hypertens*. 2007; 25: 1573-1575. https://journals.lww.com/jhypertension/

95 Rizzoni D, Porteri E, Platto C, Rizzardi N, De Ciuceis C, Boari GE, Muiesan ML, Salvetti M, Zani F, Miclini M, Paiardi S, Castellano M, Rosei EA. Morning rise of blood pressure and subcutaneous small resistance artery structure. *J Hypertens*. 2007; 25: 1698-1703. https://journals.lww.com/jhypertension/

96 Folkow B. Physiological aspects of primary hypertension. *Physiol Rev*. 1982; 62: 347-504.

97 Schiffrin EL. Remodeling of resistance arteries in essential hypertension and effects of antihypertensive treatment. *Am J Hypertens*. 2004; 17: 1192-1200.

98 Panza JA, Epstein SE, Quyyumi AA. Circadian variation in vascular tone and its relation to alpha-sympathetic vasoconstrictor activity. *N Engl J Med*. 1991; 325: 986-990.

99 Brandenberger G, Follenius M, Goichot B, Saini J, Spiegel K, Ehrhart J, Simon C. Twenty-four-hour profiles of plasma renin activity in relation to the sleep-wake cycle. *J Hypertens*. 1994; 12: 277-283. https://journals.lww.com/jhypertension/

100 Naito Y, Tsujino T, Fujioka Y, Ohyanagi M, Iwasaki T. Augmented diurnal variations of the cardiac renin-angiotensin system in hypertensive rats. *Hypertension*. 2002; 40: 827-833. http://hyper.ahajournals.org/

101 Tissot AC, Maurer P, Nussberger J, Sabat R, Pfister T, Ignatenko S, Volk HD, Stocker H, Muller P, Jennings GT, Wagner F, Bachmann MF. Effect of immunisation against angiotensin II with CYT006-AngQb on ambulatory blood pressure: a double-blind, randomised, placebo-controlled phase IIa study. *Lancet*. 2008; 371: 821-827.

102 Tochikubo O, Kawano Y, Miyajima E, Toshihiro N, Ishii M. Circadian variation of hemodynamics and baroreflex functions in patients with essential hypertension.

Hypertens Res. 1997; 20: 157-66.
103 Eguchi K, Tomizawa H, Ishikawa J, Hoshide S, Pickering TG, Shimada K, Kario K. Factors associated with baroreflex sensitivity: association with morning blood pressure. *Hypertens Res*. 2007; 30: 723-728.
104 Kario K. Prognosis in relation to blood pressure variability: pro side of the argument. *Hypertension*. 2015; 65: 1163-1169. http://hyper.ahajournals.org/
105 Sega R, Facchetti R, Bombelli M, Cesana G, Corrao G, Grassi G, Mancia G. Prognostic value of ambulatory and home blood pressures compared with office blood pressure in the general population: follow-up results from the Pressioni Arteriose Monitorate e Loro Associazioni (PAMELA) study. *Circulation*. 2005; 111: 1777-83. http://circ.ahajournals.org/
106 Boggia J, Li Y, Thijs L, Hansen TW, Kikuya M, Bjorklund-Bodegard K, Richart T, Ohkubo T, Kuznetsova T, Torp-Pedersen C, Lind L, Ibsen H, Imai Y, Wang J, Sandoya E, O'Brien E, Staessen JA; International Database on Ambulatory blood pressure monitoring in relation to Cardiovascular Outcomes (IDACO) investigators. Prognostic accuracy of day versus night ambulatory blood pressure: a cohort study. *Lancet*. 2007; 370: 1219-1229.
107 Hoshide S, Kario K, Hoshide Y, Umeda Y, Hashimoto T, Kunii O, Ojima T, Shimada K. Associations between nondipping of nocturnal blood pressure decrease and cardiovascular target organ damage in strictly selected community-dwelling normotensives. *Am J Hypertens*. 2003; 16: 434-438.
108 Ohkubo T, Hozawa A, Yamaguchi J, Kikuya M, Ohmori K, Michimata M, Matsubara M, Hashimoto J, Hoshi H, Araki T, Tsuji I, Satoh H, Hisamichi S, Imai Y. Prognostic significance of the nocturnal decline in blood pressure in individuals with and without high 24-h blood pressure: the Ohasama study. *J Hypertens*. 2002; 20: 2183-2189. https://journals.lww.com/jhypertension/
109 O'Brien E, Sheridan J, O'Malley K. Dippers and non-dippers. *Lancet*. 1988; 2: 397.
110 Shimada K, Kawamoto A, Matsubayashi K, Ozawa T. Silent cerebrovascular disease in the elderly. Correlation with ambulatory pressure. *Hypertension*. 1990; 16: 692-699. http://hyper.ahajournals.org/
111 Kario K, Schwartz JE, Pickering TG. Changes of nocturnal blood pressure dipping status in hypertensives by nighttime dosing of alpha-adrenergic blocker, doxazosin: results from the HALT study. *Hypertension*. 2000; 35: 787-794. http://hyper.ahajournals.org/
112 Kario K, Shimada K. Risers and extreme-dippers of nocturnal blood pressure in hypertension: antihypertensive strategy for nocturnal blood pressure. *Clin Exp Hypertens*. 2004; 26: 177-189.
113 Eguchi K, Pickering TG, Schwartz JE, Hoshide S, Ishikawa J, Ishikawa S, Shimada K, Kario K. Short sleep duration as an independent predictor of cardiovascular events in Japanese patients with hypertension. *Arch Intern Med*. 2008; 168: 2225-2231.
114 Kabutoya T, Hoshide S, Ishikawa J, Eguchi K, Shimada K, Kario K. The effect of pulse rate and blood pressure dipping status on the risk of stroke and cardiovascular disease in Japanese hypertensive patients. *Am J Hypertens*. 2010; 23: 749-755.
115 Komori T, Eguchi K, Saito T, Hoshide S, Kario K. Riser pattern: another determinant of heart failure with preserved ejection fraction. *J Clin Hypertens (Greenwich)*. 2016; 18: 994-999.

116 Komori T, Eguchi K, Saito T, Hoshide S, Kario K. Riser pattern is a novel predictor of adverse events in heart failure patients with preserved ejection fraction. *Circ J*. 2017; 81: 220-226.

117 Oba Y, Kabutoya T, Hoshide S, Eguchi K, Kario K. Association between nondipper pulse rate and measures of cardiac overload: the J-HOP study. *J Clin Hypertens (Greenwich)*. 2017; 19: 402-409.

118 Nagai M, Hoshide S, Ishikawa J, Shimada K, Kario K. Ambulatory blood pressure as an independent determinant of brain atrophy and cognitive function in elderly hypertension. *J Hypertens*. 2008; 26: 1636-1641. https://journals.lww.com/jhypertension/

119 Nagai M, Hoshide S, Ishikawa J, Shimada K, Kario K. Insular cortex atrophy as an independent determinant of disrupted diurnal rhythm of ambulatory blood pressure in elderly hypertension. *Am J Hypertens*. 2009; 22: 723-729.

120 Yano Y, Inokuchi T, Hoshide S, Kanemaru Y, Shimada K, Kario K. Association of poor physical function and cognitive dysfunction with high nocturnal blood pressure level in treated elderly hypertensive patients. *Am J Hypertens*. 2011; 24: 285-291.

121 Komori T, Eguchi K, Saito T, Nishimura Y, Hoshide S, Kario K. Riser blood pressure pattern is associated with mild cognitive impairment in heart failure patients. *Am J Hypertens*. 2016; 29: 194-201.

122 Palatini P, Reboldi G, Beilin LJ, Eguchi K, Imai Y, Kario K, Ohkubo T, Pierdomenico SD, Saladini F, Schwartz JE, Wing L, Verdecchia P. Predictive value of night-time heart rate for cardiovascular events in hypertension. The ABP-International study. *Int J Cardiol*. 2013; 168: 1490-1495.

123 Komori T, Eguchi K, Tomizawa H, Ishikawa J, Hoshide S, Shimada K, Kario K. Factors associated with incident ischemic stroke in hospitalized heart failure patients: a pilot study. *Hypertens Res*. 2008; 31: 289-294.

124 Eguchi K, Pickering TG, Hoshide S, Ishikawa J, Ishikawa S, Schwartz JE, Shimada K, Kario K. Ambulatory blood pressure is a better marker than clinic blood pressure in predicting cardiovascular events in patients with/without type 2 diabetes. *Am J Hypertens*. 2008; 21: 443-450.

125 Yano Y, Hoshide S, Shimizu M, Eguchi K, Ishikawa J, Ishikawa S, Shimada K, Kario K. Association of home and ambulatory blood pressure changes with changes in cardiovascular biomarkers during antihypertensive treatment. *Am J Hypertens*. 2012; 25: 306-312.

126 Kario K, Schwartz JE, Davidson KW, Pickering TG. Gender differences in associations of diurnal blood pressure variation, awake physical activity, and sleep quality with negative affect: the work site blood pressure study. *Hypertension*. 2001; 38: 997-1002. http://hyper.ahajournals.org/

127 Kario K. Are melatonin and its receptor agonist specific antihypertensive modulators of resistant hypertension caused by disrupted circadian rhythm? *J Am Soc Hypertens*. 2011; 5: 354-358.

128 Yano Y, Hayakawa M, Kuroki K, Ueno H, Yamagishi S, Takeuchi M, Eto T, Nagata N, Nakazato M, Shimada K, Kario K. Nighttime blood pressure, nighttime glucose values, and target-organ damages in treated type 2 diabetes patients. *Atherosclerosis*. 2013; 227: 135-139.

129 Kamoi K, Miyakoshi M, Soda S, Kaneko S, Nakagawa O. Usefulness of home

blood pressure measurement in the morning in type 2 diabetic patients. *Diabetes Care*. 2002; 25: 2218-2223.

130 Ishikawa J, Shimizu M, Hoshide S, Eguchi K, Pickering TG, Shimada K, Kario K. Cardiovascular risks of dipping status and chronic kidney disease in elderly Japanese hypertensive patients. *J Clin Hypertens (Greenwich)*. 2008; 10: 787-794.

131 Watanabe N, Imai Y, Nagai K, Tsuji I, Satoh H, Sakuma M, Sakuma H, Kato J, Onodera-Kikuchi N, Yamada M, Abe F, Hisamichi S, Abe K. Nocturnal blood pressure and silent cerebrovascular lesions in elderly Japanese. *Stroke*. 1996; 27: 1319-1327.

132 Siennicki-Lantz A, Reinprecht F, Axelsson J, Elmstahl S. Cerebral perfusion in the elderly with nocturnal blood pressure fall. *Eur J Neurol*. 2007; 14: 715-720.

133 Jerrard-Dunne P, Mahmud A, Feely J. Circadian blood pressure variation: relationship between dipper status and measures of arterial stiffness. *J Hypertens*. 2007; 25: 1233-1239. https://journals.lww.com/jhypertension/

134 Viera AJ, Lin FC, Hinderliter AL, Shimbo D, Person SD, Pletcher MJ, Jacobs DR, Jr. Nighttime blood pressure dipping in young adults and coronary artery calcium 10-15 years later: the coronary artery risk development in young adults study. *Hypertension*. 2012; 59: 1157-1163. http://hyper.ahajournals.org/

135 Salles GF, Reboldi G, Fagard RH, Cardoso CR, Pierdomenico SD, Verdecchia P, Eguchi K, Kario K, Hoshide S, Polonia J, de la Sierra A, Hermida RC, Dolan E, O'Brien E, Roush GC; ABC-H Investigators. Prognostic effect of the nocturnal blood pressure fall in hypertensive patients: the Ambulatory Blood Pressure Collaboration in Patients with Hypertension (ABC-H) meta-analysis. *Hypertension*. 2016; 67: 693-700. http://hyper.ahajournals.org/

136 Kario K, Mitsuhashi T, Shimada K. Neurohumoral characteristics of older hypertensive patients with abnormal nocturnal blood pressure dipping. *Am J Hypertens*. 2002; 15: 531-537.

137 St-Onge MP, Grandner MA, Brown D, Conroy MB, Jean-Louis G, Coons M, Bhatt DL; American Heart Association Obesity, Behavior Change, Diabetes, and Nutrition Committees of the Council on Lifestyle and Cardiometabolic Health; Council on Cardiovascular Disease in the Young; Council on Clinical Cardiology; and Stroke Council. Sleep duration and quality: impact on lifestyle behaviors and cardiometabolic health: a scientific statement from the American Heart Association. *Circulation*. 2016; 134: e367-e86. http://circ.ahajournals.org/

138 Grandner MA, Alfonso-Miller P, Fernandez-Mendoza J, Shetty S, Shenoy S, Combs D. Sleep: important considerations for the prevention of cardiovascular disease. *Curr Opin Cardiol*. 2016; 31: 551-565.

139 Kario K. Sleep and circadian cardiovascular medicine. In: *Encyclopedia of Cardiovascular Research and Medicine* (Vasan R, Sawyer D, eds). Amsterdam, Netherlands: Elsevier 2018, pp. 424-437.

140 Kario K. Proposal of a new strategy for ambulatory blood pressure profile-based management of resistant hypertension in the era of renal denervation. *Hypertens Res*. 2013; 36: 478-484.

141 Ishikawa J, Hoshide S, Eguchi K, Ishikawa S, Shimada K, Kario K; Japan Morning Surge-Home Blood Pressure Study Investigators Group. Nighttime home blood pressure and the risk of hypertensive target organ damage. *Hypertension*. 2012; 60: 921-928. http://hyper.ahajournals.org/

142 Hoshide S, Kario K, Yano Y, Haimoto H, Yamagiwa K, Uchiba K, Nagasaka S, Matsui Y, Nakamura A, Fukutomi M, Eguchi K, Ishikawa J; J-HOP Study Group. Association of morning and evening blood pressure at home with asymptomatic organ damage in the J-HOP study. *Am J Hypertens.* 2014; 27: 939-947.

143 Kario K, Hoshide S, Haimoto H, Yamagiwa K, Uchiba K, Nagasaka S, Yano Y, Eguchi K, Matsui Y, Shimizu M, Ishikawa J, Ishikawa S; J-HOP Study Group. Sleep blood pressure self-measured at home as a novel determinant of organ damage: Japan Morning Surge Home Blood Pressure (J-HOP) study. *J Clin Hypertens (Greenwich).* 2015; 17: 340-348.

144 Ishikawa J, Shimizu M, Sugiyama Edison E, Yano Y, Hoshide S, Eguchi K, Kario K; J-TOP (Japan Morning Surge-Target Organ Protection) Study Investigators Group. Assessment of the reductions in night-time blood pressure and dipping induced by antihypertensive medication using a home blood pressure monitor. *J Hypertens.* 2014; 32: 82-89. https://journals.lww.com/jhypertension/

145 Kario K, Hamasaki H. Nocturnal blood pressure surge behind morning surge in obstructive sleep apnea syndrome: another phenotype of systemic hemodynamic atherothrombotic syndrome. *J Clin Hypertens (Greenwich).* 2015; 17: 682-685.

146 Shirasaki O, Kuwabara M, Saito M, Tagami K, Washiya S, Kario K. Development and clinical application of a new technique for detecting 'sleep blood pressure surges' in sleep apnea patients based on a variable desaturation threshold. *Hypertens Res.* 2011; 34: 922-928.

147 Kario K. Obstructive sleep apnea syndrome and hypertension: ambulatory blood pressure. *Hypertens Res.* 2009; 32: 428-432.

148 Kario K, Kuwabara M, Hoshide S, Nagai M, Shimpo M. Effects of nighttime single-dose administration of vasodilating vs sympatholytic antihypertensive agents on sleep blood pressure in hypertensive patients with sleep apnea syndrome. *J Clin Hypertens (Greenwich).* 2014; 16: 459-466.

149 Kuwabara M, Hamasaki H, Tomitani N, Shiga T, Kario K. Novel triggered nocturnal blood pressure monitoring for sleep apnea syndrome: distribution and reproducibility of hypoxia-triggered nocturnal blood pressure measurements. *J Clin Hypertens (Greenwich).* 2017; 19: 30-37.

150 Yoshida T, Kuwabara M, Hoshide S, Kario K. Recurrence of stroke caused by nocturnal hypoxia-induced blood pressure surge in a young adult male with severe obstructive sleep apnea syndrome. *J Am Soc Hypertens.* 2016; 10: 201-204.

151 Kario K. Obstructive sleep apnea syndrome and hypertension: mechanism of the linkage and 24-h blood pressure control. *Hypertens Res.* 2009; 32: 537-541.

152 Khan SU, Duran CA, Rahman H, Lekkala M, Saleem MA, Kaluski E. A meta-analysis of continuous positive airway pressure therapy in prevention of cardiovascular events in patients with obstructive sleep apnoea. *Eur Heart J.* 2017. [in press].

153 McEvoy RD, Antic NA, Heeley E, Luo Y, Ou Q, Zhang X, Mediano O, Chen R, Drager LF, Liu Z, Chen G, Du B, McArdle N, Mukherjee S, Tripathi M, Billot L, Li Q, Lorenzi-Filho G, Barbe F, Redline S, Wang J, Arima H, Neal B, White DP, Grunstein RR, Zhong N, Anderson CS; SAVE Investigators and Coordinators. CPAP for prevention of cardiovascular events in obstructive sleep apnea. *N Engl J Med.* 2016; 375: 919-931.

154 Kario K, Schwartz JE, Gerin W, Robayo N, Maceo E, Pickering TG. Psychological and physical stress-induced cardiovascular reactivity and diurnal blood pressure

variation in women with different work shifts. *Hypertens Res.* 2002; 25: 543-551.
155 Kario K. New insight of morning blood pressure surge into the triggers of cardiovascular disease-synergistic resonance of blood pressure variability. *Am J Hypertens.* 2016; 29: 14-16.
156 Parati G, Ochoa JE, Lombardi C, Bilo G. Assessment and management of blood-pressure variability. *Nat Rev Cardiol.* 2013; 10: 143-155.
157 Kario K, Tomitani N, Matsumoto Y, Hamasaki H, Okawara Y, Kondo M, Nozue R, Yamagata H, Okura A, Hoshide S. Research and development of information and communication technology-based home blood pressure monitoring from morning to nocturnal hypertension. *Ann Glob Health.* 2016; 82: 254-273.
158 Imaizumi Y, Eguchi K, Taketomi A, Tsuchihashi T, Kario K. Exaggerated blood pressure variability in patients with pneumoconiosis: a pilot study. *Am J Hypertens.* 2014; 27: 1456-1463.
159 Kayano H, Koba S, Matsui T, Fukuoka H, Kaneko K, Shoji M, Toshida T, Watanabe N, Geshi E, Kobayashi Y. Impact of depression on masked hypertension and variability in home blood pressure in treated hypertensive patients. *Hypertens Res.* 2015; 38: 751-757.
160 Umemoto S, Ogihara T, Matsuzaki M, Rakugi H, Ohashi Y, Saruta T; Combination Therapy of Hypertension to Prevent Cardiovascular Events COPE Trial Group. Effects of calcium channel blocker-based combinations on intra-individual blood pressure variability: post hoc analysis of the COPE trial. *Hypertens Res.* 2016; 39: 46-53.
161 Imaizumi Y, Eguchi K, Kario K. Coexistence of PM2.5 and low temperature is associated with morning hypertension in hypertensives. *Clin Exp Hypertens.* 2015; 37: 468-472.
162 Kario K, Eguchi K, Nakagawa Y, Motai K, Shimada K. Relationship between extreme dippers and orthostatic hypertension in elderly hypertensive patients. *Hypertension.* 1998; 31: 77-82. http://hyper.ahajournals.org/
163 Kario K, Eguchi K, Hoshide S, Hoshide Y, Umeda Y, Mitsuhashi T, Shimada K. U-curve relationship between orthostatic blood pressure change and silent cerebrovascular disease in elderly hypertensives: orthostatic hypertension as a new cardiovascular risk factor. *J Am Coll Cardiol.* 2002; 40: 133-141.
164 Hoshide S, Matsui Y, Shibasaki S, Eguchi K, Ishikawa J, Ishikawa S, Kabutoya T, Schwartz JE, Pickering TG, Shimada K, Kario K; Japan Morning Surge-1 Study Group. Orthostatic hypertension detected by self-measured home blood pressure monitoring: a new cardiovascular risk factor for elderly hypertensives. *Hypertens Res.* 2008; 31: 1509-1516.
165 Kario K, Pickering TG. Blood pressure variability in elderly patients. *Lancet.* 2000; 355: 1645-1646.
166 Kikuya M, Ohkubo T, Metoki H, Asayama K, Hara A, Obara T, Inoue R, Hoshi H, Hashimoto J, Totsune K, Satoh H, Imai Y. Day-by-day variability of blood pressure and heart rate at home as a novel predictor of prognosis: the Ohasama study. *Hypertension.* 2008; 52: 1045-1050. http://hyper.ahajournals.org/
167 Eguchi K, Ishikawa J, Hoshide S, Pickering TG, Schwartz JE, Shimada K, Kario K. Night time blood pressure variability is a strong predictor for cardiovascular events in patients with type 2 diabetes. *Am J Hypertens.* 2009; 22: 46-51.
168 Rothwell PM, Howard SC, Dolan E, O'Brien E, Dobson JE, Dahlof B, Sever PS,

Poulter NR. Prognostic significance of visit-to-visit variability, maximum systolic blood pressure, and episodic hypertension. *Lancet.* 2010; 375: 895-905.

169 Matsui Y, O'Rourke MF, Hoshide S, Ishikawa J, Shimada K, Kario K. Combined effect of angiotensin II receptor blocker and either a calcium channel blocker or diuretic on day-by-day variability of home blood pressure: the Japan Combined Treatment with Olmesartan and a Calcium-Channel Blocker versus Olmesartan and Diuretics Randomized Efficacy study. *Hypertension.* 2012; 59: 1132-1138. http://hyper.ahajournals.org/

170 Nagai M, Hoshide S, Ishikawa J, Shimada K, Kario K. Visit-to-visit blood pressure variations: new independent determinants for cognitive function in the elderly at high risk of cardiovascular disease. *J Hypertens.* 2012; 30: 1556-1563. https://journals.lww.com/jhypertension/

171 Kawai T, Ohishi M, Ito N, Onishi M, Takeya Y, Yamamoto K, Kamide K, Rakugi H. Alteration of vascular function is an important factor in the correlation between visit-to-visit blood pressure variability and cardiovascular disease. *J Hypertens.* 2013; 31: 1387-1395; discussion 1395. https://journals.lww.com/jhypertension/

172 Fukui M, Ushigome E, Tanaka M, Hamaguchi M, Tanaka T, Atsuta H, Ohnishi M, Oda Y, Hasegawa G, Nakamura N. Home blood pressure variability on one occasion is a novel factor associated with arterial stiffness in patients with type 2 diabetes. *Hypertens Res.* 2013; 36: 219-225.

173 Endo K, Kario K, Koga M, Nakagawara J, Shiokawa Y, Yamagami H, Furui E, Kimura K, Hasegawa Y, Okada Y, Okuda S, Namekawa M, Miyagi T, Osaki M, Minematsu K, Toyoda K. Impact of early blood pressure variability on stroke outcomes after thrombolysis: the SAMURAI rt-PA registry. *Stroke.* 2013; 44: 816-818.

174 Wei FF, Li Y, Zhang L, Xu TY, Ding FH, Wang JG, Staessen JA. Beat-to-beat, reading-to-reading, and day-to-day blood pressure variability in relation to organ damage in untreated Chinese. *Hypertension.* 2014; 63: 790-796. http://hyper.ahajournals.org/

175 Nagai M, Hoshide S, Nishikawa M, Masahisa S, Kario K. Visit-to-visit blood pressure variability in the elderly: associations with cognitive impairment and carotid artery remodeling. *Atherosclerosis.* 2014; 233: 19-26.

176 Kagitani H, Hoshide S, Kario K. Optimal indicators of home BP variability in perimenopausal women and associations with albuminuria and reproducibility: the J-HOT home BP study. *Am J Hypertens.* 2015; 28: 586-594.

177 Rakugi H, Ogihara T, Saruta T, Kawai T, Saito I, Teramukai S, Shimada K, Katayama S, Higaki J, Odawara M, Tanahashi N, Kimura G; COLM Investigators. Preferable effects of olmesartan/calcium channel blocker to olmesartan/diuretic on blood pressure variability in very elderly hypertension: COLM study subanalysis. *J Hypertens.* 2015; 33: 2165-2172. https://journals.lww.com/jhypertension/

178 Shibasaki S, Hoshide S, Eguchi K, Ishikawa J, Kario K; Japan Morning Surge-Home Blood Pressure (J-HOP) Study Group. Increase trend in home blood pressure on a single occasion is associated with B-type natriuretic peptide and the estimated glomerular filtration rate. *Am J Hypertens.* 2015; 28: 1098-1105.

179 Nagai M, Hoshide S, Ishikawa J, Shimada K, Kario K. Visit-to-visit blood pressure variations: new independent determinants for carotid artery measures in the elderly at high risk of cardiovascular disease. *J Am Soc Hypertens.* 2011; 5: 184-192.

180 Nagai M, Hoshide S, Nishikawa M, Shimada K, Kario K. Sleep duration and

insomnia in the elderly: associations with blood pressure variability and carotid artery remodeling. *Am J Hypertens*. 2013; 26: 981-989.

181 Sakakura K, Ishikawa J, Okuno M, Shimada K, Kario K. Exaggerated ambulatory blood pressure variability is associated with cognitive dysfunction in the very elderly and quality of life in the younger elderly. *Am J Hypertens*. 2007; 20: 720-727.

182 Cho N, Hoshide S, Nishizawa M, Fujiwara T, Kario K. Relationship between blood pressure variability and cognitive function in elderly patients with good blood pressure control. *Am J Hypertens*. 2018; 31: 293-298.

183 Matsui Y, Ishikawa J, Eguchi K, Shibasaki S, Shimada K, Kario K. Maximum value of home blood pressure: a novel indicator of target organ damage in hypertension. *Hypertension*. 2011; 57: 1087-1093. http://hyper.ahajournals.org/

184 Johansson JK, Niiranen TJ, Puukka PJ, Jula AM. Prognostic value of the variability in home-measured blood pressure and heart rate: the Finn-Home study. *Hypertension*. 2012; 59: 212-218. http://hyper.ahajournals.org/

185 Hoshide S, Yano Y, Mizuno H, Kanegae H, Kario K. Day-by-day variability of home blood pressure and incident cardiovascular disease in clinical practice: the J-HOP study (Japan Morning Surge-Home Blood Pressure). *Hypertension*. 2018; 71: 177-184. http://hyper.ahajournals.org/

186 Matsui Y, Eguchi K, Shibasaki S, Shimizu M, Ishikawa J, Shimada K, Kario K. Association between the morning-evening difference in home blood pressure and cardiac damage in untreated hypertensive patients. *J Hypertens*. 2009; 27: 712-720. https://journals.lww.com/jhypertension/

187 Matsui Y, Eguchi K, Shibasaki S, Ishikawa J, Shimada K, Kario K. Morning hypertension assessed by home monitoring is a strong predictor of concentric left ventricular hypertrophy in patients with untreated hypertension. *J Clin Hypertens (Greenwich)*. 2010; 12: 776-783.

188 Shibuya Y, Ikeda T, Gomi T. Morning rise of blood pressure assessed by home blood pressure monitoring is associated with left ventricular hypertrophy in hypertensive patients receiving long-term antihypertensive medication. *Hypertens Res*. 2007; 30: 903-911.

189 Eguchi K, Matsui Y, Shibasaki S, Hoshide S, Kabutoya T, Ishikawa J, Ishikawa S, Shimada K, Kario K; Japan Morning Surge-1 (JMS-1) Study Group. Controlling evening BP as well as morning BP is important in hypertensive patients with pre-diabetes/diabetes: the JMS-1 study. *Am J Hypertens*. 2010; 23: 522-527.

190 Kario K. Orthostatic hypertension: a measure of blood pressure variation for predicting cardiovascular risk. *Circ J*. 2009; 73: 1002-1007.

191 Hoshide S, Parati G, Matsui Y, Shibazaki S, Eguchi K, Kario K. Orthostatic hypertension: home blood pressure monitoring for detection and assessment of treatment with doxazosin. *Hypertens Res*. 2012; 35: 100-106.

192 Kario K. Systemic hemodynamic atherothrombotic syndrome: a blind spot in the current management of hypertension. *J Clin Hypertens (Greenwich)*. 2015; 17: 328-331.

193 Ito S, Nagasawa T, Abe M, Mori T. Strain vessel hypothesis: a viewpoint for linkage of albuminuria and cerebro-cardiovascular risk. *Hypertens Res*. 2009; 32: 115-121.

194 Briet M, Boutouyrie P, Laurent S, London GM. Arterial stiffness and pulse pressure in CKD and ESRD. *Kidney Int*. 2012; 82: 388-400.

195 Matsui Y, Eguchi K, Shibasaki S, Ishikawa J, Hoshide S, Shimada K, Kario K; Japan morning Surge-1 Study Group. Impact of arterial stiffness reduction on urinary albumin excretion during antihypertensive treatment: the Japan morning Surge-1 study. *J Hypertens*. 2010; 28: 1752-1760.

196 Toriumi S, Hoshide S, Nagai M, Kario K. Day-to-day blood pressure variability as a phenotype in a high-risk patient. *Geriatr Gerontol Int*. 2014; 14: 1005-1006.

197 Eguchi K, Murakami A, Horaguchi T, Kato M, Miyashita H, Kario K. Percutaneous transluminal angioplasty for peripheral artery disease confers cardiorenal protection. *J Hum Hypertens*. 2014; 28: 51-55.

198 Yingchoncharoen T, Limpijankit T, Jongjirasiri S, Laothamatas J, Yamwong S, Sritara P. Arterial stiffness contributes to coronary artery disease risk prediction beyond the traditional risk score (RAMA-EGAT score). *Heart Asia*. 2012; 4: 77-82.

199 Ohkuma T, Ninomiya T, Tomiyama H, Kario K, Hoshide S, Kita Y, Inoguchi T, Maeda Y, Kohara K, Tabara Y, Nakamura M, Ohkubo T, Watada H, Munakata M, Ohishi M, Ito N, Nakamura M, Shoji T, Vlachopoulos C, Yamashina A; Collaborative Group for J-BAVEL (Japan Brachial-Ankle Pulse Wave Velocity Individual Participant Data Meta-Analysis of Prospective Studies). Brachial-ankle pulse wave velocity and the risk prediction of cardiovascular disease: an individual participant data meta-analysis. *Hypertension*. 2017; 69: 1045-1052. http://hyper.ahajournals.org/

200 Townsend RR, Wilkinson IB, Schiffrin EL, Avolio AP, Chirinos JA, Cockcroft JR, Heffernan KS, Lakatta EG, McEniery CM, Mitchell GF, Najjar SS, Nichols WW, Urbina EM, Weber T; American Heart Association Council on Hypertension. Recommendations for improving and standardizing vascular research on arterial stiffness: a scientific statement from the American Heart Association. *Hypertension*. 2015; 66: 698-722. http://hyper.ahajournals.org/

201 McEniery CM, Cockcroft JR, Roman MJ, Franklin SS, Wilkinson IB. Central blood pressure: current evidence and clinical importance. *Eur Heart J*. 2014; 35: 1719-1725.

202 Wang KL, Cheng HM, Chuang SY, Spurgeon HA, Ting CT, Lakatta EG, Yin FC, Chou P, Chen CH. Central or peripheral systolic or pulse pressure: which best relates to target organs and future mortality? *J Hypertens*. 2009; 27: 461-467. https://journals.lww.com/jhypertension/

203 Kabutoya T, Hoshide S, Ogata Y, Iwata T, Eguchi K, Kario K. The time course of flow-mediated vasodilation and endothelial dysfunction in patients with a cardiovascular risk factor. *J Am Soc Hypertens*. 2012; 6: 109-116.

204 Kabutoya T, Hoshide S, Ogata Y, Eguchi K, Kario K. Masked hypertension defined by home blood pressure monitoring is associated with impaired flow-mediated vasodilatation in patients with cardiovascular risk factors. *J Clin Hypertens (Greenwich)*. 2013; 15: 630-636.

205 Welsh P, Poulter NR, Chang CL, Sever PS, Sattar N; ASCOT Investigators. The value of N-terminal pro-B-type natriuretic peptide in determining antihypertensive benefit: observations from the Anglo-Scandinavian Cardiac Outcomes Trial (ASCOT). *Hypertension*. 2014; 63: 507-513. http://hyper.ahajournals.org/

206 Kim JB, Kobayashi Y, Moneghetti KJ, Brenner DA, O'Malley R, Schnittger I, Wu JC, Murtagh G, Beshiri A, Fischbein M, Miller DC, Liang D, Yeung AC, Haddad F, Fearon WF. GDF-15 (Growth Differentiation Factor 15) is associated with lack of

ventricular recovery and mortality after transcatheter aortic valve replacement. *Circ Cardiovasc Interv*. 2017. [in press].
207 Edison ES, Yano Y, Hoshide S, Kario K. Association of electrocardiographic left ventricular hypertrophy with incident cardiovascular disease in Japanese older hypertensive patients. *Am J Hypertens*. 2015; 28: 527-534.
208 Ishikawa J, Ishikawa S, Kabutoya T, Gotoh T, Kayaba K, Schwartz JE, Pickering TG, Shimada K, Kario K; Jichi Medical School Cohort Study Investigators Group. Cornell product left ventricular hypertrophy in electrocardiogram and the risk of stroke in a general population. *Hypertension*. 2009; 53: 28-34. http://hyper.ahajournals.org/
209 Ishikawa J, Ishikawa S, Kario K. Prolonged corrected QT interval is predictive of future stroke events even in subjects without ECG-diagnosed left ventricular hypertrophy. *Hypertension*. 2015; 65: 554-560. http://hyper.ahajournals.org/
210 Lastra G, Manrique C, McFarlane SI, Sowers JR. Cardiometabolic syndrome and chronic kidney disease. *Curr Diab Rep*. 2006; 6: 207-212.
211 Faraco G, Iadecola C. Hypertension: a harbinger of stroke and dementia. *Hypertension*. 2013; 62: 810-817. http://hyper.ahajournals.org/
212 Eguchi K, Kario K, Shimada K. Greater impact of coexistence of hypertension and diabetes on silent cerebral infarcts. *Stroke*. 2003; 34: 2471-2474.
213 Kario K, Matsuo T, Hoshide S, Umeda Y, Shimada K. Effect of thrombin inhibition in vascular dementia and silent cerebrovascular disease. An MR spectroscopy study. *Stroke*. 1999; 30: 1033-1037.
214 Kario K, Ishikawa J, Hoshide S, Matsui Y, Morinari M, Eguchi K, Ishikawa S, Shimada K. Diabetic brain damage in hypertension: role of renin-angiotensin system. *Hypertension*. 2005; 45: 887-893. http://hyper.ahajournals.org/
215 Eguchi K, Tomizawa H, Ishikawa J, Hoshide S, Fukuda T, Numao T, Shimada K, Kario K. Effects of new calcium channel blocker, azelnidipine, and amlodipine on baroreflex sensitivity and ambulatory blood pressure. *J Cardiovasc Pharmacol*. 2007; 49: 394-400.
216 Nakano M, Eguchi K, Sato T, Onoguchi A, Hoshide S, Kario K. Effect of intensive salt-restriction education on clinic, home, and ambulatory blood pressure levels in treated hypertensive patients during a 3-month education period. *J Clin Hypertens (Greenwich)*. 2016; 18: 385-392.
217 Matsui Y, Kario K. Differential impacts of antihypertensive drugs on central blood pressure and their clinical significance. *Curr Hypertens Rev*. 2012; 8: 114-119.
218 Ettehad D, Emdin CA, Kiran A, Anderson SG, Callender T, Emberson J, Chalmers J, Rodgers A, Rahimi K. Blood pressure lowering for prevention of cardiovascular disease and death: a systematic review and meta-analysis. *Lancet*. 2016; 387: 957-967.
219 Uzu T, Kimura G. Diuretics shift circadian rhythm of blood pressure from nondipper to dipper in essential hypertension. *Circulation*. 1999; 100: 1635-1638. http://circ.ahajournals.org/
220 Eguchi K, Kario K, Hoshide Y, Hoshide S, Ishikawa J, Morinari M, Ishikawa S, Shimada K. Comparison of valsartan and amlodipine on ambulatory and morning blood pressure in hypertensive patients. *Am J Hypertens*. 2004; 17: 112-117.
221 Kario K, Kimura K, Node K. Nearly half of uncontrolled hypertensive patients could be controlled by high-dose titration of amlodipine in the clinical setting: the

ACHIEVE study. *Curr Hypertens Rev*. 2011; 7: 102-110.
222 Kario K, Shimada K. Differential effects of amlodipine on ambulatory blood pressure in elderly hypertensive patients with different nocturnal reductions in blood pressure. *Am J Hypertens*. 1997; 10: 261-268.
223 Wang JG, Kario K, Lau T, Wei YQ, Park CG, Kim CH, Huang J, Zhang W, Li Y, Yan P, Hu D; Asian Pacific Heart Association. Use of dihydropyridine calcium channel blockers in the management of hypertension in Eastern Asians: a scientific statement from the Asian Pacific Heart Association. *Hypertens Res*. 2011; 34: 423-430.
224 Zhang Y, Agnoletti D, Safar ME, Blacher J. Effect of antihypertensive agents on blood pressure variability: the Natrilix SR versus candesartan and amlodipine in the reduction of systolic blood pressure in hypertensive patients (X-CELLENT) study. *Hypertension*. 2011; 58: 155-160. http://hyper.ahajournals.org/
225 Mizuno H, Hoshide S, Tomitani N, Kario K. Comparison of ambulatory blood pressure-lowering effects of higher doses of different calcium antagonists in uncontrolled hypertension: the Calcium Antagonist Controlled-Release High-Dose Therapy in Uncontrolled Refractory Hypertensive Patients (CARILLON) study. *Blood Press*. 2017; 26: 284-293.
226 Kario K, Ando S, Kido H, Nariyama J, Takiuchi S, Yagi T, Shimizu T, Eguchi K, Ohno M, Kinoshita O, Yamada T. The effects of the L/N-type calcium channel blocker (cilnidipine) on sympathetic hyperactive morning hypertension: results from ACHIEVE-ONE. *J Clin Hypertens (Greenwich)*. 2013; 15: 133-142.
227 Kario K, Nariyama J, Kido H, Ando S, Takiuchi S, Eguchi K, Niijima Y, Ando T, Noda M. Effect of a novel calcium channel blocker on abnormal nocturnal blood pressure in hypertensive patients. *J Clin Hypertens (Greenwich)*. 2013; 15: 465-472.
228 Kario K, Uehara Y, Shirayama M, Takahashi M, Shiosakai K, Hiramatsu K, Komiya M, Shimada K. Study of sustained blood pressure-lowering effect of azelnidipine guided by self-measured morning and evening home blood pressure: subgroup analysis of the At-HOME study. *Drugs R D*. 2013; 13: 75-85.
229 Nonaka H, Emoto N, Ikeda K, Fukuya H, Rohman MS, Raharjo SB, Yagita K, Okamura H, Yokoyama M. Angiotensin II induces circadian gene expression of clock genes in cultured vascular smooth muscle cells. *Circulation*. 2001; 104: 1746-1748. http://circ.ahajournals.org/
230 Kuroda T, Kario K, Hoshide S, Hashimoto T, Nomura Y, Saito Y, Mito H, Shimada K. Effects of bedtime vs. morning administration of the long-acting lipophilic angiotensin-converting enzyme inhibitor trandolapril on morning blood pressure in hypertensive patients. *Hypertens Res*. 2004; 27: 15-20.
231 Eguchi K, Kario K, Shimada K. Comparison of candesartan with lisinopril on ambulatory blood pressure and morning surge in patients with systemic hypertension. *Am J Cardiol*. 2003; 92: 621-624.
232 Kario K, Hoshide S, Shimizu M, Yano Y, Eguchi K, Ishikawa J, Ishikawa S, Shimada K. Effect of dosing time of angiotensin II receptor blockade titrated by self-measured blood pressure recordings on cardiorenal protection in hypertensives: the Japan Morning Surge-Target Organ Protection (J-TOP) study. *J Hypertens*. 2010; 28: 1574-1583. https://journals.lww.com/jhypertension/
233 Fukuda M, Yamanaka T, Mizuno M, Motokawa M, Shirasawa Y, Miyagi S, Nishio T, Yoshida A, Kimura G. Angiotensin II type 1 receptor blocker, olmesartan, restores nocturnal blood pressure decline by enhancing daytime natriuresis. *J Hypertens*.

2008; 26: 583-588. https://journals.lww.com/jhypertension/

234 Kario K, Saito I, Kushiro T, Teramukai S, Ishikawa Y, Hiramatsu K, Kobayashi F, Shimada K. Effect of the angiotensin II receptor antagonist olmesartan on morning home blood pressure in hypertension: HONEST study at 16 weeks. *J Hum Hypertens*. 2013; 27: 721-728.

235 Kario K, Saito I, Kushiro T, Teramukai S, Yaginuma M, Mori Y, Okuda Y, Kobayashi F, Shimada K. Persistent olmesartan-based blood pressure-lowering effects on morning hypertension in Asians: the HONEST study. *Hypertens Res*. 2016; 39: 334-341.

236 Kario K, Saito I, Kushiro T, Teramukai S, Ishikawa Y, Kobayashi F, Shimada K. Effects of olmesartan-based treatment on masked, white-coat, poorly controlled, and well-controlled hypertension: HONEST study. *J Clin Hypertens (Greenwich)*. 2014; 16: 442-450.

237 Kario K, Saito I, Kushiro T, Teramukai S, Mori Y, Hiramatsu K, Kobayashi F, Shimada K. Enhanced blood pressure-lowering effect of olmesartan in hypertensive patients with chronic kidney disease-associated sympathetic hyperactivity: HONEST study. *J Clin Hypertens (Greenwich)*. 2013; 15: 555-561.

238 Rakugi H, Kario K, Enya K, Igeta M, Ikeda Y. Effect of azilsartan versus candesartan on nocturnal blood pressure variation in Japanese patients with essential hypertension. *Blood Press*. 2013; 22 Suppl 1: 22-28.

239 Rakugi H, Kario K, Enya K, Sugiura K, Ikeda Y. Effect of azilsartan versus candesartan on morning blood pressure surges in Japanese patients with essential hypertension. *Blood Press Monit*. 2014; 19: 164-169.

240 Kario K, Hoshide S. Age-related difference in the sleep pressure-lowering effect between an angiotensin II receptor blocker and a calcium channel blocker in Asian hypertensives: the ACS1 study. *Hypertension*. 2015; 65: 729-735. http://hyper.ahajournals.org/

241 Kario K, Hoshide S. Age- and sex-related differences in efficacy with an angiotensin II receptor blocker and a calcium channel blocker in Asian hypertensive patients. *J Clin Hypertens (Greenwich)*. 2016; 18: 672-678.

242 Pickering TG, Levenstein M, Walmsley P. Nighttime dosing of doxazosin has peak effect on morning ambulatory blood pressure. Results of the HALT study. Hypertension and Lipid Trial Study Group. *Am J Hypertens*. 1994; 7: 844-847.

243 Kario K, Matsui Y, Shibasaki S, Eguchi K, Ishikawa J, Hoshide S, Ishikawa S, Kabutoya T, Schwartz JE, Pickering TG, Shimada K; Japan Morning Surge-1 (JMS-1) Study Group. An alpha-adrenergic blocker titrated by self-measured blood pressure recordings lowered blood pressure and microalbuminuria in patients with morning hypertension: the Japan Morning Surge-1 study. *J Hypertens*. 2008; 26: 1257-1265. https://journals.lww.com/jhypertension/

244 Shibasaki S, Eguchi K, Matsui Y, Ishikawa J, Hoshide S, Ishikawa S, Kabutoya T, Pickering TG, Shimada K, Kario K; Japan Morning Surge-1 (JMS-1) Study Group. Adrenergic blockade improved insulin resistance in patients with morning hypertension: the Japan Morning Surge-1 study. *J Hypertens*. 2009; 27: 1252-1257. https://journals.lww.com/jhypertension/

245 Kario K. The Sacubitril/valsartan, a first-in-class, angiotensin receptor neprilysin inhibitor (ARNI): potential uses in hypertension, heart failure, and beyond. *Curr Cardiol Rep*. 2018; 20: 5.

246 McMurray JJ, Packer M, Desai AS, Gong J, Lefkowitz MP, Rizkala AR, Rouleau JL, Shi VC, Solomon SD, Swedberg K, Zile MR; PARADIGM-HF Investigators and Committees. Angiotensin-neprilysin inhibition versus enalapril in heart failure. *N Engl J Med*. 2014; 371: 993-1004.

247 Bavishi C, Messerli FH, Kadosh B, Ruilope LM, Kario K. Role of neprilysin inhibitor combinations in hypertension: insights from hypertension and heart failure trials. *Eur Heart J*. 2015; 36: 1967-1973.

248 Ruilope LM, Dukat A, Bohm M, Lacourciere Y, Gong J, Lefkowitz MP. Blood-pressure reduction with LCZ696, a novel dual-acting inhibitor of the angiotensin II receptor and neprilysin: a randomised, double-blind, placebo-controlled, active comparator study. *Lancet*. 2010; 375: 1255-1266.

249 Kario K, Sun N, Chiang FT, Supasyndh O, Baek SH, Inubushi-Molessa A, Zhang Y, Gotou H, Lefkowitz M, Zhang J. Efficacy and safety of LCZ696, a first-in-class angiotensin receptor neprilysin inhibitor, in Asian patients with hypertension: a randomized, double-blind, placebo-controlled study. *Hypertension*. 2014; 63: 698-705. http://hyper.ahajournals.org/

250 Ito S, Satoh M, Tamaki Y, Gotou H, Charney A, Okino N, Akahori M, Zhang J. Safety and efficacy of LCZ696, a first-in-class angiotensin receptor neprilysin inhibitor, in Japanese patients with hypertension and renal dysfunction. *Hypertens Res*. 2015; 38: 269-75.

251 Kario K, Tamaki Y, Okino N, Gotou H, Zhu M, Zhang J. LCZ696, a first-in-class angiotensin receptor-neprilysin inhibitor: The first clinical experience in patients with severe hypertension. *J Clin Hypertens (Greenwich)*. 2016; 18: 308-314.

252 Supasyndh O, Sun N, Kario K, Hafeez K, Zhang J. Long-term (52-week) safety and efficacy of Sacubitril/valsartan in Asian patients with hypertension. *Hypertens Res*. 2017; 40: 472-476.

253 Wang TD, Tan RS, Lee HY, Ihm SH, Rhee MY, Tomlinson B, Pal P, Yang F, Hirschhorn E, Prescott MF, Hinder M, Langenickel TH. Effects of sacubitril/valsartan (LCZ696) on natriuresis, diuresis, blood pressures, and NT-proBNP in salt-sensitive hypertension. *Hypertension*. 2017; 69: 32-41. http://hyper.ahajournals.org/

254 Supasyndh O, Wang J, Hafeez K, Zhang Y, Zhang J, Rakugi H. Efficacy and safety of sacubitril/valsartan (LCZ696) compared with olmesartan in elderly Asian patients (≥65 Years) with systolic hypertension. *Am J Hypertens*. 2017; 30: 1163-1169.

255 Wang JG, Yukisada K, Sibulo A, Jr., Hafeez K, Jia Y, Zhang J. Efficacy and safety of sacubitril/valsartan (LCZ696) add-on to amlodipine in Asian patients with systolic hypertension uncontrolled with amlodipine monotherapy. *J Hypertens*. 2017; 35: 877-885. https://journals.lww.com/jhypertension/

256 Williams B, Cockcroft JR, Kario K, Zappe DH, Brunel PC, Wang Q, Guo W. Effects of sacubitril/valsartan versus olmesartan on central hemodynamics in the elderly with systolic hypertension: The PARAMETER study. *Hypertension*. 2017; 69: 411-420. http://hyper.ahajournals.org/

257 Solomon SD, Zile M, Pieske B, Voors A, Shah A, Kraigher-Krainer E, Shi V, Bransford T, Takeuchi M, Gong J, Lefkowitz M, Packer M, McMurray JJ; Prospective comparison of ARNI with ARB on Management Of heart failUre with preserved ejectioN fracTion (PARAMOUNT) Investigators. The angiotensin receptor neprilysin inhibitor LCZ696 in heart failure with preserved ejection fraction: a phase 2 double-blind randomised controlled trial. *Lancet*. 2012; 380: 1387-1395.

258 Zinman B, Wanner C, Lachin JM, Fitchett D, Bluhmki E, Hantel S, Mattheus M, Devins T, Johansen OE, Woerle HJ, Broedl UC, Inzucchi SE; EMPA-REG OUTCOME Investigators. Empagliflozin, cardiovascular outcomes, and mortality in Type 2 diabetes. *N Engl J Med*. 2015; 373: 2117-2128.

259 Neal B, Perkovic V, Mahaffey KW, de Zeeuw D, Fulcher G, Erondu N, Shaw W, Law G, Desai M, Matthews DR; CANVAS Program Collaborative Group. Canagliflozin and cardiovascular and renal events in Type 2 diabetes. *N Engl J Med*. 2017; 377: 644-657.

260 Ferrannini E. Sodium-glucose co-transporters and their inhibition: clinical physiology. *Cell Metab*. 2017; 26: 27-38.

261 Weber MA, Mansfield TA, Cain VA, Iqbal N, Parikh S, Ptaszynska A. Blood pressure and glycaemic effects of dapagliflozin versus placebo in patients with type 2 diabetes on combination antihypertensive therapy: a randomised, double-blind, placebo-controlled, phase 3 study. *Lancet Diabetes Endocrinol*. 2016; 4: 211-220.

262 Kario K, Weber MA, Ferrannini E. Nocturnal hypertension in diabetes: Potential target of sodium/glucose cotransporter 2 (SGLT2) inhibition. *J Clin Hypertens*. 2018. [in press].

263 Williams B, Poulter NR, Brown MJ, Davis M, McInnes GT, Potter JF, Sever PS, Thom SM; BHS Guidelines Working Party for the BHS. British Hypertension Society guidelines for hypertension management 2004 (BHS-IV): summary. *BMJ*. 2004; 328: 634-40.

264 Kario K. Proposal of RAS-diuretic vs. RAS-calcium antagonist strategies in high-risk hypertension: insight from the 24-hour ambulatory blood pressure profile and central pressure. *J Am Soc Hypertens*. 2010; 4: 215-218.

265 Kario K. Hypertension: Benefits of strict blood-pressure lowering in hypertension. *Nat Rev Cardiol*. 2016; 13: 125-126.

266 Matsui Y, Eguchi K, O'Rourke MF, Ishikawa J, Miyashita H, Shimada K, Kario K. Differential effects between a calcium channel blocker and a diuretic when used in combination with angiotensin II receptor blocker on central aortic pressure in hypertensive patients. *Hypertension*. 2009; 54: 716-723. http://hyper.ahajournals.org/

267 Matsui Y, Eguchi K, Ishikawa J, Shimada K, Kario K. Urinary albumin excretion during angiotensin II receptor blockade: comparison of combination treatment with a diuretic or a calcium-channel blocker. *Am J Hypertens*. 2011; 24: 466-473.

268 Eguchi K, Hoshide S, Kabutoya T, Shimada K, Kario K. Is very low dose hydrochlorothiazide combined with candesartan effective in uncontrolled hypertensive patients? *Blood Press Monit*. 2010; 15: 308-311.

269 Yano Y, Hoshide S, Tamaki N, Nagata M, Sasaki K, Kanemaru Y, Shimada K, Kario K. Efficacy of eplerenone added to renin-angiotensin blockade in elderly hypertensive patients: the Jichi-Eplerenone Treatment (JET) study. *J Renin Angiotensin Aldosterone Syst*. 2011; 12: 340-347.

270 Fukutomi M, Hoshide S, Eguchi K, Watanabe T, Shimada K, Kario K. Differential effects of strict blood pressure lowering by losartan/hydrochlorothiazide combination therapy and high-dose amlodipine monotherapy on microalbuminuria: the ALPHABET study. *J Am Soc Hypertens*. 2012; 6: 73-82.

271 Mizuno H, Hoshide S, Fukutomi M, Kario K. Differing Effects of aliskiren/amlodipine combination and high-dose amlodipine monotherapy on ambulatory blood

pressure and target organ protection. *J Clin Hypertens (Greenwich)*. 2016; 18: 70-78.

272 Fukutomi M, Hoshide S, Mizuno H, Kario K. Differential effects of aliskiren/amlodipine combination and high-dose amlodipine monotherapy on endothelial function in elderly hypertensive patients. *Am J Hypertens*. 2014; 27: 14-20.

273 Kario K, Hoshide S, Uchiyama K, Yoshida T, Okazaki O, Noshiro T, Aoki H, Mizuno H, Matsumoto Y. Dose timing of an angiotensin II receptor blocker/calcium channel blocker combination in hypertensive patients with paroxysmal atrial fibrillation. *J Clin Hypertens (Greenwich)*. 2016; 18: 1036-1044.

274 Fujiwara T, Hoshide S, Yano Y, Kanegae H, Kario K. Comparison of morning vs bedtime administration of the combination of valsartan/amlodipine on nocturnal brachial and central blood pressure in patients with hypertension. *J Clin Hypertens (Greenwich)*. 2017; 19: 1319-1326.

275 Kario K, Tomitani N, Kanegae H, Ishii H, Uchiyama K, Yamagiwa K, Shiraiwa T, Katsuya T, Yoshida T, Kanda K, Hasegawa S, Hoshide S. Comparative effects of an angiotensin II receptor blocker (ARB)/diuretic vs. ARB/calcium-channel blocker combination on uncontrolled nocturnal hypertension evaluated by information and communication technology-based nocturnal home blood pressure monitoring - The NOCTURNE study. *Circ J*. 2017; 81: 948-957.

276 Fujiwara T, Tomitani N, Kanegae H, Kario K. Comparative effects of valsartan plus either cilnidipine or hydrochlorothiazide on home morning blood pressure surge evaluated by information and communication technology-based nocturnal home blood pressure monitoring. *J Clin Hypertens (Greenwich)*. 2018. [in press].

277 Daugherty SL, Powers JD, Magid DJ, Tavel HM, Masoudi FA, Margolis KL, O'Connor PJ, Selby JV, Ho PM. Incidence and prognosis of resistant hypertension in hypertensive patients. *Circulation*. 2012; 125: 1635-1642. http://circ.ahajournals.org/

278 Pedrosa RP, Drager LF, Gonzaga CC, Sousa MG, de Paula LK, Amaro AC, Amodeo C, Bortolotto LA, Krieger EM, Bradley TD, Lorenzi-Filho G. Obstructive sleep apnea: the most common secondary cause of hypertension associated with resistant hypertension. *Hypertension*. 2011; 58: 811-817. http://hyper.ahajournals.org/

279 Pimenta E, Gaddam KK, Oparil S, Aban I, Husain S, Dell'Italia LJ, Calhoun DA. Effects of dietary sodium reduction on blood pressure in subjects with resistant hypertension: results from a randomized trial. *Hypertension*. 2009; 54: 475-481. http://hyper.ahajournals.org/

280 Uzu T, Ishikawa K, Fujii T, Nakamura S, Inenaga T, Kimura G. Sodium restriction shifts circadian rhythm of blood pressure from nondipper to dipper in essential hypertension. *Circulation*. 1997; 96: 1859-1862. http://circ.ahajournals.org/

281 Nishizaka MK, Zaman MA, Calhoun DA. Efficacy of low-dose spironolactone in subjects with resistant hypertension. *Am J Hypertens*. 2003; 16: 925-930.

282 Williams B, MacDonald TM, Morant S, Webb DJ, Sever P, McInnes G, Ford I, Cruickshank JK, Caulfield MJ, Salsbury J, Mackenzie I, Padmanabhan S, Brown MJ; British Hypertension Society's PATHWAY Studies Group. Spironolactone versus placebo, bisoprolol, and doxazosin to determine the optimal treatment for drug-resistant hypertension (PATHWAY-2): a randomised, double-blind, crossover trial. *Lancet*. 2015; 386: 2059-2068.

283 Krum H, Schlaich M, Whitbourn R, Sobotka PA, Sadowski J, Bartus K, Kapelak B, Walton A, Sievert H, Thambar S, Abraham WT, Esler M. Catheter-based renal

sympathetic denervation for resistant hypertension: a multicentre safety and proof-of-principle cohort study. *Lancet.* 2009; 373: 1275-1281.

284 Symplicity HTN-2 Investigators, Esler MD, Krum H, Sobotka PA, Schlaich MP, Schmieder RE, Bohm M. Renal sympathetic denervation in patients with treatment-resistant hypertension (The Symplicity HTN-2 Trial): a randomised controlled trial. *Lancet.* 2010; 376: 1903-1909.

285 Bhatt DL, Kandzari DE, O'Neill WW, D'Agostino R, Flack JM, Katzen BT, Leon MB, Liu M, Mauri L, Negoita M, Cohen SA, Oparil S, Rocha-Singh K, Townsend RR, Bakris GL; SYMPLICITY HTN-3 Investigators. A controlled trial of renal denervation for resistant hypertension. *N Engl J Med.* 2014; 370: 1393-1401.

286 Kario K, Ogawa H, Okumura K, Okura T, Saito S, Ueno T, Haskin R, Negoita M, Shimada K; SYMPLICITY HTN-Japan Investigators. SYMPLICITY HTN-Japan - first randomized controlled trial of catheter-based renal denervation in Asian patients. *Circ J.* 2015; 79: 1222-1229.

287 Kario K, Bhatt DL, Brar S, Cohen SA, Fahy M, Bakris GL. Effect of catheter-based renal denervation on morning and nocturnal blood pressure: insights from SYMPLICITY HTN-3 and SYMPLICITY HTN-Japan. *Hypertension.* 2015; 66: 1130-1137. http://hyper.ahajournals.org/

288 Kario K, Bhatt DL, Kandzari DE, Brar S, Flack JM, Gilbert C, Oparil S, Robbins M, Townsend RR, Bakris G. Impact of renal denervation on patients with obstructive sleep apnea and resistant hypertension - insights from the SYMPLICITY HTN-3 Trial. *Circ J.* 2016; 80: 1404-1412.

289 Kario K, Ikemoto T, Kuwabara M, Ishiyama H, Saito K, Hoshide S. Catheter-based renal denervation reduces hypoxia-triggered nocturnal blood pressure peak in obstructive sleep apnea syndrome. *J Clin Hypertens (Greenwich).* 2016; 18: 707-709.

290 Mahfoud F, Bakris G, Bhatt DL, Esler M, Ewen S, Fahy M, Kandzari D, Kario K, Mancia G, Weber M, Bohm M. Reduced blood pressure-lowering effect of catheter-based renal denervation in patients with isolated systolic hypertension: data from SYMPLICITY HTN-3 and the Global SYMPLICITY Registry. *Eur Heart J.* 2017; 38: 93-100.

291 Mahfoud F, Schlaich M, Kindermann I, Ukena C, Cremers B, Brandt MC, Hoppe UC, Vonend O, Rump LC, Sobotka PA, Krum H, Esler M, Bohm M. Effect of renal sympathetic denervation on glucose metabolism in patients with resistant hypertension: a pilot study. *Circulation.* 2011; 123: 1940-1946. http://circ.ahajournals.org/

292 Mahfoud F, Cremers B, Janker J, Link B, Vonend O, Ukena C, Linz D, Schmieder R, Rump LC, Kindermann I, Sobotka PA, Krum H, Scheller B, Schlaich M, Laufs U, Bohm M. Renal hemodynamics and renal function after catheter-based renal sympathetic denervation in patients with resistant hypertension. *Hypertension.* 2012; 60: 419-424. http://hyper.ahajournals.org/

293 Brandt MC, Mahfoud F, Reda S, Schirmer SH, Erdmann E, Bohm M, Hoppe UC. Renal sympathetic denervation reduces left ventricular hypertrophy and improves cardiac function in patients with resistant hypertension. *J Am Coll Cardiol.* 2012; 59: 901-909.

294 Kandzari DE, Kario K, Mahfoud F, Cohen SA, Pilcher G, Pocock S, Townsend R, Weber MA, Bohm M. The SPYRAL HTN Global Clinical Trial Program: Rationale and design for studies of renal denervation in the absence (SPYRAL HTN OFF-

MED) and presence (SPYRAL HTN ON-MED) of antihypertensive medications. *Am Heart J.* 2016; 171: 82-91.
295 Mahfoud F, Tunev S, Ewen S, Cremers B, Ruwart J, Schulz-Jander D, Linz D, Davies J, Kandzari DE, Whitbourn R, Bohm M, Melder RJ. Impact of lesion placement on efficacy and safety of catheter-based radiofrequency renal denervation. *J Am Coll Cardiol.* 2015; 66: 1766-1775.
296 Townsend RR, Mahfoud F, Kandzari DE, Kario K, Pocock S, Weber MA, Ewen S, Tsioufis K, Tousoulis D, Sharp ASP, Watkinson AF, Schmieder RE, Schmid A, Choi JW, East C, Walton A, Hopper I, Cohen DL, Wilensky R, Lee DP, Ma A, Devireddy CM, Lea JP, Lurz PC, Fengler K, Davies J, Chapman N, Cohen SA, DeBruin V, Fahy M, Jones DE, Rothman M, Bohm M; SPYRAL HTN-OFF MED trial investigators. Catheter-based renal denervation in patients with uncontrolled hypertension in the absence of antihypertensive medications (SPYRAL HTN-OFF MED): a randomised, sham-controlled, proof-of-concept trial. *Lancet.* 2017; 390: 2160-2170.
297 Kario K, Okura A, Okawara Y, Tomitani N, Ikemoto T, Hoshide S. Impact of introducing catheter-based renal denervation into Japan for hypertension management: estimation of number of target patients and clinical relevance of ambulatory blood pressure reduction. *Curr Hypertens Rev.* 2016; 12: 156-163.
298 Mauri L, Kario K, Basile J, Daemen J, Davies J, Kirtane AJ, Mahfoud F, Schmieder RE, Weber M, Nanto S, Azizi M. A multinational clinical approach to assessing the effectiveness of catheter-based ultrasound renal denervation: The RADIANCE-HTN and REQUIRE clinical study designs. *Am Heart J.* 2018; 195: 115-129.
299 Kario K. PREFACE: Is renal denervation effective option for management of hypertension in Asia? *Curr Hypertens Rev.* 2017; 13: 2-5.
300 Kario K. The HOPE Asia network for "zero" cardiovascular events in Asia. *J Clin Hypertens (Greenwich).* 2018; 20: 212-214.
301 Weber MA, Lackland DT. Hypertension: cardiovascular benefits of lowering blood pressure. *Nat Rev Nephrol.* 2016; 12: 202-204.
302 Campbell NR, Khalsa T; World Hypertension League Executive;, Lackland DT, Niebylski ML, Nilsson PM, Redburn KA, Orias M, Zhang XH; International Society of Hypertension Executive;, Burrell L, Horiuchi M, Poulter NR, Prabhakaran D, Ramirez AJ, Schiffrin EL, Touyz RM, Wang JG, Weber MA; World Stroke Organization; International Diabetes Federation; International Council of Cardiovascular Prevention and Rehabilitation; International Society of Nephrology. High blood pressure 2016: why prevention and control are urgent and important. The World Hypertension League, International Society of Hypertension, World Stroke Organization, International Diabetes Foundation, International Council of Cardiovascular Prevention and Rehabilitation, International Society of Nephrology. *J Clin Hypertens (Greenwich).* 2016; 18: 714-717.
303 Weber MA, Lackland DT. Contributions to hypertension public policy and clinical practice: a review of recent reports. *J Clin Hypertens (Greenwich).* 2016; 18: 1063-1070.
304 Chia YC, Buranakitjaroen P, Chen CH, Divinagracia R, Hoshide S, Park S, Shin J, Siddique S, Sison J, Soenarta AA, Sogunuru GP, Tay JC, Turana Y, Wang JG, Wong L, Zhang Y, Kario K; HOPE Asia Network. Current status of home blood pressure monitoring in Asia: statement from the HOPE Asia Network. *J Clin Hypertens (Greenwich).* 2017; 19: 1192-1201.

305 Hoshide S, Wang JG, Park S, Chen CH, Cheng HM, Huang QF, Park CG, Kario K. Treatment considerations of clinical physician on hypertension management in Asia. *Curr Hypertens Rev*. 2016; 12: 164-168.

306 Yano Y, Briasoulis A, Bakris GL, Hoshide S, Wang JG, Shimada K, Kario K. Effects of antihypertensive treatment in Asian populations: a meta-analysis of prospective randomized controlled studies (CARdiovascular protectioN group in Asia: CARNA). *J Am Soc Hypertens*. 2014; 8: 103-116.

307 Park JB, Kario K, Wang JG. Systolic hypertension: an increasing clinical challenge in Asia. *Hypertens Res*. 2015; 38: 227-236.

308 Wang JG, Kario K, Park JB, Chen CH. Morning blood pressure monitoring in the management of hypertension. *J Hypertens*. 2017; 35: 1554-1563. https://journals.lww.com/jhypertension/

309 Kario K, Chen CH, Park S, Park CG, Hoshide S, Cheng HM, Huang QF, Wang JG. Consensus document on improving hypertension management in Asian patients, taking into account Asian characteristics. *Hypertension*. 2018; 71: 375-382. http://hyper.ahajournals.org/

310 Ueshima H, Sekikawa A, Miura K, Turin TC, Takashima N, Kita Y, Watanabe M, Kadota A, Okuda N, Kadowaki T, Nakamura Y, Okamura T. Cardiovascular disease and risk factors in Asia: a selected review. *Circulation*. 2008; 118: 2702-2709. http://circ.ahajournals.org/

311 Perkovic V, Huxley R, Wu Y, Prabhakaran D, MacMahon S. The burden of blood pressure-related disease: a neglected priority for global health. *Hypertension*. 2007; 50: 991-997. http://hyper.ahajournals.org/

312 Lawes CM, Rodgers A, Bennett DA, Parag V, Suh I, Ueshima H, MacMahon S; Asia Pacific Cohort Studies Collaboration. Blood pressure and cardiovascular disease in the Asia Pacific region. *J Hypertens*. 2003; 21: 707-716. https://journals.lww.com/jhypertension/

313 Ishikawa Y, Ishikawa J, Ishikawa S, Kayaba K, Nakamura Y, Shimada K, Kajii E, Pickering TG, Kario K; Jichi Medical School Cohort Investigators Group. Prevalence and determinants of prehypertension in a Japanese general population: the Jichi Medical School cohort study. *Hypertens Res*. 2008; 31: 1323-1330.

314 Greenlund KJ, Croft JB, Mensah GA. Prevalence of heart disease and stroke risk factors in persons with prehypertension in the United States, 1999-2000. *Arch Intern Med*. 2004; 164: 2113-2118.

315 Katsuya T, Ishikawa K, Sugimoto K, Rakugi H, Ogihara T. Salt sensitivity of Japanese from the viewpoint of gene polymorphism. *Hypertens Res*. 2003; 26: 521-525.

316 Powles J, Fahimi S, Micha R, Khatibzadeh S, Shi P, Ezzati M, Engell RE, Lim SS, Danaei G, Mozaffarian D; Global Burden of Diseases Nutrition and Chronic Diseases Expert Group (NutriCoDE). Global, regional and national sodium intakes in 1990 and 2010: a systematic analysis of 24 h urinary sodium excretion and dietary surveys worldwide. *BMJ Open*. 2013; 3: e003733.

317 Omboni S, Aristizabal D, De la Sierra A, Dolan E, Head G, Kahan T, Kantola I, Kario K, Kawecka-Jaszcz K, Malan L, Narkiewicz K, Octavio JA, Ohkubo T, Palatini P, Siegelova J, Silva E, Stergiou G, Zhang Y, Mancia G, Parati G, Investigators A. Hypertension types defined by clinic and ambulatory blood pressure in 14 143 patients referred to hypertension clinics worldwide. Data from the ARTEMIS study. *J Hypertens*. 2016; 34: 2187-2198. https://journals.lww.com/jhypertension/

318 Hoshide S, Kario K, de la Sierra A, Bilo G, Schillaci G, Banegas JR, Gorostidi M, Segura J, Lombardi C, Omboni S, Ruilope L, Mancia G, Parati G. Ethnic differences in the degree of morning blood pressure surge and in its determinants between Japanese and European hypertensive subjects: data from the ARTEMIS study. *Hypertension*. 2015; 66: 750-756. http://hyper.ahajournals.org/
319 Kario K, Bhatt DL, Brar S, Bakris GL. Differences in dynamic diurnal blood pressure variability between Japanese and American treatment-resistant hypertensive populations. *Circ J*. 2017; 81: 1337-1345.
320 Li Y, Wang JG, Gao P, Guo H, Nawrot T, Wang G, Qian Y, Staessen JA, Zhu D. Are published characteristics of the ambulatory blood pressure generalizable to rural Chinese? The JingNing population study. *Blood Press Monit*. 2005; 10: 125-134.
321 Kario K, Park S, Buranakitjaroen P, Chia YC, Chen CH, Divinagracia R, Hoshide S, Shin J, Siddique S, Sison J, Soenarta A, Sogunuru GP, Tay JC, Turana Y, Wong L, Zhang Y, Wang JG. Practice points for home blood pressure monitoring in Asia: guidance from the HOPE Asia Network. *J Clin Hypertens (Greenwich)*. 2018. [in press].
322 Fujiwara T, Hoshide S, Kanegae H, Nishizawa M, Kario K. Reliability of morning, before-dinner, and at-bedtime home blood pressure measurements in patients with hypertension. *J Clin Hypertens (Greenwich)*. 2018. [in press].
323 Park S, Buranakitjaroen P, Chen CH, Chia YC, Divinagracia R, Hoshide S, Shin J, Siddique S, Sison J, Soenarta AA, Sogunuru GP, Tay JC, Turana Y, Wang JG, Zhang Y, Kario K. Expert panel consensus recommendations for home blood pressure monitoring in Asia: the Hope Asia Network. *J Hum Hypertens*. [in press].
324 Kario K, Tomitani N, Buranakitjaroen P, Chen CH, Chia YC, Divinagracia R, Park S, Shin J, Siddique S, Sison J, Soenarta AA, Sogunuru GP, Tay JC, Turana Y, Wang JG, Wong L, Zhang Y, Wanthong S, Hoshide S, Kanegae H; Network HA. Rationale and design for the Asia BP@Home study on home blood pressure control status in 12 Asian countries and regions. *J Clin Hypertens (Greenwich)*. 2018; 20: 33-38.
325 Kario K. Disaster hypertension - its characteristics, mechanism, and management. *Circ J*. 2012; 76: 553-562.
326 Kario K, Matsuo T, Shimada K, Pickering TG. Factors associated with the occurrence and magnitude of earthquake-induced increases in blood pressure. *Am J Med*. 2001; 111: 379-384.
327 Kario K, Matsuo T, Ishida T, Shimada K. "White coat" hypertension and the Hanshin-Awaji earthquake. *Lancet*. 1995; 345: 1365.
328 Kario K, Matsuo T, Kobayashi H, Yamamoto K, Shimada K. Earthquake-induced potentiation of acute risk factors in hypertensive elderly patients: possible triggering of cardiovascular events after a major earthquake. *J Am Coll Cardiol*. 1997; 29: 926-933.
329 Kario K, McEwen BS, Pickering TG. Disasters and the heart: a review of the effects of earthquake-induced stress on cardiovascular disease. *Hypertens Res*. 2003; 26: 355-367.
330 Kario K, Nishizawa M, Hoshide S, Shimpo M, Ishibashi Y, Kunii O, Shibuya K. Development of a disaster cardiovascular prevention network. *Lancet*. 2011; 378: 1125-1127.
331 Nishizawa M, Hoshide S, Shimpo M, Kario K. Disaster hypertension: experience from the great East Japan earthquake of 2011. *Curr Hypertens Rep*. 2012; 14: 375-

381.
332 Kario K. Management of high casual blood pressure in a disaster situation: the 1995 Hanshin-Awaji earthquake. *Am J Hypertens*. 1998; 11: 1138-1139.
333 Nishizawa M, Hoshide S, Okawara Y, Shimpo M, Matsuo T, Kario K. Aftershock triggers augmented pressor effects in survivors: follow-up of the great East Japan earthquake. *Am J Hypertens*. 2015; 28: 1405-1408.
334 Nishizawa M, Hoshide S, Okawara Y, Matsuo T, Kario K. Strict blood pressure control achieved using an ICT-based home blood pressure monitoring system in a catastrophically damaged area after a disaster. *J Clin Hypertens (Greenwich)*. 2017; 19: 26-29.
335 Sabbahi A, Arena R, Elokda A, Phillips SA. Exercise and hypertension: Uncovering the mechanisms of vascular control. *Prog Cardiovasc Dis*. 2016; 59: 226-234.
336 Oktay AA, Lavie CJ, Kokkinos PF, Parto P, Pandey A, Ventura HO. The interaction of cardiorespiratory fitness with obesity and the obesity paradox in cardiovascular disease. *Prog Cardiovasc Dis*. 2017; 60: 30-44.
337 Lee DC, Brellenthin AG, Thompson PD, Sui X, Lee IM, Lavie CJ. Running as a key lifestyle medicine for longevity. *Prog Cardiovasc Dis*. 2017; 60: 45-55.
338 Reilly JP, White CJ. Renal denervation for resistant hypertension. *Prog Cardiovasc Dis*. 2016; 59: 295-302.

Index

Note: Page number followed by f indicates figure.

A
ABC-H study, 93f, 94
ABP-International study, 84, 85f
ABPM, *see* ambulatory blood pressure monitoring (ABPM)
ACE inhibitors, *see* angiotensin-converting enzyme (ACE) inhibitors
ACHIEVE-ONE, *see* Ambulatory Blood Pressure Control and Home Blood Pressure (Morning and Evening) Lowering by N-Channel Blocker Cilnidipine (ACHIEVE-ONE) trial
ACROBAT study, *see* ARB and CCB Longest Combination Treatment on Ambulatory and Home BP in Hypertension with Atrial Fibrillation - Multicenter Study on Time of Dosing (ACROBAT)
Actisensitivity, 43, 45f–47f
AHA/ACC guidelines, 1, 10, 12f, 18f
alpha-adrenergic activity, 59
alpha/beta-adrenergic blockers, 199–201
ALPHABET study, 217, 218f
Ambulatory Blood Pressure Control and Home Blood Pressure (Morning and Evening) Lowering by N-Channel Blocker Cilnidipine (ACHIEVE-ONE) trial, 187–188, 187f, 189f
ambulatory blood pressure monitoring (ABPM), 10f, 11–12, 13f, 29–50
  24-hour BP, 29–30
  daytime BP, 29–30
  daytime BP parameters, 33f
  MBPS parameters, 30–31, 31f, 33f
  morning BP parameters, 30, 30f, 32f
  multi-sensor ABPM, *see* ICT-based multi-censor ABPM (IMS-ABPM)
  nighttime BP, 29–30
  nighttime BP dipping parameters, 31, 31f
  nighttime BP parameters, 30, 30f, 32f
  nighttime BP surge parameters, 31, 31f, 33f
AML, *see* amlodipine (AML)
amlodipine (AML), 181–184, 182f–184f
angiotensin-converting enzyme (ACE) inhibitors, 188

angiotensin-receptor blockers (ARB)
  azilsartan, 197–199, 197f–199f
  candesartan, 190–191, 191f
  olmesartan, 192–197, 192f–196f
  telmisartan, 190, 217–219, 220f
  valsartan, 176f, 190, 201–205, 206f, 214f, 219–221, 221f, 222–223, 225f
angiotensin receptor neprilysin inhibitor (ARNI), 201–204, 201f–206f
anticipation medicine, 269, 270f
antihypertensive drugs, 176f, 177–179, 178f–180f
  alpha/beta-adrenergic blockers, 199–201
  amlodipine (AML), 181–184, 182f–185f
  angiotensin-converting enzyme (ACE) inhibitors, 188, 190f
  angiotensin-receptor blockers (ARB), 190–199, 191f–199f
  azelnidipine, 188
  calcium channel blockers (CCB), 181–188
  carvedilol, 115, 116f, 117f, 121–122
  cilnidipine, 187–188, 187f, 189f, 222–223, 225f
  diuretics, 180f, 181
  doxazosin, 115, 116f, 144f, 199–201, 200f
  nifedipine, 115, 116f, 117f, 185–187
  RAS inhibitor-based combination, 214-215, 215f–218f
AOBP, *see* automated office BP (AOBP)
ARB, *see* angiotensin-receptor blockers (ARB)
ARB and CCB Longest Combination Treatment on Ambulatory and Home BP in Hypertension with Atrial Fibrillation - Multicenter Study on Time of Dosing (ACROBAT), 217–219, 220f
ARNI, *see* angiotensin receptor neprilysin inhibitor (ARNI)
ARTEMIS (International Ambulatory Blood Pressure Registry: Telemonitoring of Hypertension and Cardiovascular Risk Project) study, 255–256, 256f
arterial stiffness type, 211–212, 213f, 228f
ASCOT-BPLA, 128, 129f
Asia BP@Home study, 258
Asian, 249, 252f, 256f

assessment, morning hypertension
  ambulatory blood pressure monitoring
    (ABPM), 10f, 11–14, 13f
  home blood pressure monitoring (HBPM),
    11–14, 13f, 17–19, 17f, 20f
atmospheric sensitivity, 42f, 43
atrial fibrillation, 33, 42f, 43f
automated office BP (AOBP), 1, 2f, 3f
average of morning and evening BPs
  (ME-ave), 137–138
azelnidipine, 188
azilsartan, 197–199, 197f–199f

B

baPWV, *see* brachial-ankle pulse wave
  velocity (baPWV)
baroreflex index (BRI), 123, 124f
baroreceptor sensitivity (BRS), 73
blood pressure (BP)
  actisensitivity, 45f–47f
  atmospheric sensitivity, 42f, 43
  average of morning and evening BPs
    (ME-ave), 137–138
  beat-by-beat, 119–124
  circadian rhythm, 75
  day-by-day variability, 136, 136f, 137f
  in disaster, 259–268, 262f, 265f, 267f
  disaster cardiovascular prevention (DCAP)
    network, 259–265, 261f, 263f–265f,
    267f
  measurement, 17–19, 17f–18f
  morning-evening difference of BPs
    (ME-dif), 7, 27, 137–138, 139f
  non-dippers, 79f, 80, 82, 87–90
  pre-wakening surges, 51, 52f, 53
  rising BP surge, 52f
  seasonality, 64f, 65f
  sleep-trough morning surge, 31f, 51, 52f
  thermosensitivity, 43–44, 46f
BP, *see* blood pressure (BP)
BP surge, 125–144
  resonance hypothesis, 125–127
BP variability, 125, 126f–129f
  ambulatory, 132, 132f
  day-by-day, 136, 136f, 137f
  determinants, 129f
  home BP, 132–134, 134f
  morning-evening difference, 137–138
  prognostic relevance, 129f
brachial-ankle pulse wave velocity (baPWV),
  157, 159f
brain natriuretic peptide (BNP), 81f

BRS, *see* baroreceptor sensitivity (BRS)

C

Calcium Antagonist Controlled-Release
  High-Dose Therapy in Uncontrolled
  Refractory Hypertensive Patients
  (CARILLON) study, 185, 186f
calcium channel blockers (CCB), 181–188
  for resistant hypertension, 227
candesartan, 190–191, 191f
CARDIA study, 92f, 93–94
cardiac reactive type, 74, 74f
Cardiovascular Prognostic Coupling study in
  Japan (Coupling Registry), 160, 160f
CARILLON study, *see* Calcium Antagonist
  Controlled-Release High-Dose
  Therapy in Uncontrolled Refractory
  Hypertensive Patients (CARILLON)
  study
carotid intima-media thickness (IMT), 56,
  56f, 128, 130f–131f
Caucasian, 249, 252f, 256f
CCB, *see* calcium channel blockers (CCB)
central pressure, 162, 163f
chronic kidney disease (CKD), 59–60, 90, 91f
chronotherapy, 175
cilnidipine, 187–188, 187f, 189f, 222–223,
  225f
circadian rhythm of BP, 75
CKD, *see* chronic kidney disease (CKD)
clinical BP measurement, 1, 3f
cognitive function, 132f
COME Asia-MHDG (Characteristics On
  the ManagEment of hypertension
  in the Asia-Morning Hypertension
  Discussion Group), 248
Continuous Positive Airway Pressure (CPAP),
  110–112, 111f–115f
COUPLING registry, *see* Cardiovascular
  Prognostic Coupling study in Japan
  (Coupling Registry)
CPAP, *see* Continuous Positive Airway
  Pressure (CPAP)
CPET (ChronotheraPy for ambulatory
  cEnTral pressure) study, 219–221,
  221f
cutting-edge, HBPM
  IT-based nighttime BP monitoring system
    (ITNP), 96f, 103f, 107, 109–110, 111f,
    112, 113f
  nighttime BP monitoring at home
    (Medinote), 22f, 97, 98f

thermosensitive hypertension, 46f, 61–63, 64f
trigger nighttime BP monitoring (TNP), 96f, 102–107, 104f, 105f

D
daytime BP, 4f, 29–30
daytime (stress-induced) hypertension, 5, 5f
DCAP network, see disaster cardiovascular prevention (DCAP) network
delta SBP, 128, 130f, 131f
diabetes, 86f, 89–90
diagnosis of hypertension, 4–5, 4f
diary-based definition, nighttime BP, 30f
dippers of nighttime BP, 37f
disaster cardiovascular prevention (DCAP) network, 259–265, 261f, 263f–265f, 267f
diuretics, 180f, 181
doxazosin, 115, 116f, 144f, 199–200, 200f
dynamic BP surge, 124f, 125–127, 127f, 269, 270f

E
Effects of Vasodilating vs. Sympatholytic Antihypertensives on Sleep Blood Pressure in Hypertensive Patients with Sleep Apnea Syndrome (VASSPS), 185–187
endothelial dysfunction, 67, 67f, 68f
ethnic differences
  Asian, 249, 252f, 256f
European Society of Hypertension/European Society of Cardiology (ESH/ESC 2013) guidelines, 1, 18f
exaggerated MBPS, 27, 51–55, 72f, 109f, 211
  vascular mechanism, 71–74, 72f
examining-room BP, 19, 20f
extreme dippers with nighttime BP, 91f, 92f, 93–94, 94f

F
first-line therapy, 211
flow-mediated dilation (FMD), 163, 165f
Folkow's principle, hypertension, 71, 72f
fourth-line therapy, 227–230
frailty, 80, 83f

G
Genki-Jichi hypertension prediction simulator, 12, 13f

Genki Plaza – Jichi Medical University Hypertension Prediction Scale, 13f
Great East Japan earthquake, 259, 264f, 265, 266, 267f

H
HALT, see Hypertension and Lipid Trial (HALT)
HAST, see home active standing test (HAST)
HBPM, see home blood pressure monitoring (HBPM)
head-up tilting test, 140f, 141, 142f
heart failure with preserved ejection fraction (HFpEF), 78, 79f, 80f
heart failure with reduced ejection fraction (HFrEF), 78, 79f, 80f
HI-JAMP study, see Home-Activity ICT-based Japan Ambulatory Blood Pressure Monitoring Prospective (HI-JAMP) study
home active standing test (HAST), 141
Home-Activity ICT-based Japan Ambulatory Blood Pressure Monitoring Prospective (HI-JAMP) study, 49, 50f
Home blood pressure measurement with Olmesartan Naive patients to Establish Standard Target blood pressure (HONEST) study, 21–27, 22f–26f, 192, 192f–196f, 194, 251f
home blood pressure monitoring (HBPM), 11–12, 13f, 17–19, 17f
  cutting-edge
    IT-based nighttime BP monitoring system (ITNP), 96f, 103f, 107, 109–110, 111f, 112, 113f
    nighttime BP monitoring at home (Medinote), 22f, 97, 98f
    thermosensitive hypertension, 46f, 61–63, 64f
    trigger nighttime BP monitoring (TNP), 96f, 102–107, 104f, 105f
    maximum home SBP, 134–136, 134f, 135f
    measurement, 17–19, 17f–18f
    morning orthostatic hypertension, 138–143, 140f, 143, 143f, 144f
home BP variability, 26f, 132–134
HOMED-BP, 21
HONEST study, see Home blood pressure measurement with Olmesartan Naive patients to Establish Standard Target blood pressure (HONEST) study

HOPE Asia (Hypertension, brain, cardiovascular and renal Outcome Prevention and Evidence in Asia) Network, 18f, 245–258
hypertension, *see also* resistant hypertension, 308
  cardiovascular risk, 22f–24f, 23
  coronary artery disease risk, 23, 23f–24f
  diabetes with, 25, 25f
  disaster hypertension management, 266f
  elderly, 82–83, 82f, 83f
  home and ambulatory BP-based combination strategies, 213–225, 213f
  masked, 4–5, 5f, 7, 10f, 11f
  morning BP surge, 8f
  morning hypertension, 5, 5f, 7, 9f, 10–11, 14, 26f, 27, 27f
    definition, 10f
  orthostatic, 138–143, 140f–144f
  prevalence, 12f
  silent cerebral infarcts, risk of, 8f
  staged management, 14, 15f
  stroke risk, 8f, 10f, 23, 23f, 24f
  subtype, 4, 5f
  thresholds for diagnosis, 4f
Hypertension and Lipid Trial (HALT), 199, 200f
hypertensive heart disease with MBPS, 55–56, 56f

I

ICT-based multi-censor ABPM (IMS-ABPM), 33, 40, 46–49, 46f–50f
ICT-based real-time anticipation medicine, 271, 271f
IDACO, *see* International Database on Ambulatory Blood Pressure in Relation to Cardiovascular Outcome (IDACO)
indices, HBPM variability, 134f
inflammatory markers, 56–57
inhibitors of sodium/glucose cotransporter 2 (SGLT2i), 205–208, 207f, 209f
insomnia, 88
International Database on Ambulatory Blood Pressure in Relation to Cardiovascular Outcome (IDACO), 53, 53f, 54, 84f
IT-based nighttime BP monitoring system (ITNP), 96f, 103f, 107, 109–110, 108f, 110f, 111f, 112, 113f
  OSAS management, 102,107–112, 111f, 113f

J

Japan Ambulatory Blood Pressure Monitoring Prospective study (JAMP study), 21f, 50f, 240, 240f
Japan Morning Surge-Home Blood Pressure (J-HOP) study, 21, 21f, 22f, 97–101, 98f–101f, 137, 138f, 139f
Japan Target Organ Protection (J-TOP) study, 101, 102f, 191, 191f
Japanese Society of Hypertension (JSH 2014) guidelines, 1, 18f
J-CORE (Japan-Combined Treatment with Olmesartan and a Calcium Channel Blocker versus Olmesartan and Diuretics Randomised Efficacy) study, 214–215, 215f–216f
JET study, 218f
Jichi Medical University Center of Excellence, Cardiovascular Research and Development (JCARD), 21f
Jichi Medical University School of Medicine (JMS-ABPM) study, 52–54, 57, 58, 59f, 169f
Joint National Committee on Prevention, Detection, Evaluation and Treatment of High Blood Pressure (JNC7) guidelines, 10–11

L

large artery diseases, 55f, 73, 150, 155
LCZ696 (sacubitril/valsartan), ARNI, 201–204, 201f–205f
left ventricular hypertrophy (LVH), 55, 56, 56f
left ventricular mass index (LVMI), 55–57, 56f
LVH, *see* left ventricular hypertrophy (LVH)
LVMI, *see* left ventricular mass index (LVMI)

M

masked hypertension, 4–5, 5f
  definition, 4
    morning, 7
    nocturnal, 7
  risk, 62f
  subtypes, 5, 5f
    daytime (stress-induced) hypertension, 5, 5f
    morning hypertension, 5, 5f
    nocturnal hypertension, 5, 5f
    white-coat, 4, 5f
maximum home SBP, 134–136, 134f, 135f

MBPS, *see* morning blood pressure surge (MBPS)
melatonin, 88, 88f
mini-mental state examination, 83f, 171
MoCA-J, Japanese version of the Montreal Cognitive Assessment, 132, 133f, 171
monitoring device, nighttime BP, 97, 98f, 102, 103f, 107–109
morning blood pressure
  cardiovascular risk, 22f–25f
  parameters, 30, 30f, 32f
  stroke risk, 23f, 24f
morning blood pressure surge (MBPS), 7, 8f
  antihypertensive drugs, 176f, 177, 178f, 179f
  cardiovascular events with, 52–54, 53f
  definitions, 51–52, 52f
  determinants, 61, 61f
  haemostatic abnormality and, 68–69, 70f
  Jichi Medical University School of Medicine (JMS-ABPM) study, 52–54, 58, 59f
  morning risk, mechanism of, 63–67, 67f, 69f
  organ damage with, 54–60, 55f
    chronic kidney disease (CKD), 59–60
    hypertensive heart disease, 55–56, 55f, 56f
    silent cerebrovascular disease, 58–59, 59f
    stroke events, 8f
    vascular disease and inflammation, 56–58, 58f
  parameters, 30–31, 31f, 33f
  vascular mechanism, 71–74, 72f
morning BP parameters, 30, 30f, 32f
  24-hour-clock-based definition, 32f
  diary-based definition, 30f
morning-evening difference of BPs (ME-dif), 7, 27, 137–138, 139f
morning hypertension, 5, 5f, 7, 9f, 10–11, 14, 26f, 27f
  antihypertensive treatment, 177–178, 178f
  blood pressure (BP) level thresholds, 4f, 176f
  definition, 7, 10f
  determinant, 61, 61f
  diagnosis guidelines, 17, 18f
  evidence, 21
    HOMED-BP, 21
    HONEST study, 21–27, 22f–26f
    Japan Morning Surge-Home Blood Pressure (J-HOP) study, 21, 22f, 97–101, 98f–101f, 137, 138f, 139f
    Ohasama study, 21
  organ damage with, 7, 9f
  perfect 24-hour BP control, 175
  prevalence, 10–11
  subtypes, 27, 27f

N

neurohumoral hypertension, 205f
NICE 2011 guidelines, 1, 18f
nifedipine, 115, 116f, 117f, 185–187
nighttime BP, 29–30, 41f
  cardiovascular prognosis, 86f
  different dipping status, 76f
  organ damage, 91f
  stroke prognosis, 85f
nighttime BP dipping parameters, 31, 31f
nighttime BP parameters, 30, 30f, 32f
  24-hour-clock-based definition, 32f
  diary-based definition, 30f
nighttime BP surge, 106f, 110f, 110–112, 113f
  antihypertensive medication, 115
nighttime BP surge parameters, 31, 31f, 33f
nocturnal hypertension, 5, 5f, 7, 75–94, 176f
  antihypertensive treatment, 176f
  associated condition
    chronic kidney disease (CKD), 86f, 90, 91f
    diabetes, 86f, 89–90
  cardiovascular risk, 76–78, 83–87, 84f, 85f
  circadian rhythm of BP, 75
  definition, 7, 11f, 83
  determinants, 89, 90f
  extreme dipper, 91f, 92f, 93–94, 94f, 140f
  mechanism, 87–88, 87f, 94f
  non-dipper/risers, 38f–39f, 75–83, 77f, 79f, 80f, 81f
NOCTURNE study, 221–222, 222f–224f
non-dipper/risers of nighttime BP, 75–83, 80f
N-terminal pro-brain natriuretic peptide (NT-proBNP), 99f, 163–167, 166f, 167f

O

obstructive sleep apnoea syndrome (OSAS), 111f, 112f, 113f, 227, 229f
  continuous positive airway pressure (CPAP), 110–115, 111f–115f
  ITNP, detection and management of, 107–110, 111f, 112, 113f
Ohasama study, 17, 21, 69, 136, 137f, 257f

olmesartan, 192–197, 192f–196f
organ damage with MBPS, 54–60, 55f
   chronic kidney disease (CKD), 59–60
   hypertensive heart disease, 55–56, 55f, 56f
   silent cerebrovascular disease, 58, 59, 59f
   stroke events, 8f
   vascular disease and inflammation, 56–58, 58f
orthostatic hypertension, 138–143, 140f–144f
   definition, 142f
   detection, 142f
   diagnostic method, 142f
   home active standing test (HAST) and, 141–143, 142f
   morning BP and, 141f
OSAS, see obstructive sleep apnoea syndrome (OSAS)
out-of-clinic BP monitoring, 4–5, 4f–5f

P

PAI-1, see plasminogen activator inhibitor-1 (PAI-1)
PARAMETER study, 203, 203f, 204f, 228–230
PATHWAY–2, 230f
perfect 24-hour BP control, 175
   by renal denervation, 231, 232f
   non-specific medication, 175, 176f
   specific treatment, 175, 176f
   triad of, xiv (Preface)
peripheral artery disease (PAD), 155, 156f
plasminogen activator inhibitor-1 (PAI-1), 68, 70f
polysomnography, 119, 120f
PREDICT (Prediction of ICT-Home blood pressure variability) registry, 21f
prehypertension, 73, 73f, 74
pre-wakening surges, 51, 52f, 53, 198
pulse wave velocity (PWV), 151f

R

ramelteon, 88, 89f
RAS, see renin-angiotensin system (RAS)
RAS inhibitor-based combination, 214–223, 215f–225f
renal denervation, 230
   evidence, 231–243, 233f–243f
   perfect 24-hour BP control, hypothesis of, 231, 232f
renin-angiotensin system (RAS), 175, 176f

resistant hypertension, see also hypertension, 306
   calcium channel blockers (CCB) for, 227
   fourth-line therapy, 227–230
   management, 227, 228f
resistive index (RI), 60, 236
'resonance hypothesis' of BP surge, 125–127, 127f
rising BP surge, 52f

S

sacubitril/valsartan, 201–204
   age-related continuum, 205f
   evidence, 201–204, 202f–204f
   mechanism, 201f
salt restriction, 177, 177f, 178f, 227, 255
salt-sensitive hypertension, 204, 205f
SAS, see sleep apnoea syndrome (SAS)
SCI, see silent cerebral infarcts (SCI)
secondary hypertension, 229f
second-line therapy, 211
SGLT2i, see inhibitors of sodium/glucose cotransporter 2 (SGLT2i)
SHATS, see systemic haemodynamic atherothrombotic syndrome (SHATS)
silent cerebral infarcts (SCI), 58–59, 168–171, 172f
sleep apnoea syndrome (SAS), 111f, 112f, 113f, 227, 229f
sleep disturbance, 96f
Sleep Pressure and disordered breathing in REsistant hypertension And cardiovascular Disease (SPREAD), 21f, 103f, 109–110, 111f, 114f
sleep-trough morning surge, 31f, 51, 52f, 53f, 56, 60
small artery remodelling, 71, 71f, 154f
SPREAD, see Sleep Pressure and disordered breathing in REsistant hypertension And cardiovascular Disease (SPREAD)
SPRINT study, see Systolic Blood Pressure Intervention Trial (SPRINT)
SPYRAL HTN-OFF MED, 239f, 242
SPYRAL HTN-ON MED, 242
strain vessels, 153f, 154f
structural hypertension, 204, 205f, 206f, 243f
SUNLIGHT (Study on Uncontrolled Morning Surge for N-type CCB and Low Dose of HCTZ, Using the Internet Through Blood Pressure Data Transmission System) study, 222, 225f

SUper ciRculation monitorinG with high
    tEchnology (SURGE) research, 95
Surge Index, 121, 124f
suvorexant, 88, 89f
sympathetic nervous activity, 61, 67
Symplicity HTN, 231–235, 257f
systemic haemodynamic atherothrombotic
    syndrome (SHATS), 145–156
  biomarkers
    cardiac, 163–167, 166f, 167f
    baroreflex sensitivity, 173, 174f
    brain, 168–171, 172f, 173f
    microalbuminuria, 168
    vascular, 157–163, 158f, 159f, 161f–163f
  case, 145–148, 146f–149f
  clinical relevance, 148–150
  mechanism of vicious cycle, 152–156, 154f
  pathological target, 150–152
  strain vessel hypothesis, 150, 153f, 154f
Systolic Blood Pressure Intervention Trial
    (SPRINT), 1, 2f

T
telemedicine, 272
telmisartan, 190, 217–219, 220f
thermosensitive hypertension, 61–63, 64f
third-line therapy, 214
thrombotic and fibrin lytic activities, 63
tissue-type plasminogen activator inhibitor-1
    (PAI-1), 68
trigger nighttime BP monitoring (TNP), 96f,
    102–107, 104f, 105f
trigger-specific BP sensitivity, 40–44, 49
TROPHY study, 14, 14f
Tochigi Salt Cardiovascular Risk Study
    (T-STARS), 255f

U
urinary albumin/creatinine ratio (UACR),
    84f, 86f, 100f, 101, 101f, 155f, 191f

V
vascular disease and inflammation with
    MBPS, 56–58
vascular mechanism, MBPS, 71–74, 72f
VASSPS, *see* Effects of Vasodilating vs.
    Sympatholytic Antihypertensives on
    Sleep Blood Pressure in Hypertensive
    Patients with Sleep Apnea Syndrome
    (VASSPS)
volume retention type, 212, 213f, 228f

W
waiting-room BP, 19, 20f
wearable surge BP monitoring (WSP), 96f,
    119, 120f, 121, 121f, 122f, 123, 123f
white-coat hypertension, 4, 5f, 35f, 55
Wi-SUN transmission, 46, 47, 48f
World Hypertension League (WHL), 245